Pharmacological Basis of Small Animal Medicine

Pharmacological Basis of Small Animal Medicine

edited by

A. T. YOXALL
MA VetMB MRCVS DVA

and

J. F. R. HIRD
MA BVSc MRCVS DVA

Blackwell Scientific Publications
OXFORD LONDON EDINBURGH
MELBOURNE

Osney Mead, Oxford OX2 0EL
8 John Street, London WC1N 2ES
9 Forrest Road, Edinburgh EH1 2QH
P.O. Box 9, North Balwyn, Victoria, Australia

ISBN 0 632 002220

First published 1979

British Library Cataloguing in Publication Data
Pharmacological basis of small animal medicine.
1. Veterinary pharmacology
I. Yoxall, A T II. Hird, J F R
636.089'5'1 SF917

ISBN 0-632-00222-0

Set by Preface Ltd, Salisbury
Printed and bound in Great Britain by
Henry Ling Ltd
Dorchester

Contents

Contributors

A. R. Austin BVetMed MRCVS
Grassland Research Institute, Hurley, Maidenhead, Berkshire

R. J. Bywater MSc PhD BVMS MRCVS
Beecham Pharmaceuticals Research Division, Walton Oaks Tadworth, Surrey

L. M. Cobb DVSc PhD MRCPath MRCVS
Department of Environmental Physiology, Huntingdon Research Centre, Huntingdon, Cambridgeshire

R. M. Connan MA PhD BVetMed MRCVS
Department of Clinical Veterinary Medicine, University of Cambridge

M. G. Dear BSc BVetMed MRCVS
The Dear Animal Hospital, Blundell Centre, Richmond, Columbia

H. F. Grundy MA MD BSc
Department of Pharmacology, University of Cambridge

Anne M. Harris BSc
Glaxo Research Ltd, Greenford, Middlesex

J. F. R. Hird MA BVSc MRCVS DVA
10 Blackwall, Halifax, West Yorkshire

P. M. Keen BVSc PhD MRCVS
Department of Pharmacology, University of Bristol

P. Lees BPharm PhD
Department of Physiology, Royal Veterinary College, London

D. V. Roberts BSc MD
Department of Physiology, University of Liverpool

H. M. Snow BSc PhD
Pharmaceuticals Division, Biology Department, ICI Ltd, Macclesfield, Cheshire

K. J. Thrower BSc DPhil MRIC CChem
Upjohn Ltd, Crawley, Sussex

Catherine A. Wilson BPharm PhD
Department of Physiology, Royal Veterinary College, London

A. T. Yoxall MA VetMB MRCVS DVA
Bramley, Surrey

Preface

This volume is the first of two books which are intended to provide both up-to-date information on small animal therapeutics, and perhaps more importantly, a link between 'basic' scientific principles, conventionally taught as preclinical subjects, and clinical small animal therapeutics.

The editors have had occasion to devise and present a course in therapeutics at the Cambridge Veterinary School. Our experiences in giving this course led us to conclude that there was a dearth of readily accessible published material which related basic pharmacological and phsyiological information to clinical veterinary therapeutics. In order to gather further information in this field, a number of expert speakers were invited to take part in a course on small animal therapeutics for practitioners in December 1976. These books are based, in part, on the papers presented on that course. It was not possible to cover the whole field of small animal therapeutics in a 3-day course, and although the course material has been considerably expanded in preparing these volumes, with substantial additions from new contributors, the contents are not intended to be comprehensive. Subjects which we consider to be fully covered in specialist works, such as ophthalmic therapeutics, are not discussed in these volumes. The material has been somewhat arbitrarily divided into pharmacological and physiological aspects of therapeutics. Endocrinological therapeutics, fluid balance and alimentary and respiratory tract therapeutics have been included in *The Physiological Basis of Small Animal Medicine*, whilst most other topics are in the present volume.

Although the books contain much information which is directly applicable to day-to-day veterinary practice, they are not merely intended to be therapeutic handbooks; neither are they intended to be pure pharmacological texts. The two volumes will, however, be of use to students both in their preclinical years, in that they demonstrate the relevance of some basic studies to clinical medicine, and in their clinical years, in that they expose the rationale upon which therapeutic procedures are based. It is our belief that an understanding of fundamental principles is the prime essential for good clinical practice, and that the mere mechanical administration of medicines is an abnegation of the clinician's duty to his patients. We hope that the increasing amount of information on the behaviour of therapeutic agents in animals and dissemination of this information to clinicians will allow the clinical use of such agents to their optimum effect.

The editors are extremely grateful to the contributors to this volume for their patience and forbearance during the prolonged gestation of the work. We are especially grateful to those who did so much to produce their chapters in a short space of time when previous authors were unable to complete their commitments. Any merit which may be found in this volume is attributable to the authors, not to the editors.

We are also grateful to Professor George Brander and Doctors Peter Keen and Peter Lees for their support and enthusiasm for the concept of veterinary clinical pharmacology and therapeutics as an integrated subject, a concept which has underlain the inception of these books.

Bob Campbell and others at Blackwell Scientific Publication have tolerated our inability to meet deadlines with good humour and infectious optimism. Such optimism in fact, that they have agreed to publish *The Pharmacological Basis of Large Animal Medicine*, based on a course held in July 1978, as a companion to the small animal volumes. We are deeply grateful to Bob and his colleagues for bringing our idea to fruition.

A.T.Y.
J.F.R.H.

August 1978

1

Pharmacokinetics

H. F. GRUNDY

While pharmacodynamics is the study of drug action, pharmacokinetics is basically concerned with how a drug reaches its site of action, and there maintains an adequate concentration to exert its effect, be it therapeutic, diagnostic or toxicological. The major factors involved in pharmacokinetics are shown diagrammatically in Fig. 1.1. They are to be itemised as follows:

1 Route of administration.
2 Plasma protein binding.
3 Activation-metabolism before acting.
4 Inactivation-metabolism and excretion of metabolites.
5 Excretion in an unchanged form.
6 Redistribution (i.e. storage at an inactive site).

Some knowledge of the mechanisms by which drugs cross membranes is an essential preliminary to the more detailed consideration of the above processes.

1.1 Passage of drugs across membranes

The body may be regarded as a series of compartments (e.g. alimentary tract, plasma, tissue fluid, renal tubular fluid, intracellular fluid, brain) which are divided from each other by biological membranes. On a simplistic view, with certain exceptions (the capillary wall, the blood-brain barrier) these cellular membranes consist of a bilaminar arrangement of protein and phospholipids, such that the centre of the membrane contains the uncharged (hydrophobic) terminals of the phospholipid molecules, whilst the charged (hydrophilic) terminals of these molecules are directed towards the inner and out surfaces of the membrane. In consequence, a degree of lipid solubility is required of molecules which are to pass through the membrane itself. However, water-filled pores (of about 2–4A diameter) may exist within the membrane, through which small molecules may pass. These pores are inconstant, and appear to move about the surface of the membrane as well as varying in size and in their physicochemical properties. They are possibly associated with the mosaic-like arrangement of globular protein molecules

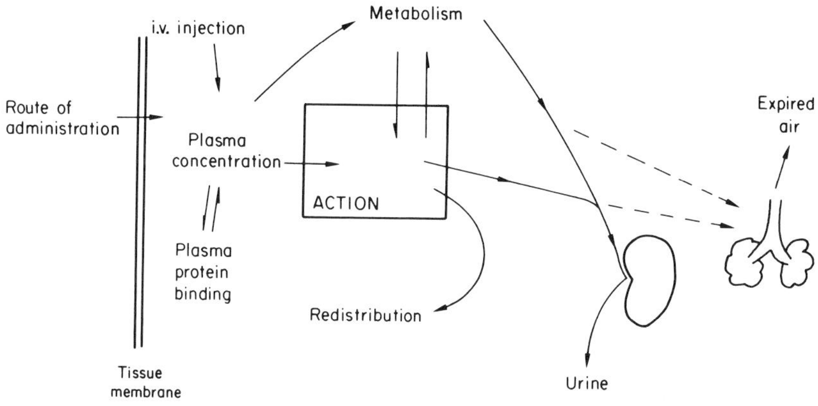

Fig. 1.1 Factors involved in pharmacokinetics.

within the membrane. The distribution of any drug within the body therefore depends, to a large extent, upon its ability to pass across this type of membrane, and there are three fundamental mechanisms by which trans-membranal movement can be achieved.

1 Active movements capable of proceeding against gradients (chemical, electrical, physical) requiring an energy supply and often a carrier (see below).
2 Facilitated diffusion; faster than simple diffusion due to the intervention of a specific, saturable, carrier system.
3 Diffusion either through water-filled pores (ultrafiltration) or through the lipoprotein cell membrane itself (simple diffusion).

Simple diffusion necessitates both a favourable concentration gradient and adequate lipid solubility. Ionised forms (either positively or negatively charged) are not significantly lipid-soluble as they attract a shell of water molecules round themselves. Unionised forms are more lipid-soluble.

Each acidic or basic group in a drug has a p*Ka* value (i.e. a pH at which there are equal numbers of its ionised and unionised forms). At other pH values the ratio of ionised to unionised forms varies as follows:

For an acid: $$\mathrm{R.COOH} \underset{\text{(add OH}')}{\overset{\text{add H}^+}{\rightleftharpoons}} \mathrm{R.COO}' \; (+\,\mathrm{H_2O})$$

(i.e. *less* of the drug is present in the ionised form as the pH falls).

For a base: $$\mathrm{R.NH_3}^+ \underset{\text{(add OH}')}{\overset{\text{add H}^+}{\rightleftharpoons}} \mathrm{R.NH_2} \; (+\,\mathrm{H_2O})$$

(i.e. *more* of the drug is present in the ionised form as the pH falls).

In the case of an acid (vice versa for a base), each *one* pH unit change to the acid side of the p*Ka* results in a tenfold increase in the unionised form relative to the ionised form; the converse occurs when shifts to the alkaline side of the p*Ka* are made.

Relatively small pH changes will therefore produce large changes in the proportion of drug present which is in a suitable (unionised) form to cross membranes.

When the acidic drug aspirin is ingested, the low pH of the stomach will cause most of the drug (which has a p*Ka* of 3·4) to be present in its unionised form in the gastric lumen (Fig. 1.2a), but within the mucosal cells, most reverts to the ionised form. The ionised drug is unable to pass out through the mucosal cell membrane, so that aspirin concentrates within these cells, and absorption into the systemic circulation is poor. This contentration of aspirin within mucosal cells may be one factor causing cell damage, and hence the

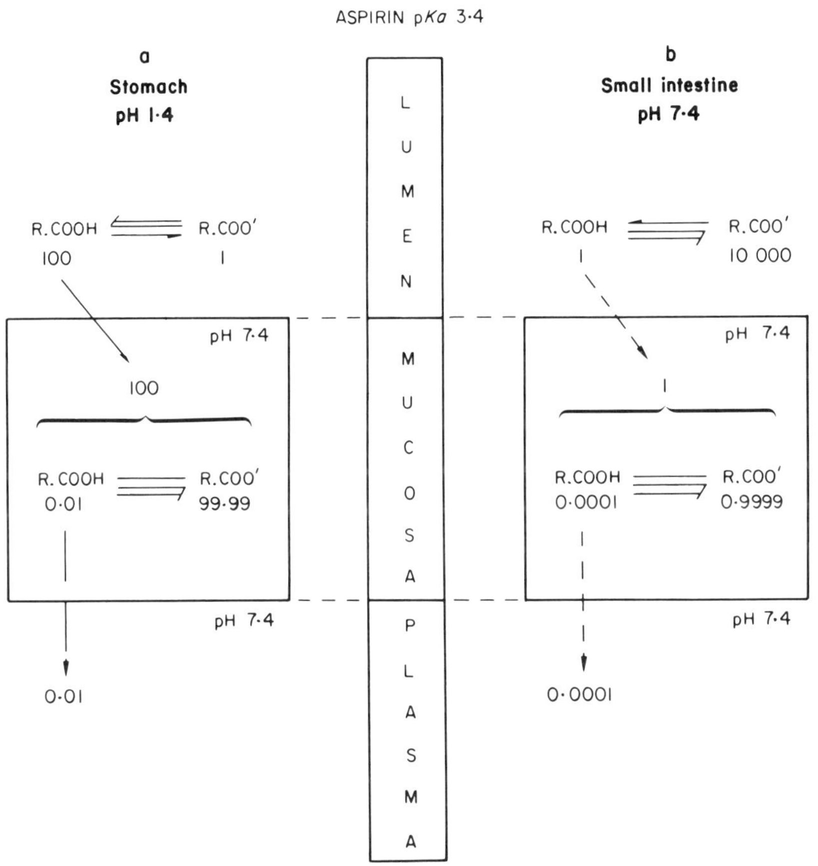

Fig. 1.2 Absorption of acetylsalicylic acid (aspirin, p*Ka* 3·4) through the mucosal cells of (a) the stomach and (b) the small intestine.

problems of gastric haemorrhage associated with the use of this drug (see Chapter 9).

The water solubility of aspirin increases as the chyme becomes less acidic and this results in a higher concentration of the drug within the lumen of the small intestine (Fig. 1.2b). Here, although the unionised form is in a much lower proportion, most of the drug entry occurs because of the large absorptive area available and, as shown, aspirin is much less concentrated in the mucosal cell. These examples show some of the interacting factors involved in the passage of substances across membranes. In particular they illustrate the general principle that lipid solubility is a prerequisite for absorption following oral drug administration. Conversely, highly charged molecules are usually not effectively absorbed when administered by this route. This property may be useful when it is required that the drug should remain within the alimentary tract, and there exert its effect.

The commonest membrane which drugs have to cross is the capillary wall. Lipid-soluble substances pass almost instantaneously through the entire surface of the capillary endothelium. However, in most tissues (brain and kidney are important exceptions, see below) water-soluble drugs up to the molecular weight of insulin, about 6000, leave the blood through pores in the capillary endothelium and then pass via the thin, surrounding basement

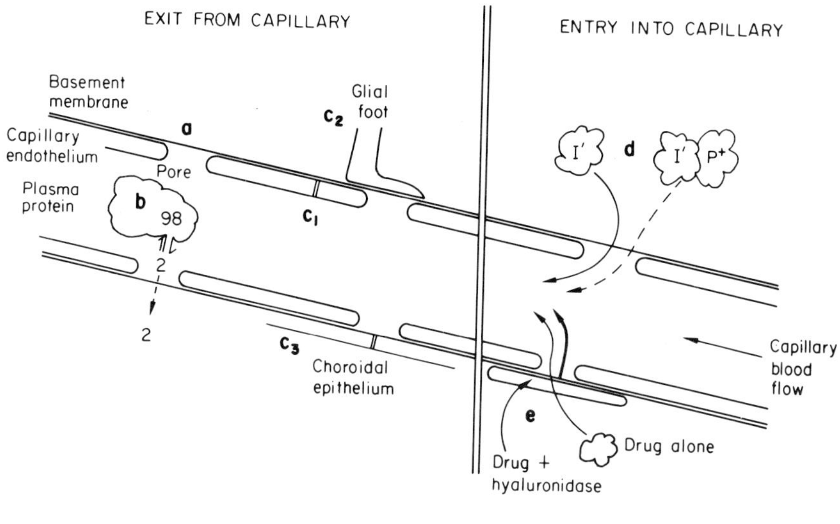

Fig. 1.3 Passage across capillary membranes (diagrammatic). Exit from capillary: (a) pore in capillary wall; (b) plasma protein binding (phenylbutazone as an example) delays passage into tissue fluid; (c) blood-brain barrier; c_1, tight junction of capillary endothelial cell; c_2, pore covered by neuroglial process (glial foot); c_3, tight junction of choroidal epithelial cell. Entry into capillary; (d) s.c. and i.m. injections — more rapidly acting soluble insulin (I′) and a depot preparation with protamine (P^+); (e) addition of hyaluronidase to increase the area of contact of the drug solution with the absorptive surface.

membrane, in a matter of minutes, into the tissue fluid (Fig. 1.3a). Thus, for practically all therapeutic agents, the only factor which significantly delays passage from the circulation into the tissue fluid is the degree of binding to the plasma proteins. A heavily protein bound drug will pass only slowly in its unbound form into the tissues (Fig. 1.3b) and thus, it acts as a 'circulating' depot preparation (e.g. sulphadimethoxine, hydroxocobalamin). The converse problem — that of passage from the tissue fluid to the plasma — is met following intramuscular or subcutaneous injections. As the capillary wall represents a negligible barrier to passage by any drug, the following are the limiting factors in these cases:

1 Aqueous solubility in order to traverse the tissue fluid.
2 Capillary blood flow.

So now, drugs which are water-soluble have the advantage of more rapid absorption and, therefore, more immediate action while the more lipid-soluble agents find a niche as depot preparations. This situation is exemplified by two well-known combinations. Soluble insulin is negatively charged at body Ph and thus acts rapidly but when combined with the positively charged protamine produces a more neutral molecule with a prolonged effect (Fig. 1.3d). Similarly, penicillin (an acid) and procaine (a base) can be united to form a depot preparation. Drug absorption from a subcutaneous or intramuscular injection site can also be retarded by the incorporation of a vasoconstrictor (e.g. local anaesthetic preparations may contain adrenaline). It must also be remembered that during shock absorption from subcutaneous and intramuscular sites will be poor, due to peripheral circulatory stasis. In the shocked patient it is almost always necessary to administer drugs intravenously. Hyaluronidase may be added to subcutaneous injections, the rationale being that this enzyme breaks down the hyaluronic acid mucopolysaccharides which are components of the intercellular ground substance, and therefore, allows a greater area of contact between the drug solution and the absorptive surface thus encouraging absorption of the drug (Fig. 1.3e).

The brain capillaries are unusual in having either close ('tight') junctions between their endothelial cells (Fig. 1.3c_1) or an investment of neuroglial tissue ('glial foot', Fig. 1.3c_2), or (in the case of the intraventricular choroid plexuses) an overlying modified ependymal lining, termed choroidal epithelium, which has close ('tight') junctions, as depicted in Fig. 1.3c_3. These collectively constitute the anatomical blood-brain barrier which allows the passage (by simple diffusion) of lipid-soluble drugs into the brain and cerebrospinal fluid, but effectively excludes highly charged molecules, which do not significantly cross these cellular elements unless they are disrupted by pathological processes (e.g. meningitis).

The kidney contains an array of membrane-transporting mechanisms. At the healthy glomerulus, where the capillary pore size is approaching that of albumin the only drugs excluded from the ultrafiltrate are the plasma protein bound moieties. From the tubular fluid, lipid-soluble substances can be reabsorbed by simple diffusion (Fig. 1.4). Two corollaries follow. Firstly, metabolism tends to render drugs more water-soluble for excretion by the kidneys. Secondly, in poisoning cases it is rational to encourage formation of the ionised forms to promote excretion. As illustrated in Fig. 1.4, at pH 6·4 aspirin (p*Ka* 3·4) shows a large differential in the ionised direction. The general rule in such circumstances, is to make the urine alkaline with potassium citrate or sodium bicarbonate if the poison is an acid (e.g. aspirin, phenobarbitone) and to acidify the urine with ammonium chloride if the poison is a base (e.g. pethidine, amphetamine). Organic acids can, in addition, be secreted into the kidney tubules by an active, carrier-mediated process so that judicious alkalinisation can achieve a clearance of aspirin, well in excess of the glomerular filtration rate. A similar, but separate mechanism exists for organic bases.

1.2 Route of administration

The factors involved here may be grouped as those necessitated by the required effect, the passage from the portal of entry to the site of action, and convenience.

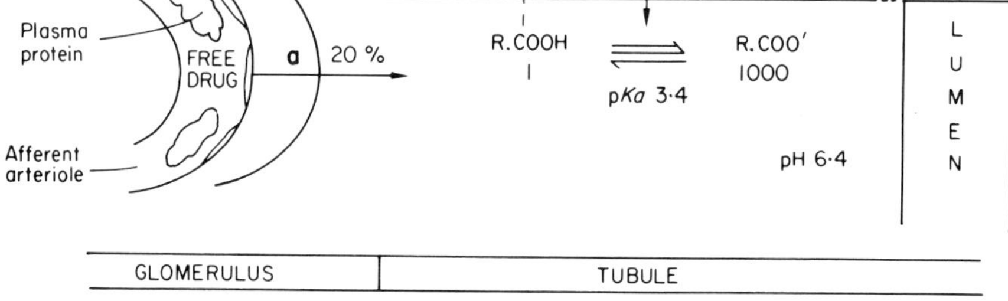

Fig. 1.4 Passage across membranes in the kidney illustrated diagrammatically for aspirin (p*Ka* 3.4): (a) glomerular ultrafiltration (about 20% of free plasma concentration); (b) passive reabsorption by simple diffusion of unionised form of the drug; (c) active secretion of organic acids (and organic bases, not shown) into the tubular fluid.

1.2.1 Dependence of drug effects on route of administration

SITE OF ACTION

Topical application is obviously indicated if circumscribed local effects are to be produced (e.g. in a skin lesion) or if an infection is difficult of access (e.g. in a fibrosed cavity).

SPEED OF ACTION

The intravenous and inhalational routes are fastest (e.g. the induction of general anaesthesia). Due to the greater vascular supply to muscle relative to the subcutaneous tissue, intramuscular injections usually have a faster onset of action than subcutaneous injections. Orally administered drugs may produce systemic effect in 20 minutes if taken on an empty stomach but appreciably longer after a meal.

CLOSE ADJUSTMENT OF DOSAGE TO EFFECT

This is again important in general anaethesia where the intravenous and inhalational routes are used.

DURATION OF ACTION

As penicillin only acts during the dividing phase of susceptible bacteria, an intravenous injection which is rapidly excreted as an organic acid by the kidney is unlikely to be as effective as an intramuscular injection, since the drug will remain in the body for a longer period of time, during which a greater number of bacteria are likely to pass through division; an even more prolonged action can be obtained by the addition of procaine (see above). Depot preparations (including subcutaneous pellet implantation) provide a convenient way of supplying small but relatively constant amounts of essential substances in chronic conditions.

ACTIVATION BY METABOLISM

Cortisone must be converted to hydrocortisone by the liver to become active. It is therefore pointless to treat a colonic condition with cortisone rectally. Similar considerations apply between prednisone (inactive) and prednisolone (active).

1.2.2 Passage from portal of entry to site of action

FORM OF THE DRUG

Gases or vapours can only be inhaled. The actual formulation of the drug preparation is a branch of pharmacy termed pharmaceutics and it can make a great deal of difference to the onset and duration of action (e.g. enteric-coated capsules, slow release preparations).

TOXICITY

This may be local or general. The former is exemplified by the rule that irritant substances must never be given orally (to avoid vomiting, colic, diarrhoea), or subcutaneously or intramuscularly (to avoid tissue necrosis). The main danger with intravenous administration is that some vital area (e.g. respiratory centre, myocardium) may suddenly be presented with a lethal concentration of the drug; to avoid this, the injection must be made sufficiently slowly and care must be taken to ensure that the needle or cannula lies freely within the lumen of the vein and *not* in an artery.

ABSORPTION

The general principles involved have been discussed in an earlier section. In the case of absorption from gastrointestinal tract, a wider variety of situations can now be explored. In the lumen calcium salts are chelated by tetracyclines with a consequently diminished absorption of both. Calcium ions are absorbed in the upper small intestine by a carrier mechanism initiated by activated vitamin D. Osteomalacia results either from antagonism of this action by adrenal glucocorticoids or by a decrease in the amount of activated vitamin D caused by phenobarbitone or phenytoin.

INACTIVATION BY METABOLISM

This will be dealt with in the next chapter, but it is obviously inappropriate to give orally insulin (a polypeptide) or adrenaline (destroyed by monoamine oxidase in the cells of the intestinal epithelium and the liver).

1.2.3 Convenience

The oral route is the most convenient. Lay-staff can give subcutaneous or intramuscular injections. The presence of a veterinary surgeon is mandatory for inhalational or intravenous administration.

1.3 Plasma protein binding

Drugs attach themselves to circulating plasma proteins, especially albumins, in varying degrees by simple ionic bonds. Heavy protein binding results in a low free plasma concentration of the drug which, however, may be disproportionally augmented as the available bonding sites become saturated. For

Table 1.1 Plasma protein binding of phenylbutazone

Daily oral dose (mg/kg)	Percentage plasma protein bound	Percentage free in plasma	Concentration free in plasma
6	98	2	1*x* mg/l
12	90	10	10*x* mg/l

example, as shown in Table 1.1, doubling the usual therapeutic dose of phenylbutazone results in a tenfold increase in the free plasma concentration which unfortunately manifests itself mainly as a proportional increase in the most serious toxic effects, rather than an increase in therapeutic effect. An interaction in the opposite direction, taking several days to develop, is that the higher dose of phenylbutazone induces enzymes which depress its concentration to that of the lower dose. Thus, the latter, except possibly for short periods, is preferably not exceeded in clinical practice. If a barbiturate anaesthetic, such as thiopentone, is administered to an animal which has been treated with phenylbutazone, the effect of the anaesthetic will, in a rather unpredictable fashion, vary from that expected due to combination of the effects of displacement of thiopentone from plasma protein and enzyme induction. Similarly, warfarin poisoning may follow an unpredictable course in animals undergoing treatment with phenylbutazone. While displacement is common, it is not inevitable as the two drugs concerned may be combining with different groups of the plasma protein molecule. In the presence of low plasma proteins, usually due to hepatic or renal disease or malnutrition, highly bound drugs should be administered in lower than normal dosage. Highly protein bound drugs generally have a prolonged action due to the hindrance of their glomerular filtration (see above).

1.4 Volume of distribution of drugs

Mention has already been made of the concept that body fluids may be divided into a number of compartments, the most important of these being plasma, total extracellular fluid and intracellular fluid. Drugs present in intracellular fluid are usually distributed throughout the entire body water. The degree to which a drug is distributed throughout these compartments can be measured and a knowledge of this is useful to determine whether a drug will be active at a given site but, more importantly, to determine the dosage to be administered and at what time intervals. It is a quantitative measurement which involves the intravenous injection of a known amount of the drug and the determination of its concentration in the plasma after an interval of time adequate to allow its dilution in the part of the total body water into which it can distribute itself. Ideally, in this connection, drugs are divisible into three

Table 1.2 Ideal volumes of distribution

Fluid compartment	Volume (l/kg)	Approximate time for equilibrium (min)	Type of substance with examples
Blood plasma	0·05	10	Fully plasma protein bound (e.g. Evans' blue)
Extracellular fluid	0·17	30	Highly ionised (e.g. hexamethonium, streptomycin)
Total body water	0·60	60	Lipid-soluble (e.g. ethanol)

groups as indicated in Table 1.2, but in practice when a drug is given by a route other than intravenous, the equilibrium concentration is rarely attained. This is because before absorption is complete, the processes of metabolism, excretion or redistribution have come into play (Fig. 1.1).

1.5 Redistribution

The secondary dispersion of drugs into active sites is particularly associated with highly lipid-soluble substances. As these drugs easily cross cell membranes, their distribution is 'blood flow limited'. Thus, organs with a high blood flow (e.g. brain, heart, liver, kidney) initially contain a high

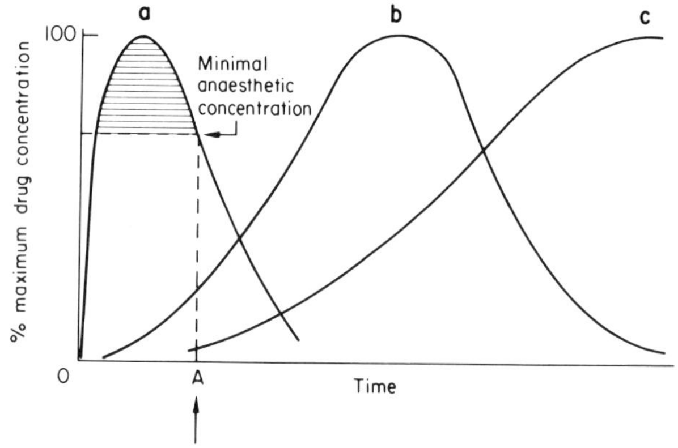

Fig. 1.5 Redistribution of a lipid-soluble substance (diagrammatic). Relative drug concentrations plotted against time for: (a) a rapidly perfused tissue (e.g. brain, heart, liver, kidney) (shaded area indicates period of anaesthesia, OA); (b) a moderately perfused tissue (e.g. skeletal muscle); (c) a slowly perfused tissue (e.g. fat).

concentration of drug but with time this is depleted as the agent redistributes into the moderately, and slowly, perfused tissues (muscle and fat, respectively, Fig. 1.5). In particular, substances acting on the central nervous system (barbiturates, see below) have their duration of effect shortened to a varying extent by redistribution into, initially, skeletal muscle and later, adipose tissue. The greater the lipid solubility of the drug, the earlier the redistribution (*A* in Fig. 1.5 is approximately 3 minutes for methohexitone but 30 minutes for thiopentone, the latter agent being more ionised, and thus less lipid-soluble).

1.6 Factors affecting the duration of action of drugs, as exemplified by the barbiturates

Within this group of drugs, an increase in lipid solubility results in:

1 Increased absorption from the gastrointestinal tract.
2 Increased redistribution (see above).
3 Increased metabolism producing metabolites which are more water-soluble and, therefore, more readily excreted by the kidney.

The general formula of the barbiturate molecule and its modifications which produce representative drugs with different durations of action are

Table 1.3 The formulae and main uses of some representative barbiturates

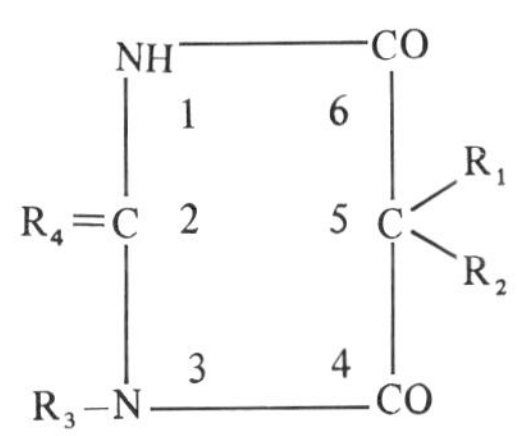

Barbiturate	R4	R3	R1	R2	Use
Methohexitone	O	*Methyl*	*allyl*	*1-methyl-2-pentynyl*	Intravenous anaesthetic
Thiopentone	*S*	H	ethyl	*1-methylbutyl*	Intravenous anaesthetic
Pentobarbitone	O	H	ethyl	*1-methylbutyl*	Oral hypnotic
Phenobarbitone	O	H	ethyl	phenyl	Oral sedative and anticonvulsant

Table 1.4 Factors affecting the duration of action of some representative barbiturates when used as indicated in Table 1.3; ++++, most; +++, moderate; ++, less; + least; 0, none.

Barbiturate	Mean duration of action	Lipid solubility	Redistribution	Metabolism	Excretion unchanged (%)	Excretion as metabolites (%)
Methohexitone	3 min	++++	++++	++++	0	100
Thiopentone	30 min	+++	+++	+++	0	100
Pentobarbitone	5 h	++	++	++	10	90
Phenobarbitone	10 h	+	+	+ (man)	25	75
				0 (dog)	*100*	0

shown in Table 1.3. The italicised groups contribute to increased lipid solubility viz.

R_4	S > 0
R_3	methyl > hydrogen
R_1	allyl > ethyl
R_2	aliphatic (optimal 5–6 carbon atoms, chain branched, unsaturated) > aromatic

Thus, the range of lipid solubilities in Table 1.4 is obtained and from this follow the amounts of redistribution, metabolism and excretory products in the same table. The parameter italicised indicates the most important, but not the only factor contributing to the duration of action of a particular barbiturate. Thus for the two intravenous anaesthetics the action is terminated by redistribution into skeletal muscle (*A* in Fig. 1.5) and, to a lesser extent, into fat. The medium length of action of pentobarbitone as an oral hypnotic is mainly determined by metabolism although redistribution and excretion in the unchanged form also play some part. Phenobarbitone in the dog is not metabolised and its prolonged action is temporally determined by the rate of renal excretion of the unchanged drug.

1.7 Kinetics of drug absorption and drug elimination

Examples of absorption and elimination processes which obey zero-order or first-order kinetics are shown in Table 1.5. A zero-order process is one which occurs at a constant rate and is not proportional to the amount of the drug present. Such a process necessitates a large excess of the drug available on the entry side (e.g. inhalational anaesthesia, intravenous infusion, roughly satisfied by slow-release preparations); or, on the exit side, a system whose

Table 1.5 Processes of drug entry and drug elimination exemplifying zero- and first-order kinetics.

	Zero-order processes	First-order processes
Drug entry	Inhalation Continuous i.v. infusion (approximately) slow-release preparations	Oral i.m. and s.c. injections (except depot preparations)
Drug elimination	Metabolism of ethanol Renal excretion (above T_{max})	Metabolism (of most drugs) Renal excretion (of most drugs) Exhalation

capacity is limited. For example, the rate-limiting step in the metabolism of ethanol is the initial change to acetaldehyde. This has a low capacity, so that a maximum rate of metabolism of about 10 ml/hour is usually achieved and the reaction is zero-order. Conversely, in the kidney tubules, the active tubular secretion of organic acids has a high capacity and, only rarely, when this is exceeded are zero-order kinetics observed.

First-order kinetics are the commonest both for drug absorption and for drug elimination (Table 1.5). Here the rate of the reaction is exponentially related to the amount of drug available and this means that a constant fraction is absorbed or eliminated in unit time. The rate constants k_{abs} and k_{el} are quantitative measurements of these fractions (e.g. k_{el} is the fraction of the drug which is eliminated in unit time).

1.8 The plateau principle

This applies when a drug undergoes zero-order absorption and first-order elimination. Under these conditions, it can be shown mathematically that the time to reach a steady-state (plateau) level is determined solely by the rate constant of elimination (k_{el}). As can be seen from Table 1.5 and Fig. 1.6, this principle can be applied to the use of inhalational general anaesthetics. For these drugs k_{el} is inversely proportional to the aqueous solubility, as shown in Table 1.6 by the Ostwald coefficient (λ). This quantifies the amount of the drug in the blood which is in equilibrium with the one unit of drug in the alveolar air. Thus for nitrous oxide, with a value for λ about 0·5, of each 1·5 units reaching the pulmonary capillaries, following cessation of anaesthesia 1·0 unit will be passed from the plasma to the alveolar air (e.g. elimination will be rapid); on the other hand, with diethyl ether this process is extremely protracted. Similar considerations apply to the onset of general anaesthesia with these agents — with nitrous oxide it is rapid, with diethyl ether slow. Halothane is intermediate in aqueous solubility but has the additional advantage with regard to onset that its distribution between brain and blood is about 2·5 : 1·0 whereas it is approximately 1·0 : 1·0 for the others and so it is readily absorbed into brain tissue and induction is medium. Although the

Table 1.6 Distribution of representative inhalational general anaesthetics between alveolar air, blood and brain (all figures are rounded to the nearest 0·5 for simplicity).

Anaesthetic gas (*G*) or vapour (*V*)	Partition coefficient blood: alveolar air (λ)	Partition coefficient brain: blood
Diethyl ether (*V*)	15·0	1·0
Halothane (*V*)	2·5	2·5
Nitrous oxide (*G*)	0·5	1·0

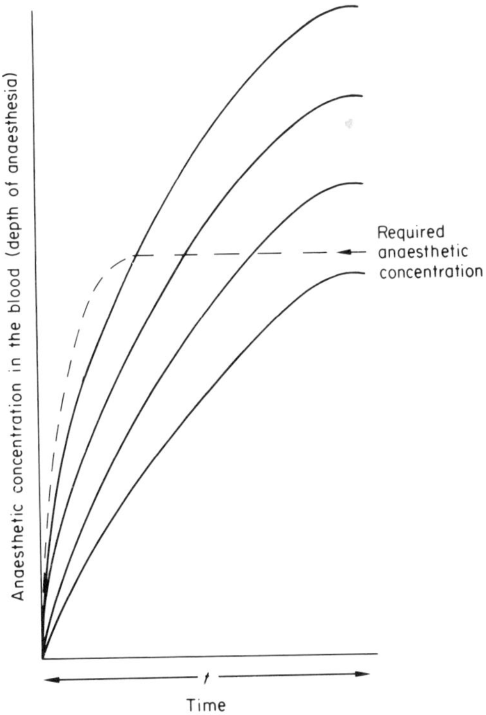

Fig. 1.6 The plateau principle as applied to the induction of general anaesthesia by inhalation. The time (t) to reach the equilibrium level depends solely upon the rate constant of elimination (k_{el}) for any given drug but the *height* of the plateau is dependent upon the concentration of the agent which is applied (solid lines depict increasing concentrations). Therefore, a high dosage of the drug is given initially and this is lessened when a satisfactory anaesthetic level has been achieved (interrupted line).

time taken to reach a plateau level depends solely on k_{el}, the *height* of the plateau reached depends upon the concentration of drug administered (Fig. 1.6). This principle is applied in practice as follows (Fig. 1.6 interrupted line). A high concentration of the drug is given at first but when the required plane of anaesthesia is attained the concentration being administered is lowered to maintain this level. Similar principles underlie the use of loading, followed by maintenance doses of digoxin, sulphonamides and other drugs.

1.9 Conclusion

Although very many pharmaceutical preparations are available to the clinician, the principles underlying their absorption and distribution within the patient, and hence their efficacy to a large extent, are relatively few. The majority of these preparations have been designed to fulfil specific functions under certain specified circumstances. In the nature of clinical practice however, situations arise in which the clinician is compelled to use therapeutic preparations outwith their usual indications. A degree of knowledge of the principles outlined above should enable the clinician to make the most appropriate decisions in such circumstances. Equally, a knowledge of pharmacokinetic principles should deter the clinician from misusing the agents available to him, so that he may obtain the maximum benefit from his therapeutic armamentarium.

2

Metabolism and excretion of drugs

R. J. BYWATER

Excretion and metabolism of a drug ensures the termination of its effect by removal or breakdown of the active agent. The rate and efficiency of these processes are clearly of great importance in ensuring that a systemically administered drug remains at the site of action for sufficiently long to produce its effect, but once that effect has been achieved, it does not remain so long that undesirable side-effects may occur, or that repeated dosage may lead to accumulation.

Many pharmacologically active drugs are lipid-soluble, non-polar and non-ionised agents which therefore cross cell membranes easily. This tends to increase the rate of absorption from the gut, and having been absorbed these agents will cross cell membranes rapidly to reach areas such as the central nervous system where their effects may be profound (see Chapter 1). Thiopentone sodium is an example of a highly active, lipid-soluble drug. These active drugs can be compared with the converse — water-soluble, ionised drugs — which may be unabsorbed from the gut, or if absorbed may not enter cells. The result will be that such drugs are likely to be pharmacologically inert. The penicillins both natural and semi-synthetic, are examples of drugs which penetrate cells to only a very limited degree. They exert their antimicrobial effect on the bacterial cell wall so it is unnecessary for them to pass through the bacterial cell membrane, which lies within the cell wall (see Chapter 5). Since they do not enter the cells of the host, the penicillins have a very low toxicity for mammals.

However, this desirable property also carries with it the penalty of somewhat poorer properties of penetration across barriers such as to the central nervous system (CNS) in comparison with other drugs whose higher toxicity may be accompanied by more rapid penetration of tissue barriers (e.g. chloramphenicol).

Metabolism of the body, often referred to as biotransformation, is likely to result in conversion of the drug to a metabolite which is less lipid-soluble, more polar, and more ionised. This is then likely to be less pharmacologically active, and is also probably in a form more easily excreted than the original, since there are often specific excretory mechanisms in the kidney for conjugates formed during biotransformation, and moreover, reabsorption in the kidney tubule will be reduced (see below).

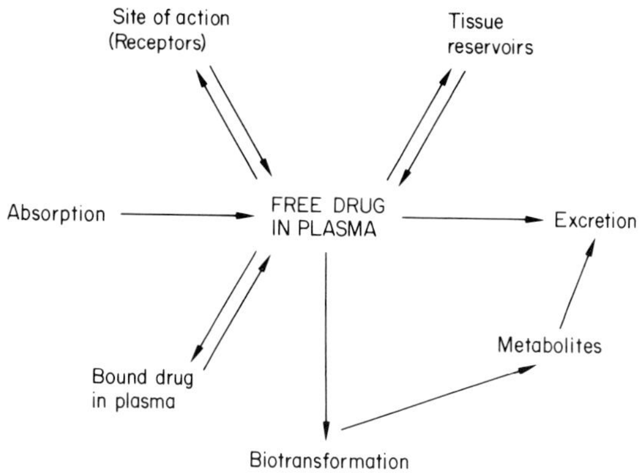

Fig. 2.1 Factors affecting plasma and tissue drug concentrations.

Excretion and biotransformation interact with other factors affecting plasma and tissue concentration as shown in Fig. 2.1.

Many drugs undergo excretion and biotransformation by more than one route (e.g. theophylline, aspirin), and the proportion of administered drug which proceeds by each route may vary with several factors, such as route of administration, and the nature of the patient's pathology, so that the overall picture of drug–patient interaction may be extremely complex. The picture may also be very different in the healthy experimental animal from that in the clinical case. Nonetheless, an understanding of the more important metabolic and excretory mechanisms is essential to a rational use of therapeutic agents.

2.1 Biotransformation or metabolism

The biochemical changes which most foreign organic compounds undergo in the animal body have been referred to as 'detoxication mechanisms' (Williams 1959). While this is often an accurate description, the term 'detoxication' does not take account of those drugs in which the metabolic change enhances the pharmacological activity, and so possibly may actually increase toxicity.

Table 2.1 Biochemical reactions which drugs may undergo.

Type		Pharmacological result
1	Inactive compound metabolised to active drug	Activation
2	Active compound changed to different active compound	Change in activity
3	Active compound inactivated	Inactivation or detoxication
4	Active compound changed to toxic metabolite	Intoxication

The biochemical reactions which drugs may undergo are summarised in Table 2.1.

2.1.1 Type 1 reactions: activation

Drugs which undergo activation are inactive *in vitro*, but show activity *in vivo*. Examples are given in Table 2.2. In some cases, when the activity was recognised as being due to a metabolite, the parent drug became obselete (e.g. prontosil was replaced by sulphanilamide).

The activation may confer useful pharmacokinetic advantages. For example talampicillin is the thiazolide carboxylic ester of ampicillin and is inactive until hydrolysed to the parent compound. The ester is however, more lipid soluble than the parent compound, and so is absorbed more rapidly from the intestine. When given orally, the hydrolysis occurs rapidly in the gut mucosa releasing the active ampicillin. The resulting blood levels are higher than with an equivalent dose of the parent ampicillin (Leigh *et al* 1976); this is an example of a 'pro-drug'. Similarly carfecillin, the phenyl ester of carbenicillin, can be given orally to achieve high concentrations of the latter drug in urine for treatment of pseudomonas infections.

Table 2.2 Examples of activation reactions.

Inactive drug	Active metabolite
Chloral hydrate	Trichlorethanol
Prontosil	Sulphanilamide
Talampicillin	Ampicillin
Carfecillin	Carbenicillin

2.1.2 Type 2 reactions: activity change

Here the parent drug is pharmacologically active, but the metabolite retains activity, although this may be qualitatively or quantitatively different. Phenacetin, which possesses some analgesic activity but can be dangerous in overdosage is being replaced by its metabolite, paracetamol, which is equally active but safer.

2.1.3 Type 3 reactions: inactivation

This is an extremely important group and includes the mechanisms for termination of activity of most drugs. The reactions involved may be non-synthetic (e.g. oxidation, reduction or hydrolysis) or may be synthetic (e.g. glucuronidation, acetylation, ethereal sulphate synthesis or methylation).

Table 2.3 Examples of oxidative biotransformation.

Amphetamine	→	p-hydroxyamphetamine
Chlorpromazine	→	chlorpromazine sulphoxide
Pentobarbitone	→	pentobarbitone alcohol
Codeine	→	morphine

NON-SYNTHETIC REACTIONS

Oxidation

An important group of oxidative enzymes is situated in the liver microsomes. These can produce a variety of reactions, including N- and O- dealkylation, aromatic ring and side-chain hydroxylation, sulphoxide formation and deamination. However, since hydroxylation is an essential step in all of these reactions, the enzymes may be grouped as hydrolases. TPNH (NADPH) and oxygen are essential cofactors. Examples of this type of reaction are given in Table 2.3.

Reduction

Liver microsomal enzymes may also catalyse reduction, as in conversion of nitro groups to amines, or of an aldehyde to an alcohol. An example of reduction is the nitro reduction of chloramphenical to primary amines.

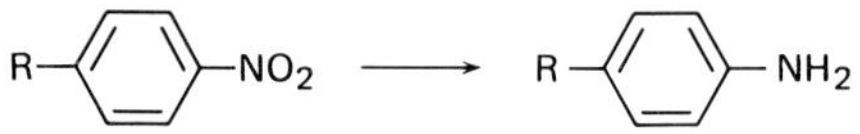

Hydrolysis

The most common hydrolysis is the de-esterification of ester linkages by esterases in plasma or tissues. There are a large number of drugs which contain ester groups (e.g. procaine, pethidine, suxamethonium, eserine, parathion, atropine, hydrocortisone acetate, pivampicillin, talampicillin etc).

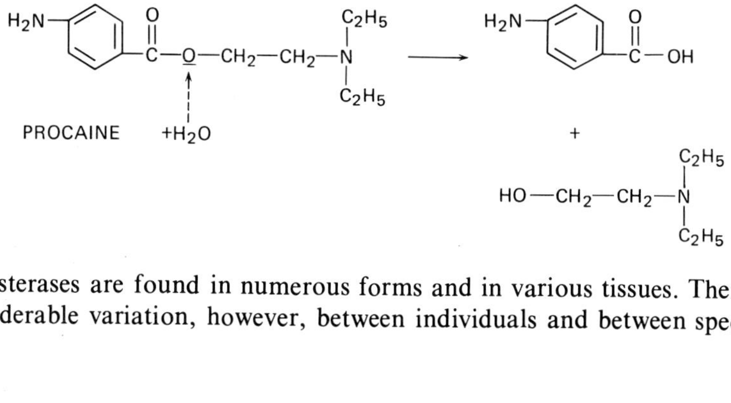

Esterases are found in numerous forms and in various tissues. There is considerable variation, however, between individuals and between species.

For instance, pseudocholinesterase is present in high amounts in horse plasma, but is low in bovine or sheep plasma. This relates to the sensitivity of the species to the depolarising muscle relaxant suxamethonium. For example cattle are considerably more sensitive to the paralysing effects of the drug than horses (Hall 1971). However the relation *in vitro* and *in vivo* between enzyme activity and hydrolysis rate for suxamethonium is probably not simple (Hansson 1957).

A further example of species difference is given by atropine, where the rabbit appears unique in having a plasma atropinesterase, guinea-pigs, and many other species, have liver atropinesterase, while men and mice do not hydrolyse atropine at all (Kalow 1961).

SYNTHETIC REACTIONS

These reactions require a source of energy. This is provided by ATP, and most of the reactions involve an active intermediate nucleotide and a conjugating enzyme.

Glucuronidation

This is an extremely important type of synthetic inactivation, and in this case the intermediate is uridinc diphosphate (UDP) glucuronic acid, and the enzyme is glucuronyl transferase. The sequence is shown in Fig. 2.2.

Glucuronides are more ionised than the parent compound, and are more water-soluble. They are therefore less pharmacologically active, and more easily excreted. In particular, kidney tubule secretion of glucuronides forms an efficient means of elimination.

As well as excretion through kidney, excretion also occurs in bile. This may be a less efficient means of elimination, since on entry into the gut, the glucuronides may be hydrolysed by intestinal glucuronidase to release the active drug. This may then be reabsorbed, so giving rise to an enterohepatic circulation. This occurs with drugs such as diethylstilboestrol, morphine, and chloramphenicol, and tends to increase persistence of these compounds in the body.

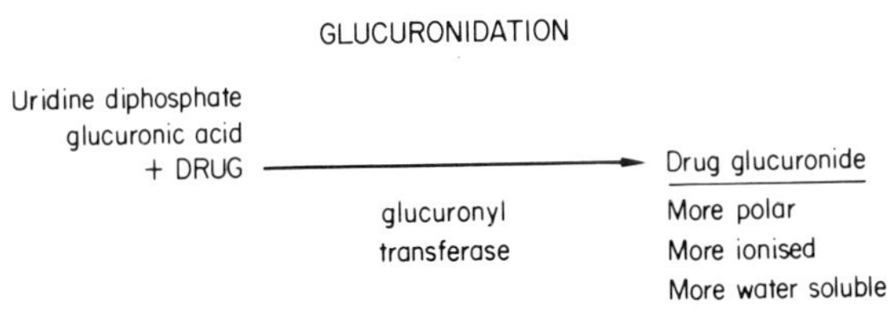

Fig. 2.2 Sequence of events in glucuronidation.

Cats appear to be deficient in the ability to form glucuronides, probably as a result of a lack of the glucuronyl transferase necessary for the reaction to occur. This increases the toxicity in cats of drugs such as chloramphenicol (Penny *et al* 1967) and salicylates, where glucuronidation is an important route of metabolism (Davis & Westfall 1972).

Acetylation

Acetylation takes place in liver, spleen, lungs, and gastrointestinal tract. This occurs in the biotransformation of sulphonamides in species other than the dog, where acetylation ability is limited (Marshall *et al* 1937).

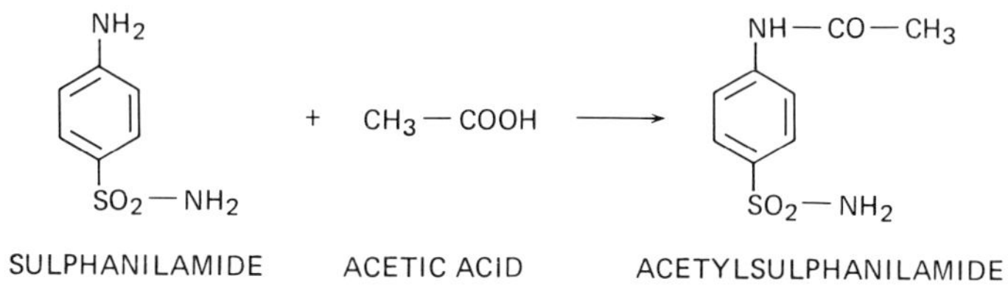

Sulphate conjugation

This occurs especially in formation of ethereal sulphates. This occurs with phenol, and to a lesser extent with ethanol and chloramphenicol.

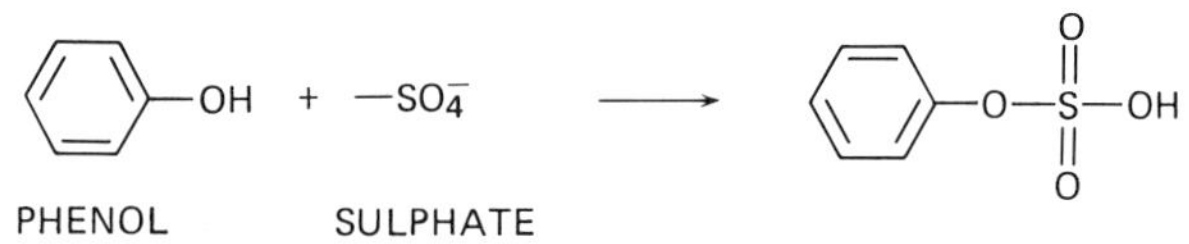

2.1.4 Type 4 reactions: intoxication

In this case metabolism results in an increase in toxicity. An example of this is carbon tetrachloride, which probably produces liver damage after enzymic conversion to intermediate products.

2.2 Excretion

Excretion of drugs or metabolites occurs principally via the urine, but significant amounts may also leave in bile or via the lungs; the latter route being especially important in removal of gaseous anaesthetics. Quantitatively insignificant amounts may be excreted in sweat, tears or saliva, although presence of drugs in these secretions may be important for therapeutic purposes.

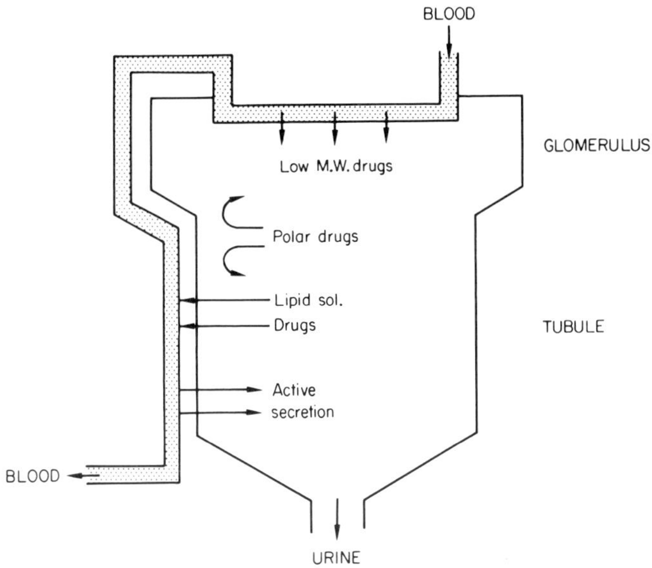

Fig. 2.3 Diagrammatic representation of a kidney tubule.

2.2.1 Excretion via the urine

The initial filtration process in the glomerulus allows most drugs to be passively transferred to the tubules (Fig. 2.3). What then occurs depends greatly on the lipid solubility of the drug. For instance, it has been calculated (Brodie 1964) that an evenly distributed compound with *low* lipid solubility, would be 50% excreted in about 5 hours. If it was also actively excreted, the time for this to occur would be reduced to about 1 hour. However, if the drug was *highly* lipid-soluble, with resulting tubular reabsorption, the time for 50% excretion would be increased to 30 days. But if, like thiopentone, localisation also occurred in tissues, the time for 50% excretion would become approximately 100 years. These figures underline the importance of metabolism which usually results in a metabolite with lowered lipid solubility, and a greater degree of ionisation, both of these characteristics reducing tubular reabsorption and increasing excretion in urine.

The degree of ionisation at a given pH will depend on the p*Ka* of the drug. This is defined as:

For acids:

$$\log \frac{\text{concentration unionised}}{\text{concentration ionised}} = \mathrm{p}Ka - \mathrm{pH}$$

For bases:

$$\log \frac{\text{concentration ionised}}{\text{concentration unionised}} = \text{p}Ka - \text{pH}$$

Many acids have their p*Ka* between 3 and 8 (e.g. salicylates, phenylbutazone, sulphadiazine, phenobarbitone). Thus salicylic acid has a p*Ka* of 3, and so in an alkaline urine, say pH 8, the log of the ratio of unionised to ionised would be minus 4. This gives a ratio of 10 000:1 in favour of the ionised form which then is excreted rather than reabsorbed. Therefore, weak acids are most rapidly excreted in an alkaline urine. Conversely weak bases (e.g. amphetamine, morphine) will be more rapidly excreted in acid urine.

Such considerations can be of importance in treatment of drug overdosage, where acidification or alkalinisation of the urine may assist in the rapid elimination of the drug.

Drugs that are less lipid-soluble, or more highly ionised at physiological pH tend to be excreted unchanged in the urine. This group includes a number of antibiotics (e.g. penicillin G, ampicillin, amoxycillin, caphaloridine and tetracycline). Since these drugs retain their antibacterial activity, they may be suitable as treatment for urinary infection, so long as the organism responsible is sensitive.

ACTIVE TUBULAR SECRETION

Active tubular secretion of drugs into the kidney tubule occurs with a number of organic acids and bases. Among the drugs excreted in this way are: penicillin G, ampicillin, amoxycillin, salicylic acid, phenylbutazone and chlorothiazide. This process occurs rapidly, and produces very high urine concentrations. Fig. 2.4 shows the concentration in calf urine of the semi-synthetic penicillin amoxycillin after oral administration. At 4 hours the concentration was approximately 100 times that in serum (Palmer *et al* 1977). This is an important factor in the treatment of urinary infections, but also implies that elimination of the drug will be relatively rapid. The tetracyclines on the other hand appear to be eliminated largely by glomerular filtration, with tubular secretion contributing much less to the drug elimination (Notari 1975).

Active secretion of a drug such as the penicillins can be delayed by administration of probenecid which probably shares the same excreting route. This results in delayed excretion (Barza *et al* 1975) and increased serum concentrations (Nauta *et al* 1974). Probenecid has been used as a means of prolonging the time for which serum levels of penicillins are maintained, but it has been suggested (Gibaldi & Schwartz 1968) that this effect may be at least partly as a result of reduced volume of distribution (i.e. by preventing access of the penicillin to the parenchyma of organs). However, Barza *et al*

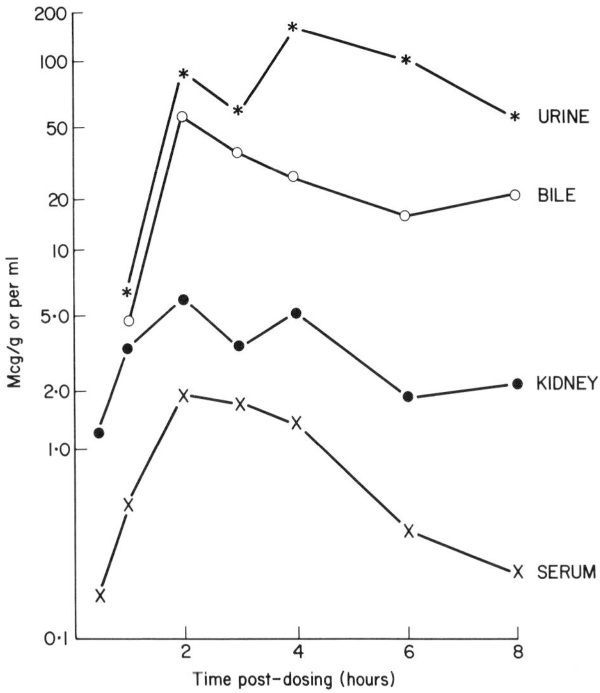

Fig. 2.4 Amoxycillin concentrations in serum, kidney, bile and urine after oral administration. Modified from Palmer *et al* (1977).

(1975) were able to show accumulation in kidney parenchyma, which was mentioned by Gibaldi and Schwartz as an example of an important tissue to which access may be limited by probenecid. The significance of the reduced volume of distribution therefore remains unclear.

2.2.2 Excretion via bile

Biliary secretion may be of drug metabolites or of the unchanged drug. Concentration of drug in the bile may be lower than that in blood (streptomycin) equal to that in blood (neomycin, bacitracin) slightly higher than that in blood (tetracyclines) or considerably higher than that in blood (novobiocin, spiramycin and semi-synthetic penicillins). The high concentration of amoxycillin in bile is shown in Fig. 2.4 (Palmer *et al* 1977).

Excretion of unchanged drug can allow reabsorption, so giving enterohepatic circulation. This will tend to delay the elimination from the body. The excretion of a drug in high concentration in the bile can also mean that parenteral administration can give rise to therapeutically active concentrations in the intestinal lumen.

2.3 Factors affecting drug metabolism and excretion

2.3.1 Previous drug therapy

This may either diminish or increase the effect of subsequent treatment. Reduction in response after repeated treatment (i.e. the phenomenon of drug tolerance) is well recognised and usually implies that as the drug is metabolised, the enzymes responsible are induced to become more active so that later doses are metabolised more rapidly. This occurs with many drugs and the barbiturates are a well-known example. Pretreatment of rats with three daily doses of pentobarbitone reduced sleeping time to less than 50% of that in control rats (Remmer 1961). However, an important point is that administration of one drug may stimulate the metabolism of a wide variety of other drugs, often unrelated to that given initially. Thus exposure to a chlorinated hydrocarbon such as DDT will shorten subsequent sleeping times due to barbiturate administration.

However, the converse can occur, and one drug may potentiate another. This is likely to be the case where the first has interfered with the metabolism of the second. An example is the potentiation of barbiturate sleeping time after chloramphenicol. Intravenous chloramphenicol increased duration of immediately subsequent pentobarbitone anaesthesia by 120% in dogs and 260% in cats (Adams & Dixit 1970). The effect has been shown after administration by oral, intramuscular or intravenous routes and was detectable for up to 24 days after the last dose (Teske & Carter 1971). Potentiation has also been identified between anaesthetics and aminoglycoside antibiotics (Adams *et al* 1976).

The implication of these observations is that there is a greater risk of anaesthetic accidents in animals undergoing chloramphenicol or aminoglycoside therapy.

2.3.2 Age

Very young animals are notably deficient in metabolic enzymes. Thus, potentially toxic drugs are more dangerous in young animals. The deficiency may be in oxidative enzymes, or in those responsible for glucuronidation.

The deficiency of oxidative enzymes is probably responsible for the unpredictable and occasionally very delayed recoveries following barbiturate anaesthesia in young animals. Hall (1976) suggested that thiopentone should be avoided in puppies and kittens below 2 or 3 months, sheep and goats below 3 months, pigs below 6 weeks and calves and foals below 8 weeks of age.

The glucuronidation deficiency in young animals means that chloramphenicol should be avoided in this age group (Fig. 2.5).

Geriatric cases, where liver function may be impaired, also require care when drugs are administered which rely on metabolism for their elimination, especially if there is inherent toxicity in prolonged exposure to the drug.

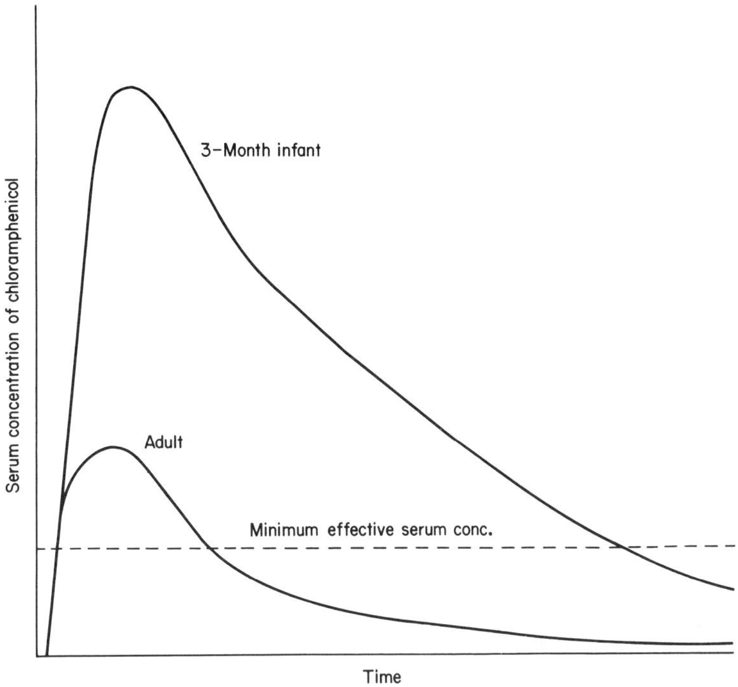

Fig. 2.5 Effect of age on persistence of chloramphenicol, following subcutaneous administration (human data). Modified from Levine (1973).

2.3.3 Disease

Where liver or kidney are diseased, biotransformation or elimination may be impaired. Repeated dosage may then give rise to grossly raised blood and tissue levels, with the danger of toxicity. In such cases, drugs should be chosen for low toxicity, so that accumulation will not induce further disease. The dosage regime may also be reduced accordingly.

Heart disease, with reduced circulation to the kidney, may allow accumulation of drugs such as tetracyclines, which in high concentrations may themselves be toxic.

2.3.4 Species and individual variation

Rates of drug metabolism and excretion are notoriously variable between species and between individuals within a species (Brodie 1964; Williams 1974). This implies that a familiar drug in an unfamiliar species must always be used with great care. Moreover, a familiar drug, even when used in a familiar species can give an unpleasant shock to the user who neglects to remember the fact of biological variation.

References

Adams H. R. & Dixit B. N. (1970) Prolongation of pentobarbital anaesthesia by chloramphenicol in dogs and cats. *J. Amer. Vet. Med. Ass.* **156**, 902.

Adams H. R., Teske R. H. & Mercer H. D. (1976) Anesthetic-antibiotic interrelationships *J. Amer. Vet. Med. Ass.* **168**, 409.

Barza M., Brusch J., Bergeron M. G., Kemmotsu O. & Weinstein L. (1975). Extraction of antibiotics from the circulation by liver and kidney: effect of probenecid. *J. Inf. Dis.* **131**, S.86.

Brodie B. B. (1964) Distribution and fate of drugs: therapeutic implications. In *Absorption and Distribution of drugs*, ed. T. B. Binns. Livingstone, London.

Davis L. E. & Westfall B. A. (1972) Species differences in biotransformation and excretion of salicylate. *Amer. J. Vet. Res.* **33**, 1253.

Gibaldi M. & Schwartz M. A. (1968) Apparent effect of probenecid on the distribution of penicillins in man. *Clin. Pharmacol. Ther.* **9**, 345.

Hall L. W. (1971) *Wright's Veterinary Anaesthesia and analgesia.* 7th edn. Baillière Tindall, London.

Hall L. W. (1976) The clinical use of thiopentone sodium. *Veterinary Review* (May and Baker) **14** 52.

Hansson C. H. (1957) Cholinesterases and Muscle Relaxants. II. Blood and muscle cholinesterase activity and domestic animals. *Acta Pharm. Tox. Kbh.* **13**, 142.

Kalow W. (1961) Esterase action. In *Proceedings of the 1st International Pharmacological Meeting Stockholm*, ed. B. Uvnas (1962) vol. 6, 159. Pergamon Press, Oxford.

Leigh D. A., Reeves D. S., Simmons K., Thomas A. L. & Wilkinson P. J. (1976) Talampicillin: a new derivative of ampicillin. *Brit. Med. J.* **1**, 1378.

Levine R. R. (1973) *Pharmacology-Drug Actions and Reactions:* 1st edn. Little Brown, Boston.

Marshall E. K., Cutting W. C. & Emerson K. (1937) Acetylation of *p*-aminobenzenosulfonamide in the animal organism. *Science* **85** 202.

Nauta E. H., Mattie H. & Goslings W. R. O. (1974) Effect of probenecid on the apparent volume of distribution and elimination of cloxacillin. *Antimicrob. Agents Chemother.* **6** 300.

Notari R. E. (1975) *Biopharmaceutics and Pharmacokinetics: Introduction.* Marcel Dekker, New York.

Palmer G. H., Bywater R. J. & Francis M. E. (1977) Amoxycillin: studies of distribution and clinical efficacy of a dispersible powder administered orally to calves. *Vet. Rec.* **100**, 487.

Penny R. H. C., Carlisle C. H., Prescott C. W. & Davidson H. A. (1967) Effects of chloramphenicol on the haemopoietic system of the cat. *Brit. Vet. J.* **123** 145.

Remmer H. (1961) Drugs as Activators of Drug Enzymes. In *Proceedings of the 1st International Pharmacological Meeting Stockholm*, ed. B. Uvnas (1962) vol. 6, 235. Pergamon Press, Oxford.

Teske R. H. & Carter G. G. (1971). Effect of chloramphenicol on pentobarbital induced anaesthesia in dogs. *J. Amer. Vet. Med. Ass.* **159**, 777.

Williams R. T. (1959) *Detoxication Mechanism.* 2nd rev. edn. Chapman & Hall, London.

Williams R. T. (1974) Interspecies variations in the metabolism of xenobiotics. *Biochem. Soc. Trans.* **2**, 359.

3

Adverse drug reactions

L. M. COBB

Adverse reactions to drugs are commonly illustrated and discussed in the literature on human medicine. In the veterinary literature there is only a handful of references; but there is no reason to think that the dog or cat has some special immunity to adverse reactions. A possible reason for the difference is because in human medicine many more drugs are used and patients frequently receive a regime of treatment in which several drugs are given at the same time. Any two of the drugs could interact and produce an unexpected effect. In addition, many of the reported effects in man are relatively mild and their counterpart in animals could go undetected; for example, abdominal discomfort, disorientation, double vision and skin rash.

Because of our limited understanding of adverse drug reactions in small animals, much of the illustration and discussion on mechanisms of action, in this chapter, is from human experience. The question is, how relevant is this experience to small animal medicine? The answer is not known; however, the human experience cannot be entirely irrelevant, for in man, streptomycin can cause ototoxicity and the same is true for the cat. Vaccines in man may cause anaphylactic shock, the same also occurs in the dog.

For the purposes of this chapter, the hypothesis has been adopted that in any adverse reaction it is *the animal* that is abnormal and is, for some reason, sensitive to the drug; *not* that the drug formulation is abnormally toxic. It is only by adopting this hypothesis that we shall eventually begin to understand what makes some animals react adversely.

3.1 Definitions

Adverse drug reaction: an unpredicted reaction produced in an animal by a drug given at the recommended dose.

Side-effect: a secondary pharmacological effect observed when a drug is given at the recommended dose. Such effects are *predictable*, for example, drowsiness with antihistamines.

An important concept when considering the side-effects of drugs is that of the therapeutic ratio (i.e. the relationship between the efficacy and the toxicity of a drug). A drug of high efficacy but also with high toxicity has as low a therapeutic ratio as a drug with low toxicity but also low efficacy. Claims that one drug has advantages over another by virtue of its lack of side-effects or greater efficacy should therefore be viewed with a degree of scepticism. Real benefit is associated with an enhanced therapeutic ratio, and ideally this enhancement should be demonstrable for all or most of the conditions for which the drug is indicated, since enhancement in the treatment of a particular condition may be accompanied by a deterioration in the therapeutic ratio with respect to other conditions.

3.2 Mechanisms of adverse drug reactions

3.2.1 Allergy

It is thought that the first step in the development of allergy to a drug is for the drug, or a metabolite of the drug, to combine with a body protein. Landsteiner (1945) referred to the drug as a hapten. When combined with a specific body protein an antigen is formed which will eventually lead to the formation of antibodies by the immune system. It is possible for foreign proteins, such as vaccines and antisera, to act as antigens giving rise to antibodies.

An animal allergic to one drug may show allergy to related drugs. This may be due to low specificity of antibody or because the hapten is a metabolite common to the drugs.

The most common result of the administration of a drug or vaccine to a hypersensitive animal is the release of vasoactive amines, including histamine, an event which precipitates the chain of reactions which constitute anaphylaxis.

In urticaria, where the anaphylactic reaction is localised to the skin, the reaction between antigen and antibody takes place on the surface of the subcutaneous mast cells. As a result of this reaction, histamine is released from the mast cells and causes dilatation of neighbouring blood vessels. Plasma leaks out from the dilated vessels leading to the skin-thickening characteristic of urticaria.

In a systemic anaphylactic reaction the vasoactive amines are released not only from mast cells but also from circulating basophils. Widespread release of histamine causes extensive peripheral vasodilation. This in turn produces hypotension and collapse of the animal. Histamine also produces contraction of the smooth muscles of the airways, observed clinically as dyspnoea and contraction of the muscle of the intestinal wall leading to colic and/or diarrhoea.

Ackroyd (1958) put forward the theory that in many instances thrombocytopenia arises when a drug, acting as a hapten, binds to the thrombocyte. Antibodies are then produced leading to the lysis of the circulating thrombocytes.

Further details of mechanisms of drug allergy are discussed by Parker (1975).

3.2.2 Secondary pharmacological effects

The definition of adverse drug reaction given in the introduction requires that the reaction is unpredictable. Generally this is because of some unusual sensitivity of the animal under treatment. There are, however, reactions in animals which are adverse but predictable because they are due to well-understood secondary pharmacological actions of the drug. Such side-effects are to be expected whenever these drugs are used. They are not, however, sufficiently deleterious to prevent the use of the drugs for their primary pharmacological effect, for example the sedative effects of many antihistamines do not detract from their value.

Oestrogens, when used for the treatment of anal adenoma or prostatic cancer in the dog, can be expected to have a feminising effect. Androgens used for the treatment of carcinoma of the mammary gland in the bitch can be expected to have a masculinising side-effect. In man, some degree of cholestasis, which may progress to frank jaundice, is to be expected during treatment with C17-substituted derivatives of testosterone (Sherlock 1967).

The secondary pharmacological effects of cortisone and related glucocorticoids are discussed in Chapter 8.

3.2.3 Photosensitisation

Photosensitisation can be classified as photoallergy or phototoxicity (Epstein 1962). In photoallergy, sunlight converts the drug, or a metabolite, into a hapten and further exposure to sunlight results in a hypersensitivity reaction, usually confined to the irradiated area. Phototoxicity arises when photoenergy from sunlight causes a drug, or a metabolite, to be converted to a toxic substance.

In man, photosensitisation has been observed with tar products (Polano 1965), sulphonamides (Schwarz & Speck 1957), promethazine (Sidi *et al* 1955) and chlorpromazine (Schulz *et al* 1956).

3.2.4 Drug interactions

IN VITRO INTERACTIONS

The mixing of drugs in a syringe or indiscriminate addition of drugs to the supply bag of an intravenous drip is a practice to be deprecated. Griffin and D'Arcy (1975) point out that *the absence of a visual incompatibility does not rule out interaction.* Although interaction usually results in reduced activity of the drugs involved, biological activity can be *increased.* Ampicillin, chlorpromazine and the soluble barbiturates should not be added to the container during infusion of dextrose injection BP or a dextran. Noradrenaline and tetracyclines should not be added to Ringer's injection.

COMPETITION FOR BINDING SITES

Many drugs bind to proteins in the blood plasma. The protein most commonly involved is albumin and to a much lesser extent the globulins. While bound to a plasma protein the drug is obviously not free to react with the cells of the target organ. If a second drug enters the blood and displaces the first drug from the binding sites on the plasma proteins a large quantity of the first drug is suddenly released. Effects due to drug overdosage may consequently arise. An example of this type of reaction in human medicine occurs when a patient who is receiving coumarin for anticoagulant therapy is treated with chloral hydrate, phenylbutazone or sulphonamides. Any of these compounds can displace the coumarin from the plasma protein and cause a massive haemorrhage as a result of the increased prothrombin time induced by excessively high levels of free (unbound) coumarin.

3.2.5 Abnormal metabolism

Under normal circumstances a drug will be excreted unchanged or metabolised by the liver in preparation for excretion. The metabolism of a drug by the body *usually* results in a less biologically active compound. It is a detoxification. The rates of metabolism and excretion do not vary greatly between individuals and therefore a drug administered on a mg/kg basis can be expected to attain approximately the same blood and tissue levels on all occasions. If, however, there is an increase or decrease in the rate of the metabolism of a drug, by whatever mechanism, unpredictable plasma and tissue levels will occur and toxicity, or reduced potency, can arise.

PHARMACOGENETICS

The appearance of an adverse drug reaction should make the clinician examine the patient rather than the drug. For instance a genetic abnormality may give rise to an adverse drug reaction. In man, approximately 1 in 2500 of the population has an atypical cholinesterase which results in prolonged apnoea after injection with succinylcholine (Kalow 1962).

Certain families have been shown to have a high predisposition to the ototoxic effects of streptomycin. There are significant differences between races in their ability to metabolise drugs; such differences also exist between populations from different parts of the country.

It would be very surprising if in animals we did not find differences between breeds in their ability to metabolise some drugs. In addition it would be advisable to give special attention to animals familiarly related to any in which unaccountable adverse drug reaction has been observed.

Different strains of both guinea-pigs (Chase 1941) and mice (McDevitt & Sela 1965) show differing ability to produce antibodies. Levine *et al* (1963) showed how susceptibility of the skin to sensitisation with dinitrochlorobenzene varied when comparing strains of guinea-pig. Adverse drug reactions of an allergic nature may therefore be caused by genetic differences.

ENZYME INDUCTION

Metabolism of a drug generally aids its excretion. Therefore, anything which stimulates the metabolism of a drug has the effect of reducing the exposure of the patient to the drug, although it should be borne in mind, that on occasions, a metabolite of a drug has itself proved to be potentially toxic.

Most drug metabolism takes place in the liver under the influence of the enzymes in the hepatocytes. Metabolism can, however, take place in the intestine, lung, and other organs.

A number of drugs are capable of stimulating (inducing) enzyme activity in the liver (e.g. barbiturates, griseofulvin and phenylbutazone). Following treatment with these drugs, the increased activity of the drug-metabolising liver enzymes causes more rapid metabolism of the drug itself (leading to tolerance), and also of many other drugs if these are administered at the same time, or soon afterwards. The effect can be that as much as twice the normal dose of a drug has to be administered in order to achieve and maintain normal tissue levels. A serious situation can arise when a treatment involves two drugs, one of which produces enzyme induction, so that increased dosage of both drugs is required. If at this stage the inducing drug is withdrawn, the activity of the drug-metabolising enzymes may return to normal, leaving the patient exposed to, perhaps, twice the normal dose of the second drug. This situation can be fatal.

AGE

Drug-metabolising enzyme activity is lower in neonates and in the elderly, and so dosage should be reduced accordingly. The neonate is also at risk from drugs administered to the nursing mother, and chloramphenicol, chlorpromazine, phenobarbitone, tetracyclines, and some sulphonamides have been reported in man to produce pharmacological effects in the neonate when injected into the mother. The elderly are more likely to suffer from the ototoxic effects of streptomycin and dihydrostreptomycin.

DIET

Starvation and abnormal diets may alter an animal's ability to metabolise drugs, and Murphy and DuBois (1958) reported that rats fed on non-protein diet have impaired drug-metabolising enzyme systems. Similarly, reduced metabolism of hexobarbitone and chlorpromazine in mice starved for 30 hours has been demonstrated (Dixon *et al* 1960). On the other hand, Kato and Gillette (1965) reported enhanced metabolism of drugs in starved female rats.

LIVER DISEASE

When the liver is directly affected by disease it is likely that detoxification of any drugs administered will be delayed; any toxic effects of such drugs will therefore be exaggerated if normal dosage is used. In such circumstances it is particularly important that drugs with a wide safety margin and minimum side-effects are used. If liver disease develops while an animal is under treatment for some other condition, it may well be necessary to reduce the dosage of any drugs in use. This point was clearly illustrated by Whelton *et al* (1968) who described how a woman, being treated with an ergot preparation for migraine, happened to develop virus hepatitis and subsequently severe gangrene of all extremities, due to ergot toxicity.

3.2.6 Abnormal excretion

The reabsorption of many drugs in the kidney tubules is influenced by urinary pH. The effective dose of quinidine and related drugs may become significantly increased if the urinary pH is increased. Urinary pH changes may arise intentionally as a result of the administration of acidifying or alkalinising agents, or may occur incidentally as a result of disease.

Kidney function dwindles with age. An apparently normal elderly person may have only half the normal kidney function of a younger adult. The effect of this reduced excretory capacity is to increase plasma levels of drugs normally excreted through the kidney, and to prolong the period for which the drug remains in the bloodstream.

Nephritis is a very common disease in dogs and cats. However, when signs indicative of this condition arise during treatment of an animal for some other disease, it would be prudent to consider whether some element of drug-induced nephritis might be present.

3.2.7 Local irritation

Local gastric irritation is encountered when aspirin is given to domestic animals (see Chapters 1 and 9). Erosion of the gastric mucosa induced in this way has been known to cause fatal haemorrhage in man.

Subcutaneous and intramuscular injections can produce severe local irritation and tissue necrosis, even though they are injected at the correct site. In many cases the mechanism of these reactions is obscure, and so such reactions may be regarded as an abnormal response by a particular animal, and not as a failing of the injected drug. *A manufacturer's instructions must not be ignored.* When there is a risk that subcutaneous injection will produce a reaction (e.g. with certain long-acting penicillin derivatives) intramuscular injection is usually recommended. On the other hand, pain is more likely to occur with intramuscular injections, and there is always a risk that an irritant preparation when given by this route, will cause damage to a nerve trunk, or that it will be inadvertently injected into a blood vessel, or that injection will be made into the fascial planes between muscle masses. These adverse effects of intramuscular injection of certain drugs may be minimised if injection is made slowly into the quadriceps muscle mass in small animals. With good technique, pain is minimal and not unacceptable.

In some cases, the local irritation or pain due to administration of drugs can be minimised by attention to the particular formulation used. Local anaesthetics have been added in small quantities to tetracycline preparations for this reason, although most modern tetracycline preparations have been designed to ensure that pain associated with their intramuscular use should be minimal. Much less discomfort is associated with the injection of a large volume of dilute crystalline penicillin than with the injection of a small volume of the concentrated solution, due to osmotic effects.

A corollary to the problem of local irritation is the absorption of drugs applied to normal or abraded surfaces, since enhanced absorption through an abraded surface may lead to subsequent production of adverse effects in distant organs. For example, ointments containing salicylates or neomycin when applied to abraded human skin may be followed by deafness attributable to the ototoxic effects of these two compounds. In the case of salicylates the deafness disappears when the treatment is stopped. Equally, the application of potent fluorinated corticosteroids may lead to suppression of the hypothalamic-pituitary-adrenal axis (see Chapter 7).

3.2.8 Carcinogenesis

The problem of identifying cancer as an adverse drug reaction is that the lesion may well arise many years after the administration of the drug has ceased. Oestrogen administered to pregnant women has induced vaginal adenocarcinoma in their daughters some 25 years later (Herbst & Sculley 1970). Oestrogens have also been shown to produce tumours in dogs, hamsters, mice, rabbits and rats. Usually the endocrine and hormone-responsive tissues are affected.

Griseofulvin fed at very high dose levels (0.5–2.5% of the diet for 400 days) produced liver tumours in mice (Hurst & Paget 1963). Experiments of this nature are difficult to relate to clinical practice, but they should not be dismissed as unrealistic, if only because there may exist within the population highly susceptible individuals who will succumb to low levels of the compound.

3.3 Specific organotoxicity

3.3.1 Eye

There have been a number of reports of corneal damage in dogs following vaccination with infectious canine hepatitis virus (ICHV) (Carmichael 1964; Curtis & Barnett 1973). The lesion is first seen 10–15 days after vaccination, usually only in one eye, but occasionally in both. Inflammation and photophobia are rapidly followed by corneal oedema, which gives the eye a bluish tinge. In mild cases the blue tinge disperses and the eye returns to normal within a few days. In more serious cases corneal ulceration and other forms of keratopathy arise. Rarely, permanent loss of vision may occur following persistently raised intraocular pressure (Curtis & Barnett 1973).

The eye has also been shown to be affected by chlorpromazine. Barron *et al* (1972a, 1972d) gave chlorpromazine orally for 10 days to dogs and produced corneal stromal granularity.

3.3.2 Central nervous system

One of the most severe adverse drug reactions affecting the central nervous system results from administration of halogenated oxyquinolines to dogs. The drug is used as an antidiarrhoeal drug in man and animals. The problem is most commonly encountered when owners dose their animals with the formulation they had purchased for their own use. Lannek (1973) and Lannek and Jöhnsson (1974) have reported 100 such cases in dogs. The animals show hyperexcitability and convulsions and at post mortem examination there are degenerative neuronal changes in the brain and spinal cord. There is also extensive focal necrosis of the heart and hydropic degeneration of the liver.

3.3.3 Liver

Adverse drug reactions involving the liver are not uncommon in man and they have been sufficiently closely studied to allow classification of the reactions and associated pathology. The same does not apply in small animal medicine where few reports have reached the literature. Because of the paucity of information on the extent of the problem in the dog and the cat one can merely be aware of those drugs which produce liver pathology in man and are used in small animal practice.

In man, drugs in the phenothiazine group including the promazines (chlorpromazine), produce cholestatic jaundice, as do the C17-substituted testosterone compounds. Drugs used in the treatment of cancer — methotrexate, 6-mercaptopurine and busulphan — and the tetracycline antibiotics may also produce liver injury.

There is now little doubt that halothane can cause hepatitis in man (Davidson *et al* 1966; Klion *et al* 1969) and it would be surprising if the same were not also true for the dog.

3.3.4 Bone marrow

A drug-induced reduction of cells in the peripheral blood may be caused by destruction of the cells as they circulate or by destruction of immature cells in the bone marrow. The cytotoxicity may be allergic or simply a direct cytotoxic destruction of the cells.

In the allergic cytopenias studied in man an antibody is formed with the drug, or a metabolite, acting as the hapten. Of the drugs commonly used in small animal practice phenacetin, chlorpromazine and penicillin have produced allergic haemolytic anaemia. Sulphadimidine, phenylbutazone and digitoxin may produce an allergic thrombocytopenia, and chlorpromazine an allergic leucopenia.

Neither direct cytotoxic cytopenia nor allergic cytopenia have been recorded very often in veterinary practice. Penny *et al* (1970) have reported depression of bone marrow by chloramphenicol in cats. The depression was predominantly of erythroid elements of the bone marrow. The clinical picture was of depression and inappetence.

3.4 Treatment

Mild anaphylactic reactions can be treated with antihistamines. However, if an animal is in a critical state of anaphylactic shock, then adrenaline should be given, followed by antihistamines.

Whenever an adverse drug reaction occurs an attempt should be made to find a replacement drug. It is as well, particularly in hypersensitivity reactions, to search for a drug which is chemically unrelated to the offending drug. In a hypersensitivity reaction it is not sufficient simply to reduce the dosage, because even very low doses can produce a severe reaction.

3.5 Notification of adverse drug reaction

The Medicines Act 1968 requires the holder of a Product Licence for a veterinary medicinal product to keep a record of reports of adverse effects in animals, or in people exposed to the veterinary products. The Licensing Authority has access to these records.

No pharmaceutical company would wish to keep on the market an unsuitable product. The decision of whether or not to withdraw a product may depend heavily on information from veterinary surgeons in practice. For this reason it is essential that a detailed history and findings of clinical examination are recorded when an adverse drug reaction is suspected.

3.6 Conclusions

When an adverse drug reaction is suspected the following should be checked:

1 Is this indeed an adverse drug reaction or are these the signs of an unassociated disease?
2 Were the lesions I am now observing in fact present, even mildly, before the drug was administered?
3 Has the animal reacted to this or a related compound previously?
4 Has a similar reaction been seen in related animals?
5 Is there only one drug involved? (The owner also may be administering a compound or altering the diet.)
6 Could anything be altering the plasma level of the drug and raising it to toxic levels? (e.g. Enteritis producing ultrarapid absorption, kidney disease reducing excretion.)
7 Were the manufacturer's instructions for dosage followed correctly by (a) the owner? (b) the veterinary surgeon?
8 Has the compound been stored correctly? Antibiotic preparations have been known to deteriorate and give rise to toxic products if incorrectly stored.
9 Am I reasonably sure that this is an adverse drug reaction and do I have the information to convince someone else?

References

Ackroyd J. F. (1958) Thrombocytopenic purpura due to drug hypersensitivity. In *Sensitivity Reactions in Drugs*, eds. M. L. Rosenheim & R. Moulton, p.28. Blackwell Scientific Publications, Oxford.

Barron C. N., Rubin L. F. & Steelman R. L. (1972a) Chlorpromazine and the eye of the dog. III. Natural daylight versus artificial light. *Exp. Mol. Pathol.* **16**, 158.

Barron C. N., Rubin L. F. & Steelman R. L. (1972b) Chlorpromazine and the eye of the dog. IV. Reversibility of ocular lesions. *Exp. Mol. Pathol.* **16**, 163.

Barron C. N., Rubin L. F. & Steelman R. L. (1972c) Chlorpromazine and the eye of the dog. V. An attempt to produce lenticular lesions. *Exp. Mol. Pathol.* **16**, 169.

Barron C. N., Murchison T. E., Rubin L. F., Rubin M. L., Herron W., Muscarella M. & Birkhead H. (1972d) Chlopromazine and the eye of the dog. VI. A comparison of phenothiazine tranquilizers. *Exp. Mol. Pathol.* **16**, 172.

Carmichael I. E. (1964) Ocular lesions of infectious canine hepatitis. *Path. Vet.* **1**, 73.

Chase M. W. (1941) Inheritance in guinea-pigs of the susceptibility to skin sensitization with simple chemical compounds. *J. Exp. Med.* **73**, 711.

Curtis R. & Barnett K. C. (1973) The ocular lesions of infectious canine hepatitis. I. Clinical features. *J. Small Anim. Pract.* **14**, 375.

Davidson C. S., Babior B. & Popper H. (1966) Concerning the hepatotoxicity of halothane. *New Eng. J. Med.* **275**, 1497.

Dixon R. L., Shultice R. & Fouts J. R. (1960) Factors affecting drug metabolism by liver microsomes. IV. Starvation. *Biol. Med.* **103**, 333.

Epstein S. (1962) Photoallergy versus phototoxicity In *Dermatoses due to Environmental and Physical Factors*, ed. R. B. Rees, p.119. C. C. Thomas, Springfield, Ill.

Griffin J. P. & D'Arcy P. F. (1975) *A Manual of Adverse Drug Interactions.* John Wright, Bristol.

Herbst A. L. & Sculley R. E. (1970) Adenocarcinoma of the vagina in adolescence: a report of 7 cases including 6 clear cell carcinoma. *Cancer, N.Y.* **25**, 745.

Hurst E. W. & Paget G. E. (1963) Protoporphyrin, cirrhosis and hepatoma in the livers of mice given griseofulvin. *Brit. J. Derm.* **75**, 105.

Kalow W. (1962) *Pharmacogenetics: Heredity and the Response to Drugs.* W. B. Saunders, Philadelphia.

Kato R. & Gillette J. R. (1965) Effect of starvation on NADPH — dependent enzymes in liver microsomes of male and female rats. *J. Pharmac. Exp. Ther.* **150**, 279.

Klion F. M., Schaffner F. & Popper H. (1969) Hepatitis after exposure to halothane. *Ann. Intern. Med.* **71**, 467.

Landsteiner K. (1945) *The Specificity of Serological Reactions.* Harvard University Press, Cambridge, Mass.

Lannek B. (1973) Toxicity of halogenated oxyquinolines in dogs. A clinical study. I. A survey of cases. *Acta. Vet. Scand.* **14**, 723.

Lannek B. & Jöhnsson L. (1974) Toxicity of halogenated oxyquinolines in dogs. A clinical study. V. Pathological findings. *Acta. Vet. Scand.* **15**, 1.

Levine B. B., Ojeda A. & Benacerraf B. (1963) The genetic control of the immune response to hapten-poly-l-lysine conjugates in guinea-pigs. *J. Exp. Med.* **118**, 953.

McDevitt H. O. & Sela M. (1965) Genetic control of the antibody. *J. Exp. Med.* **122**, 517.

Murphy S. D. & DuBois K. P. (1958) The influence of various factors on the enzymatic conversion of organic thiophosphates to anticholinesterase agents. *J. Pharmac. Exp. Ther.* **124**, 453.

Parker C. W. (1975) Drug allergy. *New Eng. J. Med.* **292**, 511.

Penny R. H. C., Carlisle C. H., Prescott C. W. & Davidson H. A. (1970) Further observations of the effects of chloramphenicol on the haemopoietic system of the cat. *Brit. Vet. J.* **126**, 453.

Polano M. K. (1965) Photosensitivity due to drugs. In *Drug Induced Diseases*, eds. L. Mayler & H. M. Peck, p.102. Excerpta Medica Foundation, Amsterdam.

Schulz K. H., Wiskemann A. & Wulf K. (1956) Klinische und experimentelle Untersuchungen über die Photodynamische Wirksamkeit von Phenothiazinderivaten insbesondere von Megaphen. *Arch. Klin. Exp. Derm.* **202**, 285.

Schwarz K. & Speck M. (1957) Experimentelle untersuchungen zur Frage der Photoallergie der Sulfonamides. *Dermatologica (Basel)* **114**, 232.

Sherlock S. (1967) The prediction of hepatotoxicity due to therapeutic agents in man. In *Drug Responses in Man*, eds. G. E. W. Wolstenholme & R. Porter, Churchill, London.

Sidi E., Hincky M. & Gervais A. (1955) Allergic sensitization and photosensitization to phenergan cream. *J. Invest. Derm.* **24**, 345.

Whelton M. J., Allaway A., Stewart A. & Kreel L. M. (1968) Ergot poisoning in acute hepatic necrosis. *Gut* **9**, 287.

4

Bacterial sensitivity to antibiotics

ANNE M. HARRIS

At the beginning of this century, Paul Ehrlich defined the weapons for the battle against bacterial disease. He suggested that we should look for medicaments attacking receptor sites on bacteria which were not present in the host. These could then 'strike the parasites with full force in the manner of magic bullets seeking out the enemy' (Ehrlich 1959).

Today we have a number of 'magic bullets', the antibiotics, which can be used against bacterial infection. In general, they behave as Ehrlich proposed and act on specific bacterial sites which are not found in animal cells.

4.1 Modes of action of antibiotics

Antibiotic action is usually directed against essential bacterial functions (Table 4.1) and may be lethal to micro-organisms; this type of activity is usually termed bactericidal. In other cases, antibiotics have a bacteriostatic action and only prevent multiplication of bacterial cells. The bacteriostatic effect is maintained whilst adequate concentrations of antibiotic are in contact with the organisms. If the level falls, bacteria may multiply again. Successful use of bacteriostatic compounds usually depends on maintenance of effective antibiotic levels for long enough to allow the organisms to be killed by host defence mechanisms.

The first antibacterial compound which satisfactorily fulfilled Ehrlich's criteria were the sulphonamides, discovered in 1932 (Domagk 1935). The sulphonamides are completely synthetic agents, whilst the true antibiotics such as penicillin, are by definition derived from naturally produced substances. The sulphonamides are, however, usually classed together with the antibiotics because they have similar antibacterial activity.

Several folic acid derivatives are necessary cofactors in the biosynthesis of the nucleotides required for nucleic acid synthesis, and for other aspects of cellular metabolism. Para-aminobenzoic acid (PABA) is utilised by many bacterial cells as the first precursor in folic acid synthesis, since they are unable to take up preformed folate, which is normally utilised by mammalian cells. PABA is thus an essential nutrient for many bacteria, and sulphonamides, which are chemically similar to PABA, compete with this nutrient

Table 4.1 Sites of antibiotic action.

Bacterial function	Antibiotic
Energy metabolism	Sulphonamides, trimethoprim
Protein synthesis	Chloramphenicol
	Tetracycline
	Erythromycin
	Streptomycin
Nucleic acid synthesis	Nalidixic acid, acridines
Cell wall synthesis	Penicillins and cephalosporins
Membrane function	Nystatin, amphotericin

for an attachment site on the bacterial enzyme which converts it to folic acid. The sulphonamide is attached preferentially to PABA in sulphonamide-sensitive strains, so that the nucleotide-synthetic pathway is blocked, cell multiplication is prevented, and a bacteriostatic effect is obtained (Fig. 4.1). Trimethoprim was discovered comparatively recently, and has a similar effect later in the same pathway, inhibiting the conversion of folic acid to folinic acid (Bushby & Hitchings 1968). Selective toxicity against bacteria is obtained by virtue of the fact that the enzyme involved in this conversion, dihydrofolate reductase, is several thousand times more sensitive to inhibition by trimethoprim when it occurs in bacteria than when it occurs in mammalian cells (Hitchings 1969). Trimethoprim is not usually used alone, but is frequently used in combination with a sulphonamide to obtain an additive and often bactericidal action. Moreover, some organisms which are insensitive to either drug alone, may be killed by the combination (Lawrence 1973).

A number of antibiotics act against bacterial protein synthesis (Table 4.1). Their action may be directed against several different points in the process as shown in Fig. 4.2. Several types of antibiotic affect attachment or movement of proteins on the ribosome. The effect is specific to bacterial ribosomes which comprise two subunits, 30S and 50S, so named from their sedimentation properties during ultracentrifugation. Animal robosomes separate into subunits of different weight, 40S and 60S, and are not affected by antibiotic action.

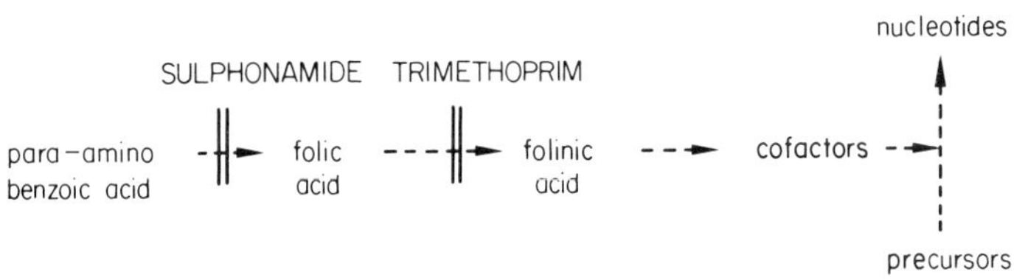

Fig. 4.1 Mode of action of sulphonamide compounds and trimethoprim.

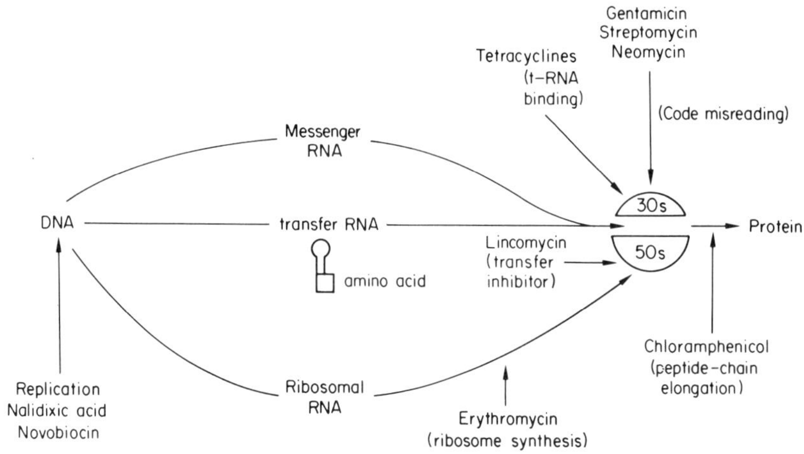

Fig. 4.2 The action of antibiotics on protein and DNA synthesis in bacterial cells. Messenger RNA, transfer RNA, and ribosomal RNA are constructed by the cell on the DNA template. Messenger RNA codes the ribosome for the amino acid sequence required for the construction of a particular protein, and the requisite amino acids are then transported to the ribosome by specific transfer RNAs. The amino acid chain is assembled on the ribosome by a series of enzymic processes, to form the new protein.
Reproduced with kind permission of Dr. G. W. Ross.

Erythromycin and other macrolide antibiotics effect ribosome synthesis particularly at the 50S site; lincomycin prevents transfer RNA attachment to the same part of the ribosome whilst tetracyclines affect the 30S subunit, and prevent binding of t-RNA (Weisblum & Davies 1968). All these compounds have a bacteriostatic action. Chloramphenicol is another bacteriostatic antibiotic which affects the growing peptide chain, preventing elongation and production of a functional protein, probably by inhibiting peptidyl-transferase (for reviews of antibiotics acting on ribosomes, see Weisblum & Davies 1968; Franklin & Snow 1971; Gale *et al* 1972).

Aminoglycosides (e.g. streptomycin, neomycin, gentamicin, kanamycin, framycetin), in contrast to most other antibiotics affecting protein synthesis, have a bactericidal effect on bacteria. They frequently cause code misreading early in the synthetic process, perhaps by distorting the ribosomes to which the drug is bound (Leon & Brock 1967), and may also have secondary effects on cell respiration and metabolism.

Antibiotics may also affect DNA replication in the bacterial cell, usually with a bacteriostatic result. Novobiocin, nalidixic acid and the acridine group of compounds all affect DNA synthesis (Smith & Davis 1967).

The penicillins and cephalosporins act on the bacterial cell wall. These antibiotics both have a similar nucleus which contains a β-lactam ring. Semi-synthetic antibiotics (e.g. ampicillin, cloxacillin, amoxycillin, and cephalexin, cephoxazole, and cephalonium) can be made by changing chemical substituents at sites on the penicillin or cephalosporin nucleus. β-lactam antibiotics exert their effect by becoming intercalated in the cell walls of *growing* bacteria in place of natural cross-linking compounds. The integrity of the cell wall is thereby destroyed and bacteria exposed to β-lactam antibiotics show conformational changes such as elongation, due to osmotic effects. Lysis of the bacteria eventually occurs, and the antibiotic effect is thus bactericidal (see Gale *et al* 1972, for a review of mode of action).

Some antibiotics are able to intercalate into the cell membranes of bacteria, rather than the cell walls. Permeability is affected, and the cells lose the ability to take up essential nutrients, whilst essential intracellular components may be lost. The polyene compounds, amphotericin and nystatin, have this effect on fungal cells, and the peptide polymyxins have a similar action on bacteria (Newton 1965; Weissman & Sessa 1967; Gale *et al* 1972).

Another antibiotic often used in small animal practice is griseofulvin. This compound acts only against fungi, and has a specific role in clinical use against dermatophyte fungi which cause ringworm, although its exact mode of action is unclear. Griseofulvin deposits in the keratin layer of skin, hair, and nail following oral administration, and causes the hyphal tips of the fungi to curl and die. Fungi cannot grow in griseofulvin-protected hair, and so new hair grows out unaffected by the dermatophyte (Blank 1960; Huber & Gottlieb 1968).

4.2 The spectrum of antibacterial activity

The spectrum of action varies from those antibiotics active against very small groups of organisms to compounds which can affect many different species. One way of classifying antibiotics is to group them according to their action against Gram-positive and Gram-negative bacteria (Table 4.2). Narrow-

Table 4.2 Antibacterial spectrum.

Gram +ve	Broad-spectrum	Gram − ve
Penicillin	Sulphonamides	Polymyxin
Cloxacillin	Tetracyclines	Carbenicillin
Methicillin	Streptomycin	
Lincomycin	Neomycin	
Erythromycin	Gentamicin	
Fusidic acid	Ampicillin	
Novobiocin	Amoxycillin	
	Cephaloridine	
	Chloramphenicol	

spectrum compounds act principally against either Gram-positive or Gram-negative organisms. Broad-spectrum antibiotics have activity against both groups. The differences in cell wall structure which give rise to the staining characteristics of Gram-positive and Gram-negative bacteria reflect general biochemical intracellular differences between these two general classes of micro-organism. The Gram-positive bacteria tend to metabolise relatively complex preformed nutrients from the environment, whilst the Gram-negative species are much less selective, and have well-developed synthetic mechanisms, which allow them to utilise very simple nutrients. This renders Gram-negative organisms much more adaptable. In addition, Gram-negative organisms tend not to concentrate osmotically active nutrients within the cytoplasm, as Gram-positive bacteria do, and therefore do not need a rigid cell wall. They have, instead, a multilayered, flexible wall, which is capable of exercising considerable selectivity over uptake of foreign molecules, such as antibiotics (Franklin & Snow 1971).

When antibacterial spectrum is considered in relation to therapy, attention is usually centred on the minimum inhibitory concentration (MIC) of an antibiotic which can be used to achieve a bactericidal or bacteriostatic effect *in vitro*.

Tables 4.3 and 4.4 show the MICs of a range of antibiotics for several commonly encountered pathogens. Levels of antibiotic required to kill Gram-positive strains (Table 4.3) are frequently lower than levels which affect Gram-negative organisms, but Gram-negative strains are often killed more quickly. The MIC value can only be used as a guide to therapy and it is important to consider the site of infection to decide whether satisfactory antibiotic levels are likely to be attained. In addition, the nature of the suspected or known pathogen should be considered. Some species include many strains which are antibiotic-resistant *in vitro* but may respond satisfactorily to antibiotic treatment *in vivo*. *Pseudomonas* spp. are frequently opportunist pathogens taking advantage of pathological changes, but if the

Table 4.3 Minimal inhibitory concentrations (μg/ml).

Antibiotic	*Staph. aureus*	*Strept. pyogenes*
Sulphonamides	8·0 – 64·0	0·25 – 16·0
Tetracyclines	0·12	0·25
Chloramphenicol	4·0	2·0
Erythromycin	0·12	0·03
Lincomycin	0·5 – 2·0	0·12
Streptomycin	2·0	32·0
Penicillin	0·01 – >1000	0·006
Ampicillin	0·01 – >1000	0·03
Cloxacillin	0·25	0·06
Cephaloridine	0·12	0·01

Table 4.4 Minimal inhibitory concentrations (μg/ml). R = Resistant.

Antibiotic	*E. coli*	*Salmonella* spp.	*Pseudomonas*
Sulphonamides	4·0 – 64·0	16·0 – 128	128
Tetracyclines	1·0	1·0	32 – R
Chloramphenicol	2·0 – 8·0	2·0	R
Streptomycin	2·0	2·0	16·0
Neomycin	2·0	2·0	8·0
Gentamicin	0·5	0·25	1·0
Penicillin	32·0	4·0 – 16·0	R
Ampicillin	8·0	1·0 – 8·0	R
Cephaloridine	4·0	2·0	R
Polymyxin	0·25	0·25	0·5

number of pseudomonas can be reduced sufficiently, the normal flora may be able to reestablish.

4.3 Bacterial resistance

Since the advent of bacterial therapy with antibiotics, a number of resistance mechanisms have been reported. Organisms able to resist antibiotic action seem to have been present in bacterial populations before the use of antibiotics (Gardner *et al* 1969) but have apparently been selected more stringently in the last 30 years. Resistance to antiseptics was recognised by Kossiakoff in 1887 and Ehrlich realised in 1914 that bacteria might become resistant to antibacterial compounds.

If organisms are grown in the presence of an antibiotic over a period of time, they may appear to become resistant to it, but when the antibiotic is removed, such cultures usually revert to sensitivity. Resistance developed in this way is usually acquired at the expense of viability or virulence and is an expression of drug tolerance rather than drug resistance (Garrod *et al* 1973).

Antibiotic resistance is more likely to arise within bacterial populations because of selection pressures from the environment. Widespread or prolonged use of an antibiotic may favour the growth of naturally occurring resistant organisms within a bacterial population and these strains may become a problem unless steps are taken to change the pattern of antibiotic usage.

Mechanisms of bacterial resistance to antibiotics include:

1 Changes in affinity of bacterial enzymes.
2 Changes in cell permeability.
3 Production of destructive enzymes.
4 Other mechanisms.

Organisms resistant to sulphonamide compounds show a change in the affinity of a target enzyme in the folic acid pathway. Sulphonamides are no longer bound preferentially to the enzyme and the natural substrate, para-aminobenzoic acid (PABA), attaches to the enzyme instead. Alternatively, the bacteria may be able to increase PABA production, thus nullifying the effects of the sulphonamide (White & Woods 1965). Tetracycline resistant cultures are able to transport the antibiotic out of their cells and so the antibiotic has no effect on protein synthesis (Franklin 1967).

The most familiar drug resistance mechanism is production, by resistant bacteria, of enzymes which are able to destroy antibiotics. Phosphorylating, adenylating and acetylating enzymes produced by bacteria destroy the aminoglycoside group of antibiotics. β-lactamases made by many Gram-positive and Gram-negative bacteria destroy β-lactamase-sensitive penicillins and/or cephalosporins.

Staphylococcal penicillinase was the first β-lactamase to be discovered (Abraham & Chain 1940). Since then, β-lactamases with widely different specificities for β-lactam compounds have been described, some destroy only penicillins, others predominantly cephalosporins. The enzyme breaks down compounds which have a β-lactam ring to form chemicals which have no antibacterial activity (see review by Sykes & Matthew 1976, for properties of β-lactamases).

If highly sensitive detection methods are used, β-lactamase can be demonstrated in most bacterial species and it has been suggested that the enzyme may play some part in normal bacterial physiology (Matthew & Harris 1976). The clinical significance of β-lactamase depends to a considerable extent upon the type and quantity of the enzyme produced by a bacterial strain and also the frequency with which a particular enzyme type occurs in clinical disease. A survey by the present author and colleagues of β-lactamases produced by isolates from animals show that in general, β-lactamases are produced in smaller quantities from veterinary sources compared with strains from humans.

In the last 15 years, a number of β-lactamase-resistant, semi-synthetic cephalosporins and penicillins have become available. These compounds have chemical substituents which make them resistant to β-lactamase attack. An alternative approach is to inhibit the enzymes using β-lactam compounds which bind to β-lactamase and inactivate the enzyme. This effect has been reported using a combination of the inhibitory cephalosporin, cephoxazole, together with penicillin. In this combination, penicillin is protected from β-lactamase attack by the inhibitory action of cephoxazole (Harris *et al* 1976). Fig. 4.3 illustrates this situation with a penicillin-resistant *Staphylococcus aureus*.

Bacterial resistance may sometimes occur by DNA mutation as described above, but this form of resistance is relatively rare. In the last 15 years, resistance mediated by Resistance (R) factors has been widely discussed. R-factors are extrachromosomal elements (plasmids) found in some bacterial

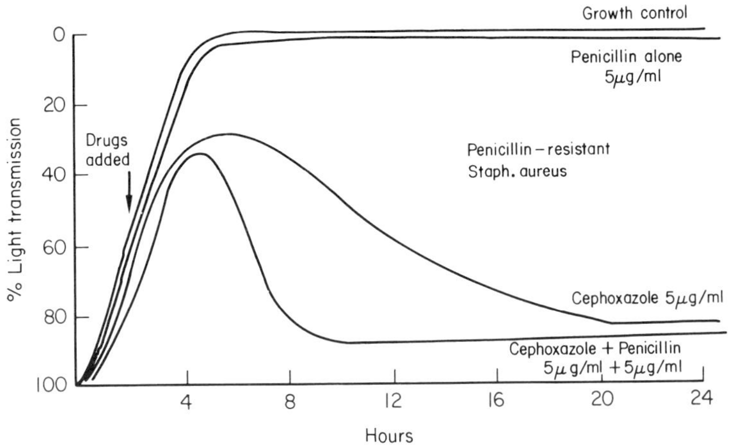

Fig. 4.3 Growth curves of *Staph. aureus* in a nutrient medium (Control) and in a medium containing penicillin or cephoxazole or a combination of the two antibiotics.

cells. These small, circular pieces of DNA are distinct from the bacterial chromosome and can be transferred independently to recipient bacteria via hair-like pili or tubes present on the surface of donor cells (Curtis 1969). R-factors may carry markers specifying antibiotic resistance and usually specify resistance to a range of antibiotics, rather than single agents. They can be transferred between bacterial species and genera (e.g. *Escherichia coli* to *Salmonella* spp.). This form of resistance is potentially alarming because normal commensal organisms may acquire resistance. In addition, R-factors mediating resistance to antibiotics which are usually used for therapy may be introduced into dangerous pathogens like *Salmonella typhi*, and organisms commensal in the gut may become significant genitourinary pathogens. The process of conjugation, as described above, does not seem to occur in Gram-positive organisms, but plasmids do exist, and these are transferred from organism to organism by bacteriophages (Datta 1973), a process known as transduction.

Lacey (1975) reviewed the *in vivo* importance of R-factors and concluded that although the use of antibiotics has selected R-factor-carrying organisms, such strains are often at a disadvantage because they grow more slowly. Populations of resistant organisms tend to lose their R-factors in the absence of antibiotics, although administration of a single antibiotic may select R-factors capable of transferring resistance to several antimicrobial agents (Whitehead 1973). Transfer of R-factors is relatively easy to accomplish *in vitro* but appears to occur rarely *in vivo*, possibly because of competition from the normal flora. It is possible that transfer may occur more easily in topical infections or in food or water. Lacey suggests that antibiotic policies should be formulated to exploit the loss of R-factors from important pathogens.

4.4 Measurement of bacterial sensitivity

Bacterial sensitivity to antibiotics can be measured by several methods, of which the minimal inhibitory concentration (MIC) is probably the most widely used. The MIC is measured by growing organisms in a range of antibiotic dilutions. The least concentration which prevents visible growth in a suitable medium is recorded as the MIC. This figure is of course only a guide to antibiotic activity and may vary for a given organism depending on the inoculum concentration added to the antibiotic dilutions. Inocula of 10^5 or 10^6 organisms are usually used but these concentrations of organisms may be significantly greater than the numbers which may be encountered in an *in vivo* infection.

If more than one antibiotic is used for therapy it is often useful to assess their effects in combination. Jawetz and Gunnison (1952) defined the principles for combined antibiotic therapy. They postulated that two or more bacteriostatic antibiotics may have an additive effect; two bactericidal antibiotics usually have an additive or sometimes a synergistic action. Bactericidal and bacteriostatic antibiotics used together may be antagonistic. The last possibility arises because bactericidal antibiotics usually act on cells which are multiplying, whilst bacteriostatic antibiotics prevent multiplication. Thus the two actions may impede each other, with an antagonistic result. The additive activity of penicillin and streptomycin, two bactericidal antibiotics often used in combination, is shown in Table 4.5. Additive or synergistic activity of two antibiotics can be demonstrated *in vitro* using several different antibiotic combinations and for a wide range of bacterial species. But whenever combined antibiotic therapy is used *in vivo*, it is most important that the formulation is designed to ensure that all components of the preparation reach the target site in the host at the correct concentration and in appropriate proportions.

Table 4.5 The activity of penicillin and streptomycin alone and in combination against common veterinary pathogens.

Organism	Strain number	MIC (μg/ml)		
		Penicillin	Streptomycin	Penicillin/ streptomycin
Staph. aureus	898	0·01	2·0	0·01 + 0·01
Staph. aureus	953E	250	31·0	1·0 + 1·0
Staph. aureus	1214E	250	16·0	0·5 + 0·5
Strept. agalactiae	849E	0·06	12·5	0·04 + 0·04
C. pyogenes	7	0·03	12·5	0·03 + 0·03
E. coli	741	25·0	6·2	3·1 + 3·1

Bacterial sensitivity is frequently assessed quantitively using paper discs impregnated with antibiotic. The diameter of the growth-inhibition zone around the disc is used to indicate sensitivity or resistance to an antibiotic. Salient factors in disc sensitivity testing were reviewed recently by Linton (1976). It is important to remember that discs contain antibiotic at a fixed level which is decided by the way in which an antibiotic diffuses in agar. The level does not relate to antibiotic dosage or to expected blood levels. In order to obtain useful results from disc tests, the test conditions, particularly the inoculum, must be standardised and zone sizes should be measured. Very light, or very heavy inocula may give false indications of sensitivity, or of resistance. In addition, it is valuable to correlate sensitivity results with *in vivo* performance of an antibiotic. Sensitivity to an antibiotic *in vitro* does not necessarily imply that a compound will be effective. In a recent study of a small number of clinical isolates we showed that 15 out of 15 organisms associated with mastitis, which were resistant to penicillin and streptomycin, responded to treatment with the antibiotic combination whilst on this occasion 5 out of 23 sensitive strains failed to respond (Evans *et al* 1975).

Bacterial sensitivity to antibiotics can also be assessed by growing the organisms in liquid culture, and then comparing the growth rates of the

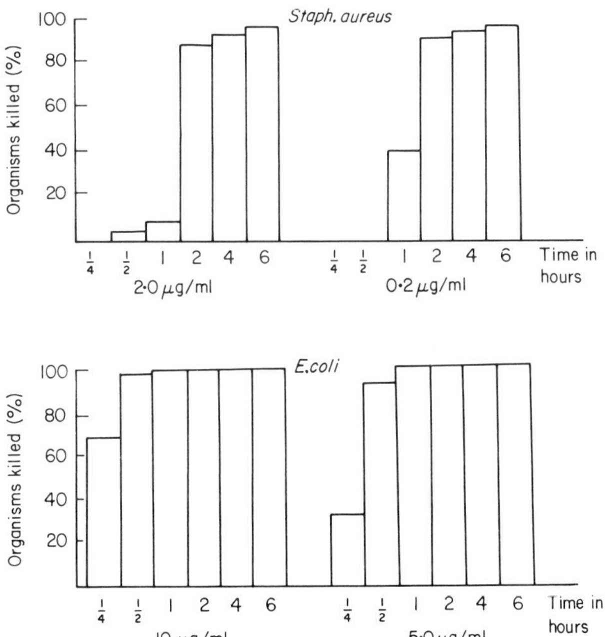

Fig. 4.4 The percentage of organisms killed after contact with cephalonium in milk for different periods of time.

organisms in the presence of various concentrations of antibiotic. The bactericidal effect of a cephalosporin compound on *Staphylococcus aureus* and *Escherichia coli* is shown in Fig. 4.4. The percentage of organisms killed after contact with the antibiotic for different periods of time was calculated by comparison with the initial count. A higher antibiotic concentration was used for the Gram-negative organisms, but these were killed more quickly than the *Staph. aureus* culture under these conditions. No organisms could be recovered in either test after 6 hours of incubation in the presence of antibiotic. This type of test provides much more information about the nature of the sensitivity of the organisms tested than does the plate test, and it has the additional advantage that it can be carried out using appropriate body fluids as the culture medium. Serum, urine or milk may have a considerable effect on antibiotic activity, and it is important to ensure that an antibiotic will maintain effective activity *in vivo* in the relevant fluid.

4.5 Practical use of antibiotics

The choice of antibiotic depends chiefly upon a knowledge of which pathogens are likely to be causing the condition to be treated. Initially the choice must often be empirical because prior bacteriological information is not available. Antibiotic selection is therefore frequently based on past experience in treating apparently similar conditions, or on known epidemiology. The problems of antibiotic selection are discussed at some length in Chapter 6, but in the present context various points relating to the identification of the causal organisms may be considered.

In selecting a suitable antibiotic for use in a particular situation, it may be reasonable to adopt an empirical approach initially, and subsequently to seek further bacteriological support. It will often be worthwhile to do a simple Gram stain to assess the prevalence of Gram-positive or Gram-negative organisms at the outset. Such an approach is particularly useful in conditions such as septic otitis, in which fungal infection may be a complication. Swabs and samples should be taken carefully to avoid contamination with unwanted organisms (e.g. urine samples by sterile catheter); and specimens should then be sent as quickly as possible to the laboratory. Transport medium is invaluable for preserving organisms on swabs which may otherwise die in transit, if laboratory facilities are not immediately available. If isolation is to be carried out in the practice laboratory, the organisms should be cultured as soon as possible on blood agar and preferably also on MacConkey's medium, and single colonies may subsequently be removed from these cultures for sensitivity testing. Attempts to assess antibiotic sensitivity on mixed cultures of primary isolates are fraught with problems, and the results are likely to be of questionable value. Special media for the specific identification of organisms are unlikely to be used in most practice laboratories, but the 'dip-slide' technique for the evaluation of bacterial infection in urine may be of particular value, since it allows rough identification of the organisms in primary culture, and aids differentiation between bacterial infection and contamination.

Anaerobic organisms may be highly significant in small animal infections, and these will be missed unless anaerobic cultures are also carried out. Certain anaerobic organisms, such as *Bacteroides* (*Fusiformis*) species, are particularly fragile, and will not survive for more than an hour or two on a swab. They will survive for rather longer in pus or other biological material, and where it is thought that such organisms may be present (they are common in oral lesions, for example), a sample of pus or debris should be submitted for anaerobic culture as soon as possible. Microaerophilic organisms can be extremely difficult to grow in culture, and the importance of examining an immediate Gram-stained preparation in addition to attempting to culture specimens cannot be overemphasised.

It is important to supply case histories and details of previous and current antibiotic therapy, when specimens are sent to distant laboratories, in order to assist the laboratory staff in subsequent tests. The veterinary surgeon has considerable influence on the final laboratory report because he or she decides the way in which samples are taken and transported; both of these factors have a profound effect upon bacterial survival.

4.6 Conclusion

A wide range of antibiotics is now available to the veterinary surgeon and the mode of action and activity of the compounds against known or likely pathogens must be carefully assessed. However, these aspects of therapy cannot be considered in isolation. The veterinary surgeon in practice has to assume the roles of pharmacologist, microbiologist and clinician in order to apply the available information effectively in the treatment of bacterial disease.

References

Abraham E. P. & Chain E. (1940) Enzyme from bacteria able to destroy penicillin, *Nature* **146**, 837.

Blank H. (ed.) (1960) Symposium on griseofulvin. *Arch. Dermatol.* **81**, 649.

Bushby S. R. M. & Hitchings G. H. (1968) Trimethoprim, a sulphonamide potentiator. *Brit. J. Pharmac. Chemother.* **33**, 72.

Curtis R. (1969) Bacterial conjugation. *Ann. Rev. Microbiol.* **23**, 69.

Datta N. (1973) Transmissible antibiotic resistance. In *Current Antibiotic Therapy*, eds. A. M. Geddes & J. D. Williams, p.31. Churchill Livingstone, Edinburgh.

Domagk G. (1935) Ein Beitrag zur Chemotherapie der bakteriellen Infektionen. *Dtsch. Med. Wschr.* **61**, 250.

Ehrlich P. (1959) *The Collected Papers of Paul Ehrlich.* Ed. F. Himmelweit, vol. III, p. 505. Pergamon Press, Oxford.

Evans J. M., Watson D. J., Harris A. M. & Llewellyn G. G. (1975) Antibiotic selection in clinical mastitis. *Vet. Rec.* **97**, 248.

Franklin T. J. (1967) Resistance of *Escherichia coli* to tetracyclines: changes in permeability to tetracyclines in *Esch. coli* bearing transmissible resistance factors. *Biochem. J.* **105**, 371.

Franklin T. J. & Snow G. A. (1971) *Biochemistry of Antimicrobial Action.* Chapman & Hall, London.

Gale E. F., Cundliffe E., Reynolds P. E., Richmond M. H. & Waring M. J. (1972) *The Molecular Basis of Antibiotic Action.* John Wiley, New York.

Gardner P., Smith D. H., Beer H. & Moellering R. C. (1969) Recovery of resistance (R) factors from a drug-free community. *Lancet* ii, 774.

Garrod L. P., Lambert H. P. & O'Grady F. (1973) *Antibiotic and Chemotherapy.* Churchill Livingstone, Edinburgh.

Harris A. M., Marshall M. J., Curtis R., Evans J. M. & Watson D. J. (1976) Cephalosporins in the prevention and treatment of mastitis. *Vet. Rec.* **99**, 128.

Hitchings G. H. (1969) Species differences among dihydrofolate reductases as a basis for chemotherapy. *Postgrad. Med. J.* **45**, (suppl. Nov.) 7.

Huber F. M. & Gottlieb D. (1968) The mechanism of action of griseofulvin. *Can. J. Microbiol.* **14**, 111.

Jawetz E. & Gunnison J. B. (1952) Studies on antibiotic synergism and antagonism: the scheme of combined antimicrobial activity. *Antibiot. Chemother.* **2**, 243.

Kossiakoff M. G. (1887) De la propriété que possèdent les microbes de s'accomoder aux milieux antiseptiques. *Ann. Inst. Pasteur* **1**, 465.

Lacy R. W. (1975) A critical appraisal of the importance of R-factors in the enterobacteriaceae *in vivo. J. Antimicrob. Chemother.* **1**, 25.

Lawrence D. R. (1973) *Clinical Pharmacology.* 3rd edn. Churchill Livingstone, Edinburgh.

Leon S. A. & Brock T. D. (1967) Effect of streptomycin and neomycin on physical properties of the ribosome. *J. Molec. Biol.* **24**, 391.

Linton A. H. (1976) The antibiotic sensitivity testing of pathogens commonly found in veterinary practice. *Vet. Rec.* **99**, 370.

Matthew M. & Harris A. M. (1976) Identification of β-lactamases by analytical isoelectric focusing: correlation with bacterial taxonomy. *J. Gen. Microbiol.* **94**, 55.

Newton B. A. (1965) Mechanisms of antibiotic action. *Ann. Rev. Microbiol.* **19**, 216.

Smith D. H. & Davis B. D. (1967) Mode of action of novobiocin in *Escherichia coli. J. Bact.* **93**, 71.

Sykes R. B. & Matthew M. (1976) The β-lactamases of Gram-negative bacteria and their role in resistance to β-lactam antibiotics. *J. Antimicrob. Chemother.* **2**, 115.

Weisblum B. & Davies J. (1968) Antibiotic inhibitors of the bacterial ribosome. *Bact. Rev.* **32**, 493.

Weissmann G. & Sessa G. (1967) The action of polyene antibiotics on phospholipid-cholesterol structures. *J. Biol. Chem.* **242**, 615.

White P. J. & Woods D. D. (1965) The synthesis of p-amino-benzoic acid and folic acid by Staphylococci sensitive and resistant to sulphonamides. *J. Gen. Microbiol.* **40**, 243.

Whitehead J. E. M. (1973) Bacterial resistance: changing patterns of some common pathogens. *Brit. Med. J.* **2**, 224.

5

Pharmacokinetics of antibacterial agents in the dog and cat

P. M. KEEN

The different types of antibacterial agent differ widely in the way in which they are absorbed, distributed, metabolised and excreted and these differences carry profound implications for the therapeutic use of these drugs.

5.1 General principles

The aim of antibacterial therapy is to obtain at the site of infection a concentration of drug sufficient to kill the invading bacteria or to inhibit their further multiplication. The concentration of drug needed to inhibit a particular organism (the minimal inhibitory concentration or MIC) can be determined *in vitro* and the usual aim is to attain a concentration in tissue fluid in excess of the MIC for the organism concerned. This makes the assumption that the physiological milieu neither potentiates nor impedes the action of the drug. The concentration of drug in blood plasma or serum may be used as an indication of the likely concentration in tissue fluid, after an allowance has been made for the amount of drug bound to plasma proteins and hence unable to diffuse into tissues (Keen 1971). Verwey and Williams (1963) showed that in the dog the level of penicillin in tissue fluid was very similar to the level of free (i.e. non-protein bound) penicillin in plasma and that levels in tissue fluid followed those in plasma with a latency of only a few minutes (Verwey *et al* 1966). Hence it would seem to be desirable to keep the concentration of *free* drug in plasma well above the MIC for the bacterium concerned. Empirical support for this view is provided by the data of Rolinson (1967) who showed that for a wide range of antibacterial drugs the *peak* free plasma concentration attained following administration of the recommended dose was at least twice the MIC for bacteria which had been found susceptible to that drug in clinical practice.

Given that these peak levels are required, is it necessary, or practicable, to maintain effective concentrations of drug in the tissues throughout the treatment period, or may levels be allowed to fall between successive doses?

Table 5.1 Classification of bactericidal and bacteriostatic agents.

Bactericidal	Bacteriostatic
Penicillins	Chloramphenicol
Cephalosporins	Tetracyclines
Streptomycin group	Erythromycin group
Nitrofurantoin (acid urine)	Lincomycin
Sulphonamide and trimethoprim	Sulphonamides

In theory at least, effective levels of bacteriostatic agents (see Table 5.1 for classification) should be maintained throughout therapy and, whilst there is no firm evidence that this is necessary, it is commonly recommended (e.g. Crofton 1969). The bacteriostatic agents chloramphenicol and erythromycin, whether given orally or by injection, maintain effective levels for approximately 6 hours and so four *equally spaced* doses need be given every 24 hours if blood levels are to be maintained. For tetracyclines the time is 8 hours requiring three equally-spaced doses per 24 hours. Repeated administration of sulphonamides carries the danger that the drug may cumulate in the body to toxic levels. To avoid this it is customary to give a loading dose and after one half-life (i.e. when half of the sulphonamide has been eliminated) to give a dose equal to one-half of the loading dose and to repeat this every half-life, thus maintaining plasma levels below toxic but above effective levels. Of the bactericidal agents, ampicillin, amoxycillin and sodium benzylpenicillin maintain effective levels for approximately 6 hours, injected streptomycin for 12 hours and procaine benzylpenicillin for 22 hours. Thus when the latter agents are combined as 'Streptopen' only one remains effective throughout therapy. It is probably less important to maintain an effective level of a bactericidal agent than it is of a bacteriostatic one. Some bactericidal agents (e.g. penicillins, cephalosporins, streptomycin group) are lethal only to dividing bacteria and for this reason intermittent therapy with these agents may be effective and has even been positively advocated in some cases (Weinstein & Perrin 1950). There is no simple rule as to how long effective levels of bactericidal drugs should be maintained — this depends on the speed of action of the drug, and even members of the penicillin-cephalosporin group differ in the speed with which they exert their bactericidal effect (Greenwood 1976).

In most tissues, as described above, unbound antibiotic in plasma is able to diffuse freely through the fenestrated walls of the capillaries to enter tissue fluid. In the brain and the eye, however, the capillaries are not fenestrated and so drugs may obtain access to the cerebrospinal fluid (CSF), the brain substance and the internal structures of the eye only by crossing an intact cell membrane. Antibacterial agents differ in the ease with which they are able to enter these compartments and values for the levels attained in aqueous

Table 5.2 Levels in aqueous humor and cerebrospinal fluid as a percentage of serum levels.

Antibiotic	Aqueous humor	Cerebrospinal fluid
Benzylpenicillin	10	2
Streptomycin	6	trace
Chloramphenicol	25	40
Tetracyclines	17	10
Erythromycin	28	6
Lincomycin	10	5
Sulphanilamide	45	50

humor and CSF, culled from a variety of sources, are shown in Table 5.2. Although these values provide a useful guide, they were obtained in healthy animals and it should be noted that the permeability of the blood-brain and blood-aqueous barriers may be increased in inflammation.

The ability of an antibacterial agent to cross cell membranes depends largely on its being lipid-soluble. On the one hand an uncharged lipid-soluble drug is likely to cross the bowel wall and so will be absorbed following oral administration; it will cross membranes to enter the brain, the eye and the fetal circulation; it will enter cells where it may produce toxic effects and may be effective against intracellular organisms; lastly it will enter liver cells to be metabolised. By contrast an ionised, and hence lipid-*insoluble*, drug is less likely to be absorbed from the bowel or, when injected, to enter the brain or eye. By the same token it will be excluded from cells, including liver cells, and so will not be metabolised. Most antibacterial drugs lie somewhere between these two extremes and so it may be worthwhile to review the pharmacological properties of the chief groups.

5.2 Pharmacokinetics of the main antibacterial agents

5.2.1 The penicillin group

The penicillins (benzylpenicillin, phenoxymethylpenicillin, ampicillin, cloxacillin, amoxycillin) attain effective plasma levels after injection or (except benzylpenicillin which is destroyed in the stomach) oral administration. Orally administered ampicillin gives fourfold higher plasma levels in fasted dogs than in fed animals (Cabana *et al* 1969). Amoxycillin gives higher blood levels than ampicillin when given orally to dogs (Palmer *et al* 1976). Like most antibiotics the penicillins diffuse well into tissue fluids (Verwey *et al* 1966) and into acute inflammatory foci (Florey *et al* 1946). In general, however, they do not diffuse well across membranes and so (a) they are not metabolised but are excreted unchanged, (b) they penetrate poorly into brain and eye, (c) they are acidic molecules which are substrates for active transport systems in the kidney, the biliary system and the choroid plexus. The levels of benzylpenicillin attained in CSF and aqueous humor of healthy animals are shown in Table 5.2. The low levels in CSF are partly attributable to the fact that benzylpenicillin is actively transported from the CSF to the blood at the choroid plexus (Pappenheimer *et al* 1961). Ampicillin penetrates better into CSF than benzylpenicillin and benzylpenicillin levels in CSF are increased in meningitis (Ruedy 1965). Because the penicillins do not diffuse well into aqueous humor, subconjunctival injection (preferably together with adrenaline) is the route of choice for the treatment of intraocular infections in the dog (Rowley & Rubin 1969). High concentrations of ampicillin are found in the bile of the dog (Brown & Acred 1961); some of the antibiotic so excreted is reabsorbed in the small intestine. This so-called 'enterohepatic circulation' of drug prolongs plasma levels and gives appreciable concentrations in the upper intestine following parenteral administration (Stewart & Harrison 1961).

The penicillins are actively secreted into the urine by the renal tubules, resulting in high urine concentrations (of clinical use only in the case of the broad-spectrum agents such as ampicillin) and rapid elimination from the body. Because of this rapid elimination the soluble salts of benzylpenicillin, which may be given intravenously, intramuscularly or subcutaneously, maintain effective blood levels for only 4 hours. Because the length of time for which effective plasma levels are maintained varies with the *logarithm* of the dose, the length of action of benzylpenicillin cannot be greatly increased by increasing the dose (Eagle 1948). English (1965) even suggests that there is a 'critical dose' of benzylpenicillin in the dog above which no advantage at all is obtained by increasing the dose. Because of the short half-life of the soluble salts of benzylpenicillin, insoluble salts are commonly used as 'depot' preparations. The insoluble procaine salt of benzylpenicillin gives lower plasma levels which remain effective for 18–24 hours. Insoluble preparations may not of course be given intravenously, but intramuscular and subcutaneous injection are equally effective (English 1959). The very insoluble benzathine and benethamine salts of benzylpenicillin last several days but plasma levels are usually inadequate for effective therapy. The greater persistence of the insoluble salts is gained at the expense of high peak blood levels and in severe infections it may be advisable to initiate treatment with a loading dose of a soluble preparation.

The antibacterial action of penicillins is exerted at the level of the bacterial cell wall (as opposed to the cell membrane). The constituents of cell walls are unique to bacteria and so penicillins have virtually no direct toxicity for mammalian cells. Two types of toxic effect may, however, be seen. Individual animals may show a hypersensitive reaction to penicillins (Clarke 1960). It is thought that the β-lactam ring of the penicillin may open to form a penicilloic acid which becomes coupled to a body protein to form an antigen; this stimulates antibody formation so that subsequent administration of a penicillin produces a hypersensitive reaction. A second type of toxic effect is manifested in the guinea-pig and related species in which consequently penicillins are contraindicated. These animals may die some hours after administration of penicillin — apparently from an enterotoxaemia resulting from the effect of the antibiotic on the bacterial flora of the bowel (Milner 1975).

5.2.2 The cephalosporin group

The cephalosporins are closely related chemically to the penicillins and so have a very similar pharmacology. They do not, however, precipitate hypersensitive reactions in penicillin-sensitive animals and do not themselves give rise to hypersensitivity. This is apparently because opening the β-lactam ring of a cephalosporin gives rise to an unstable product so that no equivalent of penicilloic acid can be formed (cf penicillins above) and hence the coupling to body proteins, which is a prerequisite of antigenicity, cannot take place.

5.2.3 The streptomycin group

Members of this group (streptomycin, neomycin, framycetin, kanamycin and gentamicin) are aminoglycosides, large charged molecules which are unable to pass freely through body membranes. Hence members of this group are not absorbed following oral administration and this route is indicated only for the treatment of bowel infections; for systemic infections they must be injected. Although the more toxic members of this group, such as neomycin, can be given systemically only with care, they may, because they are not absorbed, be administered orally without risk. Because of its poor diffusibility, streptomycin does not reach effective concentrations in CSF (Table 5.2) even in meningitis and is not metabolised by the intracellular hepatic enzymes. Unlike the penicillins, streptomycin is not secreted by the renal tubules but is cleared by glomerular filtration only, and so plasma levels are maintained for 8–12 hours following a single injection. As they are excreted unchanged, members of the group may be used to treat infections of the urinary tract.

Unlike the penicillins, which act externally to the cell membrane and on a process which is unique to bacteria, the streptomycin group affect bacterial protein synthesis. This necessitates their penetrating the bacterial cell membrane and also means that they may exert toxic effects by interfering with protein synthetic mechanisms in mammalian cells. Streptomycin is a base which, in the acid milieu of carnivore urine, is almost totally ionised; the ionised form is unable to penetrate bacteria and hence the antibacterial activity of streptomycin may be increased several hundredfold by alkalinising the urine and thus increasing the amount of streptomycin present in the undissociated lipid-soluble form (Garrod & O'Grady 1971). Prolonged administration of large doses of streptomycin may cause ataxia by damaging the vestibular branch of the eighth cranial nerve, particularly in the cat (McGee 1962). Because streptomycin is eliminated solely by renal excretion, the drug is especially liable to cumulate to toxic levels if repeated injections are given to an animal with oliguria or renal failure. Dihydrostreptomycin is less liable to produce vestibular disturbance but more likely to cause deafness by damaging the auditory branch of the eighth nerve. To lessen the risk of toxicity a mixture of streptomycin and dihydrostreptomycin is sometimes employed. Vestibular disturbances are usually reversible following withdrawal of the drug. Deafness is often delayed in onset and may be permanent. Neomycin and the remaining members of the group may cause deafness and may also be nephrotoxic. As a result they should be administered systemically only with care (Fowler 1968). Streptomycin may also cause neuromuscular blockade and may thus potentiate muscle relaxants, cause apnoea during anaesthesia and exacerbate myasthenia gravis (Adams 1975). This neuromuscular blockade is brought about by a dual mechanism; a presynaptic inhibition of acetylcholine release by chelating calcium and a postsynaptic curare-like effect (Pittinger & Adamson 1972). These effects may be antagonised by calcium and neostigmine respectively.

5.2.4 Chloramphenicol

In contrast to the previous group, chloramphenicol is a simple, non-ionised and freely diffusible molecule. It is well absorbed from the bowel; oral administration gives plasma levels similar to those following subcutaneous injection, while subcutaneous injection is preferred to the intramuscular route (Pauli & English 1971; Watson 1972). Chloramphenicol attains effective levels in the eye and CSF (Table 5.2); it enters cells and so is effective in rickettsial infections and is metabolised in the liver. Because it is excreted almost entirely as inactive metabolites, chloramphenicol is not usually considered for the treatment of urinary tract infections. Young animals of all species are deficient in chloramphenicol-metabolising enzymes and in these, and in adults with extensive liver disease, repeated dosing may lead to cumulation. The cat is particularly ill-equipped with drug-metabolising enzymes and the slow dealkylation of chloramphenicol in this species may lead to cumulation which in turn may explain the effect of repeated doses of chloramphenicol on the bone marrow (see below). Chloramphenicol diffuses well not only in the body but also in agar plates, hence the wide zones of inhibition which may lead to an overoptimistic prediction of its *in vivo* efficacy.

Chloramphenicol depresses bacterial protein synthesis, and its side-effects reflect the spread of this action to protein synthesis in mammalian cells. The fatal aplastic anaemia sometimes caused by chloramphenicol in children is not seen in domesticated animals but it may cause blood dyscrasias, especially in cats (Penny *et al* 1967). Chloramphenicol may suppress immunoglobulin synthesis and wound-healing (Caulfield & Burke 1971) and suppresses the activity of the liver enzymes responsible for the metabolism of pentobarbitone, thus prolonging the period of anaesthesia produced by this drug (Teske & Carter 1971).

5.2.5 The tetracycline group

Effective plasma levels are obtained following either oral or parenteral administration of the tetracyclines (tetracycline, oxy- and chlortetracycline and methacycline). Intramuscular injection of some preparations may cause pain and intravenous injection may cause an acidosis (McPherson *et al* 1974). Members of the group form chemical complexes with calcium, hence high calcium levels in the bowel hinder absorption and oral tetracyclines should not be given with milk. The calcium tetracycline complex formed in bones probably has little clinical significance but deposition of tetracyclines in teeth can cause permanent discolouration (Owen 1963) and so this group should be avoided in young animals and in late pregnancy. Most tetracyclines are not metabolised and are cleared by glomerular filtration. Orally administered tetracyclines may cause diarrhoea due to local irritation and to suppression of the normal bacterial flora of the alimentary tract by the broad-spectrum antibacterial activity of the tetracycline, occasionally leading to superinfection with candida or other organisms.

5.2.6 The erythromycin group and lincomycin

Lincomycin is not chemically a member of the erythromycin group (erythromycin, spiramycin and tylosin) but it has certain similarities. Therapeutic plasma levels are attained following either oral or parenteral administration of appropriate formulations. These antibiotics are partly metabolised in the body and are also excreted in the bile and undergo an enterohepatic circulation similar to that described for ampicillin. Lincomycin penetrates well into bone in the dog (Grady & Stern 1965) and so may be indicated in osteomvelitis. As explained elsewhere in this volume (see p. 3), basic drugs tend to become concentrated in any tissue fluid which is acidic relative to the blood — the so-called 'pH trap'. Canine prostatic fluid has a pH of 6·4 and hence the concentration of erythromycin (which is a basic molecule) in prostatic fluid is more than twice that in blood whereas the acidic drugs amoxycillin and benzylpenicillin together with the lipid-insoluble drugs kanamycin and oxytetracycline are totally excluded (Stamey *et al* 1970).

5.2.7 The sulphonamide group

Most members of this group may be given either orally or by injection to treat systemic infections. They diffuse well (Table 5.2) and the folic acid antagonist trimethoprim, with which sulphonamides may be combined (cotrimazine, cotrimoxine) diffuses equally well. A proportion of the sulphonamides is acetylated in the liver, except in the dog which metabolises them by other routes. The danger that sulphonamides or their metabolites may cause renal failure by precipitating in the acid urine of the dog and cat appears not to be a problem with the newer sulphonamides and with the established agents (e.g. s'diazine, s'merazine, s'pyridine) is overcome by using a triple sulphonamide combination so that alkalinisation of the urine is not usually considered necessary. The so-called 'bowel-active' sulphonamides, notably phthalylsulphathiazole, have a substituent which prevents their absorption from the bowel and so they are indicated solely for the treatment of enteric infections.

5.2.8 Nitrofurantoin

When given orally, nitrofurantoin is absorbed and, although plasma levels are inadequate for the treatment of systemic infections, effective concentrations are attained in the urine. Nitrofurantoin is an acidic molecule and so, conversely to the basic streptomycin, is more active in an acid than an alkaline urine.

5.2.9 Metronidazole

When metronidazole is given orally to dogs, it is excreted largely unmetabolised. It is active against anaerobic infections, high concentrations are present in saliva and its indications include gingivitis (Dean *et al* 1969) and tear-staining (Gale 1976).

References

Adams H. R. (1975) Acute adverse effects of antibiotics. *J. Amer. Vet. Med. Ass.* **166**, 983.

Brown D. M. & Acred P. (1961) 'Penbritin' — a new broad-spectrum antibiotic. *Brit. Med. J.* **2**, 197.

Cabana B. E., Willhite L. E. & Bierwagen M. E. (1969) Pharmacokinetic evaluation of the oral absorption of different ampicillin preparations in beagle dogs. *Antimicrob. Agents Chemother.* **1969**, 35.

Caulfield J. B. & Burke J. F. (1971) Inhibition of wound healing by chloramphenicol. *Arch. Path.* **92**, 119.

Clarke P. B. (1960) Acute allergic response to penicillin. *Vet. Rec.* **72**, 1054.

Crofton J. (1969) Some principles in the chemotherapy of bacterial infections. *Brit. Med. J.* **2**, 137.

Dean T. S., Shinn D. L. S., McFadzean J. A. & Squires S. L. (1969) Metronidazole in the treatment of gingivitis. *Vet. Rec.* **85**, 449.

Eagle H. (1948) Speculations as to the therapeutic significance of the penicillin blood level. *Ann. Intern. Med.* **28**, 260.

English P. B. (1959) Serum penicillin concentrations in the dog with fortified benzathine and benethamine penicillins. *Aust. Vet. J.* **35**, 16.

English P. B. (1965) The therapeutic use of penicillin: the relationship between dose rate and plasma concentration after parenteral administration of benzylpenicillin (Penicillin G). *Vet. Rec.* **77**, 810.

Florey M. E., Turton E. C. & Duthie E. S. (1946) Penicillin in wound exudates. *Lancet* ii, 405.

Fowler N. G. (1968) The ototoxicity of neomycin in the dog. *Vet. Rec.* **82**, 267.

Gale V. C. (1976) Use of metronidazole in treating 'tear staining' in the dog. *Vet. Rec.* **98**, 14.

Garrod L. P. & O'Grady F. (1971) *Antibiotic and Chemotherapy*. 3rd edn. Livingstone, Edinburgh.

Grady J. E. & Stern K. F. (1966) Penetration of lincomycin into bone. *Antimicrob. Agents Chemother.* **1965**, 201.

Greenwood D. (1976) Unrealistic nature of the 'MIC'. *J. Antimicrob. Chemother.* **2**, 312.

Keen P. (1971) Effect of binding to plasma proteins on the distribution, activity and elimination of drugs. *Handb. Exptl. Pharmacol.* **28**, 213.

McGee T. M. (1962) Streptomycin sulfate and dihydrostreptomycin toxicity: behavioural and histopathologic studies. *Arch. Otolaryngol.* **75**, 295.

McPherson J. C., Ellison R. G., Davis H. N., Hawkridge F. M. & Ellison L. T. (1974) The metabolic acidosis resulting from intravenous tetracycline administration. *Proc. Soc. Exp. Biol. Med.* **145**, 450.

Milner N. A. (1975) Penicillin toxicity in guinea-pigs. *Vet. Rec.* **96**, 554.

Owen L. N. (1963) The effects of administering tetracyclines to young dogs with particular reference to localisation of the drugs in the teeth. *Arch. Oral Biol.* **8**, 715.

Palmer G. H., Buswell J. F., Dowrick J. S. & Yeoman G. H. (1976) Amoxycillin: a new veterinary penicillin. *Vet. Rec.* **99**, 84.

Pappenheimer J. R., Heisey S. R. & Jordan E. F. (1961) Active transport of Diodrast and phenolsulfonphthalein from cerebrospinal fluid to blood. *Amer. J. Physiol.* **200**, 1.

Pauli J. V. & English P. B. (1971) Plasma chloramphenicol concentrations in the dog after parenteral administration of chloramphenicol sodium succinate. *J. Small Anim. Pract.* **12**, 643.

Penny R. H. C., Carlisle C. H., Prescott C. W. & Davidson H. A. (1967) Effects of chloramphenicol on the haemopoietic system of the cat. *Brit. Vet. J.* **123**, 145.

Pittinger C. & Adamson R. (1972) Antibiotic blockade of neuromuscular function. *Ann. Rev. Pharmacol.* **12**, 169.

Rolinson G. N. (1967) The significance of protein-binding of antibiotics *in vitro* and *in vivo*. In *Recent Advances in Medical Microbiology*, ed. A. P. Waterson, p. 254. Churchill, London.

Rowley R. A. & Rubin L. F. (1969) Penetration of penicillin into the aqueous humor of the dog. *Amer. J. Vet. Res.* **30**, 1945.

Ruedy J. (1965) The concentrations of penicillins in the cerebrospinal fluid and brain of rabbits with experimental meningitis. *Canad. J. Physiol. Pharmacol.* **43**, 763.

Stamey T. A., Meares E. M. & Winningham D. G. (1970) Chronic bacterial prostatitis and the diffusion of drugs into prostatic fluid. *J. Urol.* **103**, 187.

Stewart G. T. & Harrison P. M. (1961) Excretion and re-excretion of a broad-spectrum penicillin in bile. *Brit. J. Pharmacol.* **17**, 414.

Teske R. H. & Carter G. G. (1971) Effect of chloramphenicol on pentobarbital-induced anaesthesia in dogs. *J. Amer. Vet. Med. Ass.* **159**, 777.

Verwey W. F. & Williams H. R. (1963) Relationships between the concentrations of various penicillins in plasma and peripheral lymph. *Antimicrob. Agents Chemother.* **1962**, 476.

Verwey W. F., Williams H. R. & Kalsow C. (1966) Penetration of chemotherapeutic agents into tissues. *Antimicrob. Agents Chemother.* 1965, 1016.

Watson A. D. J. (1972) Chloramphenicol plasma levels in the dog: a comparison of oral, subcutaneous and intramuscular administration. *J. small Anim. Pract.* **13**, 147.

Weinstein L. & Perrin T. S. (1950) The treatment of scarlet fever with penicillin G administered orally three times a day. *J. Pediat.* **37**, 844.

6

Clinical Use of Antibiotics in Small Animal Practice

J. F. R. HIRD

The problem which faces the small animal practitioner in the consulting room is that of bridging the gap between the amount of theoretical information available to him and the actual treatment of the patient under his care. The most rational use of an antimicrobial agent is based on the result of a sensitivity test on the suspected pathogen isolated from the lesion in question. However, this procedure takes time (a minimum of 24 hours) and adds to the cost of treatment. Nonetheless, facilities for undertaking bacteriological examination and sensitivity testing are of very great value in the treatment of 'difficult' cases, and the cost and time involved may both be considerably less than that involved in administering repeated courses of different antibiotics until the lesion responds. On the other hand, the clinician frequently sees patients with conditions which merit immediate treatment, and indeed, this is usually what the owner expects. Under these circumstances, the clinician is forced to act without knowing which organism is involved or its sensitivity, and he must base his choice of treatment on his clinical experience. This chapter is designed to guide the clinician working under these circumstances to a reasonable conclusion upon which to base his treatment.

6.1 Indications for the use of antibiotics

Before he takes his decision to use an antibiotic the veterinarian *must* have reached a diagnosis, however tentative, that his patient is suffering from a bacterial infection. Although this conclusion may be clearly apparent from the clinical signs, the use of antibiotics should never be automatic. Both humans and animals recovered from bacterial infections before the advent of penicillin; antibiotics should never be used as a substitute for supportive treatment and good nursing. It may be possible to cure the complaint without recourse to an antibiotic (e.g. the treatment of canine cystitis with hexamine or mandelic acid; the use of antiseptics, such as eusol, or non-antibiotic antimicrobial agents such as clioquinol, for the treatment of superficial cutaneous infections (Anon. 1971)). This has the effect of curing the patient, usually more cheaply and with less interference with the normal body flora, whilst allowing time for natural host defence mechanisms to control the infection. Natural immunity has the very considerable advantage of persisting for a long time, if not indefinitely, whilst the response to an antibiotic only persists as long as the antibiotic is administered, or until the organisms in question are entirely eliminated.

The use of an antibiotic will inevitably cause some disruption of the normal bacterial flora of the patient, and in the case of the guinea-pig, fatal enterocolitis may ensue if the animal is treated with a narrow-spectrum antibiotic such as penicillin, which allows Gram-negative organisms resistant to the antibiotic to proliferate and cause an enterointoxication (Milner 1975). In a parallel situation, the indiscriminate use of antibiotics for the symptomatic treatment of canine diarrhoea may exacerbate, rather than improve the situation by allowing yeasts and resistant bacteria to proliferate in the colon. Similar situations may arise in other sites. The longer the course of treatment lasts, the more likely it becomes that side-effects will assert themselves, but the practitioner must balance this risk against that of failure to treat an infection for sufficient time. As a result of the potential hazards of the indiscriminate use of antibiotics, it is now general practice in human hospital practice to reserve these drugs only for patients who have a sustained pyrexia which can be attributed to microbial infection. This is sound therapeutic practice, which can be equally well applied to small animal medicine.

Once the clinician has made the decision to use an antibiotic, he faces a most difficult dilemma — which one to choose?

6.2 Antibiotic selection

In some diseases, the diagnosis alone will dictate the selection of the agent to be used; for example, the diagnosis of tetanus in the dog is an indication for the use of large doses of penicillin, but such instances are rare. In the absence of sensitivity tests the decision must be based on the clinician's experience of which organism is *likely* to be responsible for the condition present. This information in itself can only be gained by the routine culture of organisms from all infective conditions prior to treatment, over a reasonable time interval. Even this information will provide only a rough indication, and variations are to be expected in the bacteriological profile thus obtained in different animal populations. A further problem arises in that commensal organisms may be isolated from septic lesions, and their contribution to the pathogenic process may not be altogether clear. For example, Hirsh and Wiger (1977), in a study of the bacterial flora of the normal canine vagina compared with that of vaginal exudates, were unable to demonstrate any significant differences between the vaginal bacterial flora in normal and affected animals, in terms of the bacterial species present, and suggested that treatment should be directed simply against those species of bacteria present in higher than normal numbers.

Some information on the incidence of certain pathogens and their likely bacterial sensitivity is displayed in Tables 6.1 and 6.2. The information displayed in Table 6.2, and in the first column of Table 6.1 is based on the isolation and sensitivity testing of organisms from dogs carried out at The Department of Clinical Veterinary Medicine, University of Cambridge, over an 18-month period (1975–77). The choice of antibiotic (columns 2 and 3 of Table 6.1) is based both on these results and upon the data from various sources icluding Aronson and Kirk (1975), and is intended to represent current conventional views in antibacterial chemotherapy. The results obtained from the Cambridge data are in broad agreement with those obtained from bacterial isolates in general practice (A. T. Yoxall, pers. comm.). The limitations of sensitivity testing have been discussed in Chapter 4, and an organism may prove either more or less sensitive *in vivo* than expected from *in vitro* sensitivity testing. This may be due to the magnitude of the host response, failure of the antibiotic to penetrate to the site of infection in adequate concentration, or to incorrect usage (see below). Despite these reservations, sensitivity testing remains the best, if not the only guideline on which the practitioner may work.

On occasion, the choice of antibiotic may be dictated by other factors, the first of these being the condition of the patient. Bacteriostatic antibiotics arrest the multiplication of organisms, thus allowing the body's defences to overwhelm the bacteria, but this may not occur in cases of debilitating or chronic disease in which the host's defence mechanisms may be impaired. For this reason, conditions such as septicaemia, endocarditis and the chronic infections should always be treated with a bactericidal agent, if possible.

A second important factor influencing the choice of antibiotic is the differing tissue-penetrating properties of the compounds which might be used. Although ampicillin appears to have little advantage over penicillin on the basis of sensitivity testing, the penetration of ampicillin into tissues is usually better, due to its lower degree of plasma protein binding and greater lipid solubility, and this agent may therefore be the wiser clinical choice. Amoxycillin is superior to ampicillin in this respect (Yeoman 1977), but this consideration should not induce the clinician to abandon penicillin itself in favour of the semi-synthetic derivatives, since the latter are generally less active than penicillin G against Gram-positive organisms sensitive to penicillins (Weinstein 1975; and Table 6.2). Penethamate is the diethyl aminoethyl hydriodide ester of penicillin. It is stable at plasma pH, and is fat-soluble, allowing it to penetrate readily into tissues. It dissociates to yield penicillin G in areas where the pH is low, such as in septic lesions (usually), and in milk (Edwards 1965). Particular circumstances in which tissue

Table 6.1 Suggested antibiotics for use in some canine bacterial infections. Where specific data for incidence quoted, source as for Table 6.2; for other sources, see text.

Site of infection	Possible causal organisms (in order of frequency of occurrence)	First choice antibiotic	Second choice antibiotics
Bacterial infection of the skin and appendages	*1* Pure *Staph. pyogenes* (66% cases) *2* Mixed staphylococcus with β-haemolytic streptococcus (18% cases) *3* Mixed infections – including Gram –ve organisms (11% cases) *4* Pure β-haemolytic streptococcus (5% cases)	Penicillin (neomycin or framycetin for topical use)	Erythromycin, cloxacillin Amoxycillin, cotrimazine and Lincomycin may be useful by virture of their ability to penetrate into skin, but should do sensitivity test first, as range of sensitive organisms limited
Abscesses, sinuses, infected wounds	*1* *Staph. pyogenes*, and mixed infections including *Staph. pyogenes* *2* β-haemolytic streptococcus *3* Pasteurella & Pasteurella-like organisms *4* Miscellaneous Gram –ve organisms, including coliforms & *P. pyocyanea*	Penicillin	Erythromycin, cloxacillin gentamicin, framycetin (fusidate for *Nocardia* spp.)
Urinary tract infections	*1* Mixed infections, with coliforms almost invariably involved (43% cases) *2* Pure coliform infection (39% cases) *3* *Proteus* spp. *4* β-haemolytic streptococci	Cotrimazine, amoxycillin (possibly high dose penicillin G)	Nitrofurantoin (acid urine), gentamicin (alkaline urine)

Vaginitis	*1* β-haemolytic streptococci *2* Coliforms *3* Miscellaneous organisms	Cotrimazine	Ampicillin, tetracycline
Otitis externa	Most external ear infections are mixed, with various yeasts frequently present in addition to bacteria *Staph. pyogenes* in the predominent organism, with a β-haemolytic streptococci, and assorted Gram −ve organisms, of which *Pseudomonas* is usually the most difficult to eliminate	Neomycin (by topical application)	Fusidate, Framycetin, Nystatin } by topical application Cloxacillin and erthromycin are the most effective agents for parenteral use, reflecting the predominance of Gram +ve organisms in this condition Tetracycline is the best broad-spectrum agent
Lesions of the oral cavity	Nearly always mixed infections, with *Bacteroides* spp. and Pasteurella-like organisms predominating Flagellates may also be pathogenic	Penicillin Metronidazole (if flagellates present)	Tetracycline
Superficial ocular infections	*1* *Straph. pyogenes* *2* β-haemolytic streptococcus *3* Mixed infections, including coliforms	Neomycin, penicillin, (topical application) or chloramphenicol if penetration of aqueous humor is required	Framycetin

Table 6.2 Antibiotic sensitivity of the four most commonly isolated organisms (%) Data derived from 500 cases investigated at the Department of Clinical Pathology, University of Cambridge over a 12-month period.

Antibiotic	*Staph. pyogenes*	β-haemolytic streptococcus	Pasteurella and Pasteurella-like organisms	Coliforms
Penicillin	51*	98	85	0
Cloxacillin	79	90	15	0
Erythromycin	84	95	76	0
Ampicillin	48	95	85	0
Lincomycin	63	90	0	0
Streptomycin	63	0	15	20
Neomycin	84	10	31	72
Gentamicin	82	0	92	96
Framycetin	84	0	85	100
Polymixin B	2	0	15	8
Tetracycline	57	28	92	64
Chloramphenicol	71	83	85	68
Sulphafurazole	2	20	38	28
Cotrimazine	34	75	85	80
Furazolidone	74	35	100	64
Nitrofurantoin	83	98	100	92

*This figure appears low, possibly due to prior exposure to penicillin. The same may apply to ampicillin and cotrimazine.

penetration is important arise where infected lesions in bone, the central nervous system, the eye or the urinary tract require treatment.

6.2.1 Bone

In the treatment of osteomyelitis, where bone penetration by the antibiotic is of prime importance, lincomycin and sodium fusidate (fusidic acid) should be considered. In man, Gram-positive organisms are usually the significant pathogens in this condition, especially *Staphylococcus aureus* (Chalmers & Gardner 1974), and the same is likely to be true in small animals, so that the limited spectrum of these agents is not a serious drawback. Lincomycin is an extremely soluble antibiotic and penetrates extremely well into bone (Weinstein 1975), (as into other tissues). Therapy with lincomycin is only effective if started early, whilst the bone still retains its blood supply, and, since levels in bone are only about one-sixth to one-eighth of that in blood, large doses should be given in order to ensure an adequate concentration at the site of infection. Lincomycin is well absorbed when given orally, but blood levels are only maintained for 6–8 hours (Brander & Pugh 1977) so that frequent dosing is required. Frequent administration of large doses will produce a brisk diarrhoea in most dogs — whether or not this is related to the fatal colitis which has developed in some human patients following exposure to this agent remains to be seen.

Fusidic acid is a small steroid molecule, and has been shown to diffuse into bone sequestra (Chater *et al* 1972) and, indeed, is the only antimicrobial agent known to do so. Like lincomycin it has a propensity for causing gastro-intestinal upsets in man.

6.2.2 Central nervous system (CNS)

Although many antibiotics will readily cross the blood-brain barrier when the meninges are inflamed, it is desirable to use an antibiotic which readily crosses the normal blood-brain barrier, so that effective concentrations can be maintained to eliminate any residual micro-organisms when the acute, inflammatory phase of the condition has subsided. Thus erythromycin and ampicillin are both capable of attaining high cerebrospinal fluid (CSF) levels when the meninges are inflamed, but only trivial levels otherwise. Chloramphenicol is capable of crossing the blood-brain barrier, and although it takes several hours for brain concentrations to approximate blood concentrations after oral dosing in the dog, brain levels appear to remain adequate for as long as 12 hours, even though the blood level will have diminished to a minimal level in this period (Watson & McDonald 1976). There is a tendency for some clinicians to underdose with chloramphenicol. Mercer *et al* (1978) review the literature on chloramphenicol administration in animals, and it would appear that chloramphenicol is better absorbed if given orally, rather than intramuscularly, in carnivores at least, and that a dose of at least 50 mg/kg should be administered twice daily.

Although chloramphenicol can be used for treating infections of the CNS, the sulphonamides may be preferable, unless there is thought to be a real likelihood of sulphonamide resistance. Sulphonamides which are readily acetylated or plasma protein bound (such as suphadimidine) will not be free to cross the blood-brain barrier or exert a therapeutic effect within the CNS.

The CSF contains little protein, so that sulphonamide in the CNS will mostly be free, rather than protein bound, and therefore able to exert its antimicrobial action. Thus a given CSF concentration is much more effective than the same serum concentration, in terms of its ability to attack bacteria. This renders sulphonamides particularly suitable for the treatment of CNS infections. The advantages of the sulphadiazine-trimethoprim combination, discussed in Chapter 4, render this combination the treatment choice for CNS infections. This combination has the advantage of being highly effective when given orally. Sulphadiazine penetrates well into the CSF (Barber & Garrod 1963) (it is worth noting that it may penetrate better than sulphamethoxazole, the other sulphonamide often combined with trimethoprim). Up to 35% of the plasma level of trimethoprim has been found in the CSF of the normal guinea-pig (Von Tiesler & Schmitt 1973), but only 16% in the normal rabbit (Fujihara *et al* 1975). Figures for the dog do not appear to be available, but it would be wise to maintain maximal dosage, since there is some evidence that adequate CSF levels of trimethoprim may not be attained, even when the meninges are inflamed (in man) (Kirwan 1974), although this may be because the trimethoprim is all going into brain tissue, since adequate brain tissue levels may be attained with reasonable dosage (Maderazo & Quintiliani 1974).

Treatment with both chloramphenicol and sulphonamide together has been recommended for the treatment of Gram-negative CNS infections in man (Hutchinson 1971).

6.2.3 The eye

Penetration of antibiotics into the eye following topical application will only occur if the cornea has been abraded, or if the preparation is combined with a detergent, such as bezalkonium. It has been suggested that antibiotic preparations administered as eye drops may remain in the eye for no longer than 20 minutes maximum, the majority disappearing within 30 seconds. Ointment formulations should remain in the conjunctival sac for up to 1 hour (Norn 1964). However, drops have a considerable advantage in cases of purulent conjunctivitis, since ointment tends to add to the stickiness of the pus and mucus produced. In cases in which there is a penetrating lesion of the cornea or conjunctiva, ointment bases may enter the anterior chamber and produce an inflammatory lesion which may lead to permanent blindness (Wyman 1975). Drops are frequently easier for owners to administer, and should be instilled hourly initially, and a response should be expected within 48 hours. A broad-spectrum agent, such as neomycin or chloramphenicol, without addition of a corticosteroid should be the first line of approach. If there is not a great deal of pus in the conjunctival sac, subconjunctival injection of an aqueous solution of penicillin, chloramphenicol or neomycin may be preferred. This technique has the advantage of introducing the antibiotic to a site whence it achieves therapeutic concentration within the globe. Chloramphenicol is also capable of crossing the blood-aqueous barrier, when given systemically, as is kanamycin and erythromycin when given at maximal dosage. The sulphonamides also penetrate well, and sulphacetamide will penetrate the cornea, when applied topically. However, to judge from the data in Tables 6.1 and 6.2, relatively few organisms infecting the canine eye are likely to be sensitive. Recommended regimes for systemic therapy of ocular infections are given by Leopold (1974).

6.2.4 Urinary infections

When treating infections of the lower urinary tract, it is desirable to use an antimicrobial agent which is excreted and concentrated in the urine. If the agent is concentrated, relatively low systemic dosage may produce therapeutic levels in the urine. In treating renal infections, the urine antibiotic concentration is unimportant, an adequate tissue level being required in this case. The penicillins, cephalorides, streptomycin, erythromycin, gentamicin, nitrofurantoin, and the more soluble sulphonamides attain satisfactory urinary concentrations, whilst oxytetracycline is less well concentrated. Only 10% of an administered dose of chloramphenicol is excreted in an active form in the urine.

Because of the high concentration of antibiotic which may be obtained in the urine, narrow-spectrum antibiotics, such as penicillin G, may be present in urine in concentrations sufficiently high to kill even normally insensitive bacterial species such as *Escherichia coli.* The value of penicillins in this context has been discussed by Ling and Gilmore (1977). The same authors also discuss the manoeuvres which should be adopted with any antimicrobial agent, in order to ensure that a high urinary concentration is maintained, thus exposing organisms in the bladder at least, to a continuous high dose of antibiotic. The agent should be administered three or four times daily, and opportunities for urination should, if possible, be restricted to 15–20 minutes before the next dose is due to be given. Giving potassium penicillin G (110 000–165 000 units/kg), or ampicillin (77–110 mg/kg per os) in the regime described above, Ling and Gilmore were able to demonstrate a bacteriological cure in 64% of cases of canine urinary tract infections using penicillin G and 79% using ampicillin in a small series of cases. Most of the cases which failed to respond were due to *E. coli*, and had undergone previous extensive antibiotic therapy. In untreated *E. coli* cases, 80% success was achieved. Other failures were due to infection with some species of *Proteus*, and with some strains of *Klebsiella pneumoniae*, and with *Pseudomonas aeruginosa.* These are all organisms with limited antibiotic sensitivity, and sensitivity testing would normally be indicated in order to devise effective therapy. Amoxycillin achieves much higher blood levels in the dog than ampicillin for the same administered dose, but is excreted at the same rate (Pugh 1977), so that higher urine levels are attained by amoxycillin. Although the antibacterial spectrum for urinary pathogens for ampicillin and amoxycillin are similar, at least in man (Kosmidis *et al* 1972), amoxycillin should now be regarded as the drug of choice because of its more rapid bactericidal action, and because of the higher urinary concentration achieved.

In man, recurrence of urinary tract infections is often associated with the development of a chronic bacterial prostatitis. Trimethoprim is concentrated in the canine prostate (unlike most other antibacterial agents, which cannot be detected in prostatic fluid), especially when given in combination with sulphamethoxazole, or (less effectively) with sulphadiazine (Robb *et al* 1971). Such a combination may therefore be of especial value in the treatment of chronic or recurrent urinary tract infections in the male. Trimethoprim is a weakly basic drug (p*Ka* 7·3), whilst sulphadiazine is a weak acid (p*Ka* 6·8), so that variations in urinary pH in either direction will alter the ratio of the one to the other in the urine. In addition, trimethoprim appears to be extensively metabolised in the dog, unlike man, so that urine levels tend to be low (Kaplan *et al* 1970). The organisms are therefore *not* exposed to the optimum ratio of the two drugs, and the *in vivo* activity may well be less satisfactory than that predicted by *in vitro* sensitivity testing. This is particularly unfortunate in that the combination appears to be notably efficacious in this respect (Weaver & Pillinger 1977). In spite of these drawbacks, however, co-trimazine appears to be quite effective in the treatment of urinary tract infections, possibly due to the penetration of the two components into the urinary tract mucosa.

If sensitivity testing indicates that neither amoxycillin nor cotrimazine are likely to be effective, and other antibiotics need to be given, it is worth remembering that erythromycin, gentamicin and streptomycin are most effective when the urine is alkaline (pH 7·5–8·0), whilst hexamine (methenamine)mandelate, nitrofurantoin, and tetracyclines are most effective in acid urine. If hexamine mandelate is used, the urinary pH should be maintained at or below 5·5. At this pH the compound dissociates to release the two active antibacterial agents mandelic acid and formaldehyde. Hexamine is available in combination with sodium acid phosphate, which is a urinary acidifying agent, but the urine should nonetheless be tested regularly with a suitable indicator paper, to ensure that the pH is below 5·5. Although this approach has all the benefits associated with not using an antibiotic, a chemical cystitis may occur if the dose administered is excessive, and it may not be possible to lower the urinary pH sufficiently if urea-splitting organisms are present. Ascorbic acid is also a useful urinary acidifying agent which may itself inhibit bacterial growth (Gnarp *et al* 1968), but any urinary acidifier may produce systemic acidosis if given to excess in an attempt to correct alkaluria due to the presence of ammonia-producing organisms in the urine.

The excretion of many of the agents described in this section will be reduced if there is renal failure, and this may not only interfere with the treatment of urinary infections, but may lead to the accumulation of toxic levels in the body. If any degree of renal failure is suspected, a reduced dose of a non-toxic agent such as amoxycillin should be used.

6.2.5 Skin

For superficial lesions, simple antiseptics are generally preferable, and cheaper, than antibiotic preparations. There are several reasons for this. In the first place, antiseptics often have a much wider spectrum of activity than antibiotics. Secondly, it has been suggested (Hamilton-Miller 1975) that topical use of antibiotics produces particularly significant selection pressure for resistant organisms. Thirdly, there is a potential problem of inducing hypersensitivity to the antibiotic used. This may present as a failure of the lesion to resolve, or as a generalised hypersensitivity reaction when the patient is subsequently exposed to the antibiotic systemically. For these reasons, it is generally preferable to use antibiotics such as neomycin, bacitracin or polymixin B for topical application, which are not often given systemically.

For more deep-seated or persistent dermatoses, problems of non-response or recurrence may occur. Penicillin is probably the antibiotic of first choice for such infections, followed by specific therapy based on sensitivity results, if the response is inadequate. When selecting an antibiotic on such a basis, it is worth considering especially those agents with good tissue-penetrating properties, since pockets of organisms may remain walled-off in fibrosed abscesses. Facultatively anaerobic streptococci may remain sealed in areas of fibrosis when the condition is apparently cured, causing the condition to recur subsequently. There is frequently a heavy colonisation of staphylococci which may swamp the growth of the streptococci if the active lesion is subsequently cultured. Agents such as erythromycin, lincomycin and cotrimazine, which distribute well into both extracellular and intracellular fluids may be particularly valuable, although it may be necessary to continue treatment for several weeks.

The above section lists some of the circumstances in which especial care is needed in the selection of an appropriate antibiotic. Other special situations will be described in the appropriate chapters of this volume, and in *The Physiological Basis of Small Animal Medicine* (Yoxall & Hird 1979). In general, the selection of an antibiotic with a narrow spectrum of antimicrobial activity is preferable to a broad-spectrum compound, because it will cause less disruption to normal body flora, and will give fewer organisms the chance to develop resistance. In small animal practice, infections due to Gram-negative organisms are relatively uncommon, except in special sites, such as the ear. Penicillin remains the most useful first choice antibiotic, provided it is administered in adequate dose, for most situations. Indiscriminate use of broad-spectrum antibiotics, especially the tetracylines, in food animals, was one of the principal reasons for the setting up of the Swann Committee, and the excessive use of these compounds in small animal medicine is equally to be discouraged.

Once the choice of antibiotic has been made, the clinician must use it correctly in order to achieve optimum conditions for a cure, for there are many reasons why an organism sensitive *in vitro* may resist chemotherapy in the body.

6.3 Effective use of the antibiotic selected

In order to exert any effect on an organism the antibiotic must be present in sufficient concentration in the immediate vicinity of the bacterial cell. The ways in which the different antibiotics vary in their tissue-penetrating abilities have already been discussed, but it is a fundamental prerequisite of successful therapy that there should be sufficient antibiotic present within the bloodstream for it to diffuse to the site of action in the required quantity, and there remain for an adequate period of time. The principles governing the absorption and distribution of drugs have been discussed in Chapters 1 and 2, and a good deal of further discussion is to be found in Baggot's *Principles of Drug Disposition in Domestic Animals* (1977). Although a knowledge of the pharmacokinetic behaviour of a particular agent may enable the clinician to devise the most appropriate therapeutic regimes for that agent in each species, the amount of pharmacokinetic data relating to small animals is very limited, and many of the recommendations which can be made have a purely empirical basis. It is clear, however, that the desired effect is unlikely to be obtained unless an appropriate dose is administered to the patient. The manufacturers of antibiotics give specific instructions about dose rates in terms of milligrams per kilogram, but these are often not easy to follow in a busy surgery, and the weighing of patients is often impractical. Errors in antibiotic dosing often occur because the clinician does not guess the weight of his patient correctly, which commonly results in the overdosage of small patients (especially cats, with an average body weight of 3–5 kg), and the underdosing of large dogs. Overdosage is wasteful and expensive, and occasionally dangerous, but is generally less serious than underdosage, since most antibiotic preparations have a wide therapeutic ratio. Underdosage may result in a previously sensitive organism becoming resistant, without producing significant improvement in the condition under treatment. Where possible the accurate weighing of patients is very helpful, especially in cases where expensive drugs are to be used.

Once the correct dose has been selected, some thought should be given to the factors which may alter the bioavailability of the agent, defined by Sanford (1976) as 'that fraction of a dose which is actually able to exert a therapeutic effect'. Although many of these factors depend upon pharmacokinetic effects which are not generally within the clinician's control, product formulation and route of administration also have an important influence. Sanford discusses the ways in which formulation may affect availability. It is worth remembering that small changes in formulation may have a profound effect upon the efficacy of the final product, and the saving gained by using cheap preparations may be very much more apparent than real. It is also essential that the preparation used should be administered by the correct route for its maximum antibacterial activity to be achieved. Drugs administered intravenously reach their maximum serum concentration very rapidly, but are rapidly removed from the circulation, either by redistribution to tissue, or by excretion and/or metabolism. Maximum blood concentrations following intramuscular administration take longer to achieve and blood levels for many preparations given subcutaneously are often unreliable, and may never reach therapeutic levels, because clearance from the body is proceeding as rapidly as the drug is released from the injection site. This is of especial importance when antibiotics are being administered, for giving a preparation intended for intramuscular use by the subcutaneous route may fail to achieve antibacterial levels at the site of infection, not only failing to effect a cure, but also giving the organisms a chance to become resistant. Intramuscular injections are unpopular in small animal practice because they may be relatively painful, and if incorrectly administered may distress the owner more than the patient. The factors which affect absorption of a substance from an injection site are complex and extremely poorly understood (Symposium 1978). Under these conditions it is worth considering the oral route of administration when this route is appropriate and feasible. Although absorption following oral dosing with any drug is dependent upon several factors, the recommended dose rates for antibiotics, as provided by manufacturers attempt to take these into account, and, if followed correctly, should result in satisfactory blood levels. Table 6.3 lists antibiotics, the absorption of which from the gastrointestinal tract is affected by feeding.

It is theoretically desirable to ensure that the concentration of antimicrobial agent at the site of infection remains constantly above the mean inhibitory concentration of that antibiotic for the organism to be treated, although this may not always be of prime importance for some highly bactericidal antibiotics (Bywater 1978). In serious infections, it may be advisable to administer the agent three or four times daily, by the oral route, rather than relying upon once or twice daily administration (Bogan 1977). It appears that adequate tissue levels of cotrimazine are maintained for up to 24 hours following oral administration (Craig & White 1976).

Having decided upon the antibiotic itself, the dose, route and frequency of administration, the clinician must next decide upon a suitable time period for which to continue with treatment. Excessive length of treatment is more likely to lead to the emergence of side-effects, but a more serious error is the

Table 6.3 Effects of feeding on the absorption of some antimicrobial agents from the alimentary tract.

Alimentary absorption reduced in the presence of food	Absorption proceeds normally in the presence of food
Penicillin	Amoxycillin
Ampicillin	Chloramphenicol
Cephalexin	Erythromycin estolate (or stearate if enteric-coated)
Tetracyclines	Clindamycin
Lincomycin	Nitrofurantoin
	Metronidazole

cessation of treatment on the disappearance of symptoms, whilst virulent organisms are still present. Treatment should always be continued for at least 48 hours beyond apparent clinical cure in order to minimise this possibility.

If treatment with the first choice antibiotic does not appear to be successful the practitioner may wish to change to another compound. In these cases, Laurence (1973) recommends that the original treatment should be continued for a minimum of 3 days before any change is made. If a change of antibiotic is considered necessary during a course of treatment, great care must be exercised in the selection of a second drug. Whilst it is sensible to change to another drug with the same type of action, it is useless to change from a bactericidal to a bacteriostatic compound. The most logical change is from bacteristatic to bactericidal, and if bacterial resistance is suspected an antibiotic from a different family should be selected (see Chapter 4).

6.4 Antibiotic combinations

There are at present many combinations of antibiotics, put up as a single preparation, on the British veterinary market, although they have been banned from the American veterinary market, and are fast disappearing from the human medical scene. The advantages claimed for these combinations are that they have a broader spectrum of antimicrobial activity; may have synergistic actions; and by containing less of each component drug (in some cases) reduce the toxicity of each relative to the total dose. The disadvantages of such fixed-dose combinations have been mentioned by many authors (e.g. Bogan & Snow 1976). The chief disadvantage is that the proportions of each compound present is unlikely to be suitable for all susceptible infections in all the domestic species. Moreover, individual animals will modify the components to different degrees and in different ways. The practising clinician has no way of knowing exactly what interactions are taking place within the patient, and is unlikely to be able to take appropriate counter-measures. The antibiotics in the combination not infrequently have totally different pharmacokinetic characteristics, so that, for example, blood levels for one may be maintained for 24 hours, and for the other for only half that time.

Most importantly, the veterinary surgeon must beware of the feeling that 'if one antimicrobial drug is good, two should be better, and three should cure almost everybody of everything' (Jawetz 1975). The use of combinations to broaden the antibacterial spectrum may induce a false sense of security, whilst presenting to the infecting organism too low a level of each component to kill it, but enough to induce resistance. The accepted indications for the use of antibiotic combinations have been reviewed by Sanford (1976), and are listed below.

6.4.1 Indications for antibiotic combination therapy (after Jawetz 1968)

1 In overwhelming infection.
2 Mixed infections.
3 To avoid rapid emergence of resistant mutants.
4 Reduction in adverse reactions.
5 Synergism.

In cases of overwhelming infection, when an animal is being treated for a bacteraemic condition, it is certainly desirable to give a maximal dose of each component rather than to use a fixed-dose combination, in order to ensure maximum effect (Hamilton-Miller 1975). Mixed systemic infections are rare (e.g. in shock), but contamination of surface wounds by many species of bacteria is common. The use of antibiotic combinations for this type of condition (e.g. otitis externa or infected skin abrasions) is probably justified (Jawetz 1975).

True synergism between antibiotics is rare, and then only applies to a narrow range of susceptible organisms. Useful synergism can only be reliably obtained from the combination of trimethoprim with a sulphonamide; from some penicillin and cephalosporin mixtures; and, under a limited number of specified circumstances, from penicillin with streptomycin (see Chapter 3; and Jawetz 1968). This enhanced activity may make the combination more effective than when either agent is used alone, and may render the combination effective against organisms normally resistant to the individual components.

It is difficult to justify the existence of fixed-dose combinations of antibiotics with other compounds (e.g. corticosteroids) on grounds other than convenience. The danger of these products is that it makes it lethally easy to administer the combination to every case with the vague feeling that it must be doing some good, and without thinking about the specific indications for each component. If it is thought necessary to give more than one antimicrobial agent to a patient, they may be given separately.

However, the clinician should beware not only of interactions between two or more antimicrobial agents, but also those which may occur between antimicrobial agents and other therapeutic products. Some such interactions are listed in Table 6.4, and are discussed more fully by Davis (1976).

6.5 Prophylactic use of antibiotics

In general, antibiotics should not be used for prophylactic reasons, but some circumstances can arise in which their use is beneficial. Prophylactic use of a broad-spectrum agent or combination of agents will not eliminate a potentially hazardous bacterial population, but when a single potent agent is used to prevent infection by a specific organism, prohylaxis is usually successful. The emergence of resistant bacteria in human hospitals has been, perhaps,

Table 6.4 Adverse reactions and side-effects of some antibiotics in small animals. Data modified from Thornton (1975) and Yeary (1975).

Agent	Reactions reported
Sulphonamides	*1* Renal tubular damage due to precipitation of sulphonamide crystals in urine. Avoid by using slowly excreted sulphonamides which are unlikely to reach high urinary concentration (e.g. sulphadiazine), or soluble derivatives (e.g. sulphamethazine, sulphadimethoxine, sulphadoxine). If high doses are to be given, consider alkalinising urine, and in any event ensure free access to water. Using 'triple sulphonamide' preparations obtain higher therapeutic efficiency with lower risk of crystalluria *2* Depression, anorexia, nausea and vomiting
Penicillin	Unknown incidence of hypersensitivity to penicillin in animals. Yeary (1975) suggests that most reported cases may be due to procaine toxicity, when procaine penicillin given in large doses, or death due to streptomycin toxicity when given in conjunction with penicillin
Streptomycin and dihydrostreptomycin	*1* Neuromuscular blockade and respiratory failure. Especially in cats, monkeys, and neonates (toxic dose c.150 mg/kg i.v.) *2* Hearing loss. Permanent, and may occur after a single dose. Potentiated by frusemide and ethacrynic acid
Streptomycin and kanamycin	Vestibular damage and loss of equilibrium, especially in cats. In cats, kanamycin is relatively safe below 100 mg/kg daily i.m., but streptomycin is toxic at this dose.
Gentamicin	Nephrotoxic in both dog and cat. Probably safe if low dose (less than about 5 mg/kg) used for short period, and renal function otherwise normal
Tetracyclines	*1* Vomiting and diarrhoea *2* Discoloration of teeth and bones – especially in the young *3* May cause hypotension if given rapidly i.v. *4* Low grade, non-specific pyrexia, which subsides when antibiotic discontinued *5* Extensive hair-loss has been reported in cats.
Lincomycin	Diarrhoea
Erythromycin	Vomiting, tremors, at high doses
Nitrofurantoin	Gastrointestinal upsets
Most broad-spectrum agents	Anorexia and lethargy – especially following oral administration
Other antibiotics of limited indication	Nalidixic acid is very much more toxic (liver and CNS) in dog and cat than in man. Conversely, polymixin B, colistin and bacitracin may be less toxic in the small animal species.

the most serious consequence of widespread antibiotic usage in human practice. Stamp (1977) suggests that a similar problem may be emerging in some veterinary hospitals in the USA, in consequence of the habit of administering prophylactic antimicrobial therapy to hospitalised animals. Apart from the encouragement for the emergence of bacterial resistance, the other problems associated with use of antibiotics, discussed at the beginning of this chapter, also arise during prophylactic therapy. Since, under most circumstances, prophylactic therapy is not successful, it follows that in prophylaxis the risks outweigh the benefits. Stamp states that the only documented indications for prophylactic therapy are streptococcal endocarditis, chronic respiratory disease due to structural abnormalities, and in the treatment of traumatic and contaminated wounds (human data). Surgery in infected tissues may call for antibiotic prophylaxis, but broad-spectrum agents must be avoided, for there is a danger that resistant organisms will proliferate, giving rise to a complicated refractory infection, and antibiotic therapy should be based on bacteriological culture results. Antibiotics are sometimes given to sterilise the gut prior to intestinal surgery, or as a routine post-operative measure to prevent the possible development of peritonitis. Mechanical cleansing of the bowel by purgation and/or enema is more effective than attempting to sterilise the bowel prior to surgery by antimicrobial agents, as mechanical techniques will reduce the population of *all* organisms, not only those susceptible to the antibiotic in question. Indeed, it would appear that the risk of postoperative infection and prolonged morbidity follow preoperative antibiotic therapy (Altmeier *et al* 1968; Polacek & San Fellipo 1968). There is no unequivocal evidence (in man) that prophylactic antibiotic therapy will reduce the incidence of postoperative infection (Williams 1972), whether given systemically, or instilled into the wound (Jackson *et al* 1971). A possible exception is the prophylactic use of metronidazole prior to bowel surgery.

One circumstance in which antibiotic prophylaxis is indicated is where there is a distinct likelihood of bacterial secondary infection in viral diseases. Tetracyclines may be used to prevent the development of *Bordetella bronchiseptica* pneumonia in dogs suffering from distemper. The other indication for prophylactic tetracycline administration appears to be in the prevention of tropical pancyopenia (Willder 1977).

It is unwise to administer antibiotics to animals in which there is some degree of immunosuppression, since the patient will be less than usually able to cope with resistant organisms which will emerge. In this context, Rijnberk (1978) advises that antibiotic prophylaxis is not required for animals undergoing corticosteroid therapy.

6.6 Adverse reactions and interactions

Although some antibiotics, such as penicillin, are remarkably free of adverse reactions and side-effects in veterinary usage, such unwanted sequelae are

Table 6.5 Some interactions involving antimicrobial agents. Data modified from Davis (1976)

Site of interaction	Agents involved	Mechanism/comment
Pharmaceutical interactions (outside the body)	Penicillins and intravenous fluids	Penicillins stable in such fluids up to 6 hours, although ampicillin stable in simple 0.9% saline only for 10 hours. Much less stable if bicarbonate added to drip. Always unstable in amino acid preparations and fat emulsions
	Tetracyclines and intravenous fluids	Precipitation if Ca^{++} ions present (e.g. Ringer's solution). Incompatible with heparin.
In gut	Tetracyclines with any agents or foods (e.g. milk) containing calcium or magnesium	Precipitation and non-absorption of tetracycline
	Penicillins or tetracyclines with antacids	Decreased antibiotic absorption
	High molecular weight antibiotics with most antidiarrhoeals	Decreased antibiotic absorption
	Neomycin and penicillins	Decreased penicillin absorption
At receptor site of non-antibiotic agent	At acetylcholine receptors, causing neuromuscular block. All aminoglycoside antibiotics, bacitracin, colistin, interact with each other and will potentiate blocking actions of muscle-relaxants, anaesthetics, barbiturates, promethazine, quinidine, sodium citrate (blood transfusions) and organophosphorus insecticides	Aminoglycoside-induced blockade may be reversed by neostigmine
	Tetracyclines and glucocorticoids	Potentiation of catabolic effects of glucocorticoid
	Chloramphenicol with agents for active immunisation (e.g. tetanus toxoid)	Depression of antibody production
Reduced antimicrobial activity	Most bacteriostatic and bactericidal antibiotic combinations	See text, this chapter and preceding chapters
Toxic interactions	Aminoglycosides with frusemide or ethacrynic acid	Progressive, cumulative and additive effects, leading to hearing loss

Table 6.5 (*continued*)

Site of interaction	Agents involved	Mechanism/comment
	Tetracycline with methoxyflurane	Potentially fatal renal toxicity (in man)
	Aminoglycosides with cephalosporins	Nephrotoxicity (in man)
Metabolic interations	Chloramphenicol and tetracyclines with barbiturates codeine, phenytoin	These antibiotics inhibit hepatic microsomal enzymes, and thus potentiate the other agents listed – even if given some time prior to administration of agents of the latter group

occasionally seen — if less commonly recorded. A number of interactions with other agents may also occur, and the most serious and common of these side-effects and interactions are listed in Tables 6.4 and 6.5.

6.7 Possible causes of unsuccessful treatment

A proportion of cases will fail to respond to what appears to be adequate antibiotic therapy, and the following list of possible causes of treatment failure is intended as a guideline for considering what might have gone wrong in such cases.

1 Failure to start treatment early enough in the disease. Antibiotics, in general, work best during the logarithmic phase of bacterial growth.
2 Failure to select the correct antibiotic.
3 Emergence of resistance in the bacterial population.
4 Failure of the antibiotic to penetrate to the site of infection. This may be due to natural barriers (e.g. blood-aqueous and blood-brain barriers), or to pathological processes (e.g. fibrosis round an abscess, pH of pus).
5 Failure of the body's defences. This may result from the presence of chronic disease (e.g. osteomyelitis), or from the use of drugs (e.g. corticosteroids, cyotoxic agents).
6 Premature cessation of treatment. This may result in the recurrence of clinical signs or the production of a carrier state.
7 Masking of progress of treatment by corticosteroid therapy. A single large dose of corticosteroid seems to have no adverse effect on the inflammatory process, and may even be beneficial (see Chapter 8), but repeated administration will retard healing.
8 Inactivation or antagonism of antibiotic as a result of drug interaction (Table 6.5).

6.8 Conclusion

The concern over transferable drug resistance which gave rise to the Swann Report still remains. Indeed there is now a suggestion that veterinary use of antibiotics may have led to the appearance of a highly resistant *Salmonella* organism in the human population (Anon. 1978). Small animals may transmit pathogenic organisms, or non-pathogenic resistance-inducing organisms to man and there is no excuse for the irresponsible use of antibiotics in veterinary medicine, nor for their use as a cover for inadequate diagnosis. It is unlikely that the range of antibiotics available to the veterinary surgeon will increase greatly in the near future, so prudent conservation of our therapeutic resources is essential. Antibiotics should never be used as a placebo merely to satisfy an owner that some treatment is being given; but only when circumstances justify their use.

References

Altemeier W. A., Culbertson W. R. & Hummel R. P. (1968). Surgical considerations of endogenous infections — sources, types and methods of control. *Surg. Clin. N. Amer.* **48**, 227.

Anon. (1971) Topical Corticosteroids. In *Todays Drugs 2*, ed. M. Ware, p. 47. British Medical Association, London.

Anon. (1978) False friends. *Vet. Rec.* (editorial) **102**, 93.

Aronson A. L. & Kirk R. W. (1975) Use of antibiotics. In *A Textbook of Veterinary Internal Medicine*, ed. S. J. Ettinger, chapt. 7, p. 153. W. B. Saunders, Philadelphia.

Barber M. & Garrod L. P. (1963) *Antibiotic and Chemotherapy*. Livingstone, Edinburgh.

Baggot J. D. (1977). *Principles of Drug Disposition in Domestic Animals*. W. B. Saunders, Philadelphia.

Brander G. C. & Pugh D. M. (1977) *Veterinary Applied Pharmacology and Therapeutics*. 3rd edn., p. 379. Baillière Tindall, London.

Bogan J. A. (1977) Treatment of small animals with ampicillin and amoxycillin. *Vet. Rec.* **101**, 473.

Bogan J. A. & Snow D. H. (1976) Mixed blessing. *Vet. Rec.* **99**, 56.

Bywater R. J. (1978) Treatment of animals with ampicillin and amoxycillin. *Vet. Rec.* **102**, 44.

Chalmers J. & Gardner D. L. (1974) Diseases of bone. In *A Companion to Medical Studies*, eds. R. Passmore & J. S. Robson, vol. 3, chapt. 26. Blackwell Scientific Publications, Oxford.

Chater E. H., Flynn J. & Wilson A. L. (1972) Fucidin levels in osteomyelitis. *J. Irish Med. Ass.* **65**, 506.

Craig G. R. & White G. (1976) Studies in dogs and cats dosed with trimethoprim and sulphadiazine. *Vet. Rec.* **98**, 82.

Davis L. E. (1976) Important interactions of antibiotic drugs. *Clin. Pharm. Newsletter (Colorado State University)* **1**, 1.

Edwards S. J. (1965) Penicillin levels in milk following intramuscular injection. *Vet. Rec.* **78**, 583.

Fujihara M., Meshi T., Joh K., Yoshikawa M., Takahashi T. & Sato Y. (1975) Studies on sulphariethoxazole/trimethoprim. Transport into CSF of rabbits. *Pharmacometrics* **10**, 485

Gnarp H., Michaelson M. & Dreborg S. (1968) *Acta Path. Microbiol. Scand.* Quoted in Bush B. M. (1976) A review of the aetiology and consequences of urinary tract infections in the dog. *Brit. Vet. J.* **132**, 632.

Hamilton-Miller J. M. T. (1975) The logical use of antibiotics. *J. Small Anim. Pract.* **16**, 679.

Hirsch D. C. & Wiger N. (1977) The bacterial flora of the normal canine vagina compared with that of vaginal exudates. *J. Small Anim. Pract.* **18**, 25.

Hutchinson J. H. (1971) Common disorders in infancy and early childhood. In *Textbook of Medical Treatment*, 12th edn., eds. S. A. Istead, A. G. MacGregor & R. H. Girdwood. Churchill Livingstone, Edinburgh.

Jackson D. W., Pollock A. V. & Tindall D. S. (1971) The value of plastic adhesive drape in the prevention of wound infection. A controlled trial. *Brit. J. Surg.* **58**, 340.

Jawetz E. (1968) The use of combinations of antimicrobial drugs. *Ann. Rev. Pharmacol.* **8**, 151.

Jawetz E. (1975) Actions of antimicrobial drugs in combination. *Vet. Clin. N. Amer.* **5:1**, 35.

Kaplan S. A., Weinfield R. E., Cotler S., Abruzzo C. W. & Alexander K. (1970) Pharmacokinetic profile of trimethoprim in dog and man. *J. Pharm. Sci.* **59**, 131.

Kirwan W. O. (1974) Cerebrospinal fluid cotrimoxazole levels. *J. Irish Med. Assoc.* **67**, 76.

Kosmidis J., Williams J. D., Andrews J., Goodall J. A. D. & Geddes A. M. (1972) Amoxycillin—pharmacology, bacteriology and toxicology. *Brit. J. Clin. Pract.* **26**, 341.

Laurence D. R. (1973) *Clinical Pharmacology*. 4th edn., p. 7. 25. Churchill Livingstone, Edinburgh.

Leopold I. H. (1974) Drugs for ophthalmic use. In *Drugs of Choice 1974–1975*, ed. W. Modell, p. 579. C. V. Mosby, St. Louis.

Ling G. V. & Gilmore C. J. (1977) Penicillin G or ampicillin for oral treatment of canine urinary tract infections. *J. Amer. Vet. Med. Assoc.* **171**, 358.

Maderazo E. G. & Quintiliani R. (1974) Treatment of nocardial infection with trimethoprim and sulphamethoxazole. *Amer. J. Med.* **57**, 671.

Mercer H. D., Heath G. E., Long P. E., Showalter D. H. & Powers T. E. (1978) Drug residues in food animals — 1. Plasma and tissue kinetics of chloramphenicol in young cross-bred swine. *J. Vet. Pharmacol. Therap.* **1**, 19.

Milner N. A. (1975) Penicillin toxicity in guinea pigs. *Vet. Rec.* **96**, 554.

Norn M. S. (1964) Vehiklets betydning for lokalbehandling i øjet. *Dansk. Tidsskr. Farm.* **38**, 95.

Polacek M. A. & San Felippo P. (1968) Oral antibiotic bowel preparation and complications in colon surgery. *Arch. Surg.* **97**, 412.

Pugh D. M. (1977) Pharmacokinetic studies and amoxycillin. *Vet. Med. Small Anim. Clin.* **72**, 704 (suppl.).

Rijnberk A. (1978) Systemic glucocorticoid therapy in dogs and its complications. *Proc. Assoc. Vet. Clin. Pharmacol. Therap.* **2**, 39.

Robb C. A., Carroll P. T., Tippett L. O. & Langston J. B. (1971) The diffusion of selected sulphonamides, trimethoprim and diaveridine into prostatic fluid of dogs. *Invest. Urol.* **8**, 679.

Sanford J. (1976) The selection of antibiotics. *Vet. Rec.* **99**, 61.

Stamp G. L. (1976) Antibacterial prophylaxis in veterinary medicine. *Clin. Pharm. Newsletter (University of Colorado)* **1**, 5.

Symposium (1978) Intramuscular injections. *Proc. Assoc. Vet. Clin. Pharmacol. Therap.* **2**, 49.

Thornton G. W. (1975) Antimicrobial therapy in the dog and cat. *Vet. Clin. N. Amer.* **5:1**, 133.

Von Tiesler E. & Schmitt D. (1973) Serum,- liquor- und Gewebsspiegel von Trimethaprim beim Meershweinchin. *Arzneim. Forsch.* **23**, 463.

Watson A. D. J. & McDonald P. J. (1976) Distribution of chloramphenicol in some tissues and extravascular fluids of dogs after oral administration. *Amer. J. Vet. Res.* **37**, 557.

Weaver A. D. & Pillinger R. (1977) Lower urinary tract pathogens in the dog and their sensitivity to chemotherapeutic agents. *Vet. Rec.* **101**, 77.

Weinstein L. (1975) Chemotherapy of microbial diseases. In *The Pharmacological Basis of Therapeutics*, 5th edn. eds. L. S. Goodman & A. Gilman, p. 1090. Macmillan, New York.

Willder A. G. (1977) Prophylactic use of tetracycline for tropical pancytopaenia. *Vet. Rec.* **101**, 15.

Williams J. A. (1972) Prophylactic use of antibiotics in surgery. In *Current Antibiotic Therapy*, eds. A. M. Geddes & J. D. Williams, p. 142. Churchill Livingstone, Edinburgh.

Wyman M. (1975) Anti-infectives in ophthalmology. *Vet. Clin. N. Amer.* **5:1**, 71.

Yeary R. A. (1975) Systemic toxic effects of chemotherapeutic effects of chemotherapeutic agents in domestic animals. *Vet. Clin. N. Amer.* **5:1**, 51.

Yeoman G. H. (1977) Microbiology and availability of amoxycillin. *Vet. Med. Small. Anim. Clin.* **72**, suppl. *Proc. Int. Vet. Symp. on Amoxicillin*, 720.

Yoxall A. T. & Hird J. F. R. (1979) *The Physiological Basis of Small Animal Medicine* Blackwell Scientific Publications, Oxford.

7

Corticosteroids
I. Clinical pharmacology in small animals

A. R. AUSTIN

The cortex of the adrenal gland secretes a mixture of steroids, the most important being hydrocortisone, corticosterone and aldosterone. It is these three steroid hormones, together with other steroids that are closely related in structure and activity, which are termed corticosteroids. Both natural and synthetic compounds are included in this definition. The adrenal cortex also produces other steroid hormones, such as oestrogens and androgens, in small amounts but these are not included in the working definition of corticosteroids.

The physiology of the corticosteroid hormones is complex for they affect many aspects of cell function. Their pharmacology is equally complex and modern medicinal preparations are often extremely potent, so that small doses can produce profound therapeutic results. A good understanding of their physiology and pharmacology is necessary, therefore, if corticosteroids are to be used to achieve maximum therapeutic benefit with minimum side-effects.

7.1 Classification

Corticosteroids influence a multitude of physiological processes, including electrolyte balance and carbohydrate metabolism. Individual steroids are usually conveniently classified as mineralocorticoids, if their main effect is on electrolyte metabolism, or as glucocorticoids, if they mainly affect carbohydrate metabolism. Such grouping may be rather arbitrary as many corticosteroids have the ability to influence both mineral and carbohydrate metabolism, in which cases classification is according to their most important activity. In domestic mammals, cortisol is the most important natural glucocorticoid and aldosterone is the most important mineralocorticoid.

7.2 Actions of mineralocorticoids

Compounds with mineralocorticoid activity promote excretion of potassium and retention of sodium and chloride by the tubular epithelial cells of the kidney; water is retained with the sodium and chloride. Excessive amounts of such compounds cause abnormal retention of sodium, chloride and water, which may lead to oedema and associated circulatory changes. These effects may occur naturally, as in Cushing's disease, or during overdosage with steroids having mineralocorticoid actions. Cortisol and cortisone, for instance, despite having relatively weak actions on electrolyte balance, may cause considerable sodium retention, oedema and potassium excretion if administered in large, prolonged dosages. Sometimes, however, these compounds and other glucocorticoids will have the opposite effect in promoting diuresis, probably due to their ability to increase glomerular filtration rate in some situations, or to their effect in decreasing the permeability of the collecting ducts to water and thus promoting a dilute urine. Whether water retention or excretion is promoted by compounds like cortisol, which have both mineralocorticoid and glucocorticoid actions, may depend upon factors such as the activity of aldosterone in the body and the existing sodium status. During therapy of dogs and cats polydipsia and polyuria are often seen in the early stages of corticosteroid administration but these settle to normal patterns after a time. With longer courses of treatment, however, the mineralocorticoid actions of cortisol and cortisone often become apparent in the form of hypernatraemia, hypokalaemia and oedema. These later effects are rare with synthetic glucocorticoids like betamethasone and dexamethasone, although the early effects of polydipsia and polyuria are often encountered and while this extra throughput of water may be undesirable, it is not usually associated with marked electrolyte imbalance (Osbaldiston 1971).

Deficiency of mineralocorticoid hormone results in excessive loss of sodium and raised levels of potassium in plasma and extracellular fluid. When severe these changes cause dehydration, circulatory collapse and death. To some extent, the severity of the clinical signs in deficiency depends upon the dietary intake of sodium and potassium; thus less hormone is required if intake of sodium is high and that of potassium is low. Adrenalectomised rats can often be maintained on a high salt diet with no hormone administration, whereas this is difficult in dogs and cats because of higher potassium intake from meat diets.

7.3 Uses of mineralocorticoids

The only important clinical use for mineralocorticoid activity is as replacement therapy for inadequate adrenocortical functioning. Such deficiency may be due to primary disorders of the adrenal cortex, to diminished adrenocorticotrophic hormone (ACTH) in hypothalmic or pituitary disease, or to suppression of the hypothalmic-pituitary-adrenal (HPA) axis by treatment with corticosteroids.

7.4 Actions of glucocorticoids

Those corticosteroids which have potent glucocorticoid activity influence a wide variety of physiological and pathological processes, hence they have a great many uses in veterinary therapy.

7.4.1 Effects on physiological processes

GENERAL METABOLIC EFFECTS

The general effects of glucocorticoids on metabolism are to promote gluconeogenesis from protein and to increase the rate of lipolysis, that is the release of fatty acids and glycerol from adipose tissue. Gluconeogenesis is enhanced as a result of the increased release of amino acids from muscle primarily, but also from skin and connective tissue, and the subsequent conversion of these amino acids into glucose by the liver and, to a lesser extent, by the kidney. Another effect of glucocorticoids is to decrease the uptake or utilisation of glucose by peripheral tissues, thus conserving the carbohydrate. In monogastric animals these effects cause a tendency to hyperglycaemia but this is opposed by insulin and the net result is usually an increase in liver glycogen rather than marked elevation of blood glucose.

The effect of lipolysis also serves to conserve glucose; the glycerol so derived is another glucose precursor for liver gluconeogenesis and the fatty acids provide an alternative energy source to glucose.

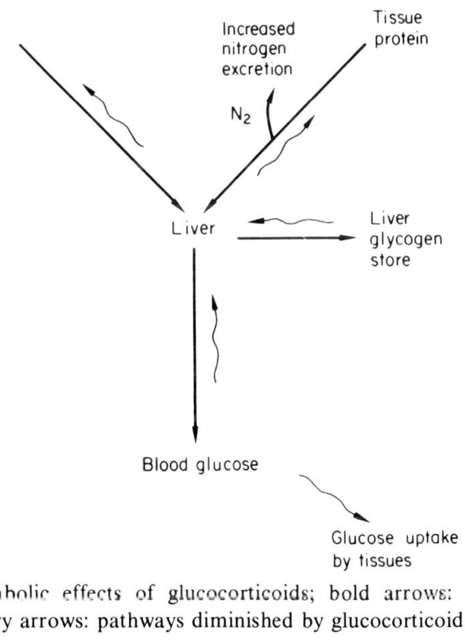

Fig. 7.1 The metabolic effects of glucocorticoids; bold arrows: pathways enhanced by glucocorticoids; wavy arrows: pathways diminished by glucocorticoids.

Whilst having these general metabolic effects, glucocorticoids affect individual tissues in various ways:

LIVER

The actions of glucocorticoids on most tissues are catabolic, but in the liver they are mostly anabolic; thus enzyme synthesis is increased and a number of functions, including gluconeogenesis, are stimulated.

MUSCLE

Glucocorticoids cause muscular wasting by increasing the mobilisation of amino acids from muscle protein and by decreasing the uptake of amino acids by muscle fibres.

BLOOD

In some species, glucocorticoids induce marked changes in the total and differential white blood cell counts; for instance, in cattle total leucocytes and neutrophils are increased while lymphocytes decrease. In contrast, an equivalent dose in dogs produces little alteration.

FAT

The lipolytic effects of glucocorticoids have already been mentioned. Additionally, the synthetic reactions in fat cells are decreased by decreasing glucose uptake. In states of glucocorticoid excess, changes in fat distribution occur. Deposition of facial fat causes the 'moon face' of Cushing's disease in man and altered distribution of adipose tissue may be a feature of cushingoid syndromes or therapeutic overdosage in dogs.

CENTRAL NERVOUS SYSTEM (CNS)

The effects of corticosteroids on the CNS are more readily discernible in man than in animals, but behavioural changes are sometimes seen in dogs undergoing treatment with these agents. In man, increased motor activity with elevation of mood and even euphoria are recognised concomitants to corticosteroid therapy, and electroencephalographic changes can be recognised in man and experimental animals. Mineralocorticoids appear to reduce brain excitability by virtue of their effects on electrolytes, whilst glucocorticoids increase excitability by some unknown mechanism (Haynes & Larner 1975).

GASTROINTESTINAL TRACT

Corticosteroids reduce gastric motility by interfering with synthesis of prostaglandins, which to some extent appear to be responsible for maintaining motility. There is also thinning of the gastric mucosa and decreased mucus production. In man they may precipitate or exacerbate gastric ulceration in some cases. Absorption of calcium from the gastrointestinal tract is reduced by corticosteroids, and this, coupled with a proteolytic effect of bone matrix, leads to loss of bone strength, and eventually to osteoporosis.

LYMPHOID TISSUE

Glucocorticoids have dramatic effects on the lymphoid tissues, generally by depressing their activity. Accordingly, they are used in the treatment of many inflammatory, immunological and lymphoproliferative diseases. There are marked species variations in the responses of these tissues. Some animals (e.g. rabbit, mouse, rat, hamster) are very sensitive and show lymphopenia, a rapid decrease in thymus weight and shrinkage of spleen and lymph nodes after systemic administration (Claman 1972). Most other species are relatively resistant with these lymphoid changes occurring only with bigger and repeated dosage.

Corresponding differences between species exist in the effects of glucocorticoids on immune mechanisms. Production of circulating antibody can be depressed in steroid-sensitive species but this is much more difficult in resistant species. Even in sensitive species, it is the primary antibody response which is mostly sensitive to inhibition by glucocorticoids; much higher doses are necessary to depress secondary responses or on-going antibody production. Apparently, antibody synthesis in mice is especially sensitive to inhibition if steroids are administered a short while before antigen; if they are given after antigen exposure antibody inhibition is much less marked (Gabrielsen & Good 1967).

The cell-mediated immune reactions are similarly affected to differing degrees, with those of resistant species being inhibited only as a result of high prolonged dosage (Makinodan *et al* 1970).

Glucocorticoids have varying effects on the different subclasses of cells within the lymphoid system. Cells in the thymus cortex of sensitive species are killed, while in resistant species there is little actual destruction of cells although their activity is decreased owing to inhibition of both glucose uptake and nucleic acid synthesis.

The fact that glucocorticoids affect the metabolism of so many diverse tissues has encouraged researchers to look for some common pathway through which these steroids might act at a cellular level. Many effects result from the stimulation of production of specific enzymes and other proteins, and one approach to the elucidation of the fundamental mode of action of glucocorticoids has been to investigate the possibility that they might regulate cellular protein synthesis by influencing messenger ribonucleic acid activity (Baxter & Forsham 1972). Details of the mechanisms of action proposed for corticosteroids are considered in Chapter 8.

7.4.2 Effects on pathological processes

INFLAMMATION

The cardinal signs of inflammation, heat, redness, swelling and pain, are all suppressed by the corticosteroids, which reduce hyperaemia, exudation, cellular infiltration, increased capillary permeability, endothelial swelling and the release of vasoactive kinins from plasma proteins. The anti-inflammatory effect of corticosteroids is apparent regardless of the cause of the inflammatory response.

The nature of the inflammatory reaction and the mechanism of the anti-inflammatory actions of the corticosteroids is discussed in some detail in Chapter 9. The anti-inflammatory activity of the various corticosteroid compounds closely parallels their potency as glucocorticoids in most cases.

The comprehensive way in which glucocorticoids suppress inflammation, besides being clinically convenient, has inherent dangers. In most cases corticosteroids do not ameliorate the underlying condition, and recurrence of clinical signs may occur when corticosteroids are withdrawn unless the underlying pathology is treated or resolves spontaneously. Effective anti-inflamatory medication may reduce the incentive to clinician and owner to search for the fundamental cause of an inflammatory lesion, with the consequent institution of unnecessary long courses of corticosteroid treatment.

When treating musculoskeletal conditions, corticosteroids should not be used unless it is clear that the benefits of inhibiting the inflammatory response will outweigh the disadvantages. Impressive as corticosteroids may be in terms of making the lame walk, they should not be automatically used as alternative to masterly inactivity or mild analgesic or non-steroidal anti-inflammatory medication, and should be regarded primarily as a treatment to be used when such alternative therapies have failed. Steroids are of minimal value in treating long-standing calcified lesions, unless accompanied by an active inflammatory reaction. There is also a possibility that long-term administration of corticosteroids may give rise to osteoporosis or myopathy which will exacerbate musculoskeletal conditions.

Another problem is that elimination of inflammation and pain in musculoskeletal conditions may permit an undesirable degree of joint movement and exercise, which may exacerbate underlying pathological changes.

Nevertheless, judicious use of anti-inflammatory medication in cases in which a precise diagnosis is impossible is justified provided that clinical management takes account of potential problems. For example, corticosteroids inhibit prostaglandin synthesis, and prostaglandins lower the threshold of skin to histamine-induced itching (Greaves & McDonald-Gibson 1973). They are therefore useful in treating skin conditions of obscure aetiology, for they offer a means of breaking the vicious cycle of itching, scratching and self-inflicted damage, which accompanies so many of these cases. Although corticosteroids have a useful role to play in the management of such cases, prolonged courses of treatment are inadvisable unless determined efforts have been made to define the aetiology of the condition and to control it by other means. A small proportion of cases, nevertheless, do require long-term therapy, sometimes for life, and these present difficult problems of management, for the benefits of treatment have to be balanced against an increasing risk of side-effects as therapy is prolonged.

HYPERSENSITIVITY REACTIONS

Glucocorticoids can have profound effects on immunologically mediated diseases: they may act directly upon the hypersensitivity reaction itself or only upon the tissue responses following such reactions Hypersensitivity reactions are often classified into four distinct types (Gell & Coombs 1968); glucocorticoids influence each type in rather different ways.

Type I reactions are those in which tissue-fixing antibodies, chiefly IgE, become attached to mast cells. Subsequent exposure of these sensitised cells to specific antigen results in reaction between the cell-attached antibody and the antigen. Release of histamine and, possibly, other chemical mediators of inflammatory reactions, then cause the clinical signs characteristic of allergic reactions. Examples of type I hypersensitivity are pollen allergy in dogs, equine respiratory allergies, food allergies in various species, drug allergies and hypersensitivity to external parasites.

Glucocorticoids do not prevent the IgE-antigen reaction in the first instance, but instead they suppress the events which take place subsequently, that is the inflammatory reaction and cellular infiltration which histamine release normally causes. Other effects may contribute to the longer term suppression of type I reactions; thus reduction in the synthesis of histamine is probably important (Jasani 1972). Additionally, reduction of mast cell concentrations in affected tissues and suppression of IgE formation may play some part (Halliwell 1971).

Type II reactions are the 'autoimmune' reactions. These are mediated by antibody combining with antigen that is associated with cells; this combination, with the aid of the complement reaction, causes damage to the cells. Examples of these reactions are canine polyarthritis, systemic lupus erythematosus and acquired haemolytic anaemia of dogs. Also, antibodies may react against tissues which have been damaged during the course of an infection thereby prolonging the disease, as may possibly occur in canine nephritis and the late demyelinating encephalitis of distemper. The mode of action of glucocorticoid suppression in these reactions is not fully understood but there is evidence suggesting that interference with the complement reaction, alteration of cell membranes and antibody depression each may be involved (Jasani 1972).

Type III reactions involve the formation of complexes between antibody and antigen (usually in conditions of antibody excess), the fixation of complement and, following later, the accumulation of polymorphonuclear leucocytes and local tissue destruction. This sequence of events may occur, for instance, in severe respiratory allergies in which hypersensitivity often begins as type I but progresses to type III with repeated exposure to the antigen. Glucocorticoids probably probably suppress type III reactions at several levels: they may depress the formation of complement-fixing antibody; they reduce the accumulation of polymorphs and, by stabilising their lysosomal membranes, they prevent these cells from liberating destructive enzymes into the surrounding area.

Type IV reactions are those which are commonly called delayed hypersensitivity reactions and are the result of specifically sensitised lymphocytes reacting with the corresponding antigen. This reaction is the basis of cell-mediated immunity. Examples occurring in veterinary medicine are contact dermatitis and the tuberculin reaction. Recent studies have indicated that glucocorticoids do not interfere with the lymphocyte-antigen reaction nor with the release of chemical mediators by the lymphocytes which brings about the characteristic tissue reaction; instead they appear to depress this type of reaction by preventing the chemical mediators from exerting their usual effects. For instance, they prevent the accumulation of macrophages which normally takes place at the site of these reactions in response to the release of macrophage aggregation factor from sensitised lymphocytes (Weston *et al* 1973).

To summarise the effects of glucocorticoids in hypersensitivity reactions: the importance of these hormones to the clinician dealing with diseases caused by immunological reactions is that they suppress all types of such reaction, regardless of cause. Thus, the glucocorticoids are the major therapeutic agents used in combating allergic diseases. The use of corticosteroids in acute hypersensitivity or anaphylactic conditions has been questioned since the full effect of systemically administered glucocorticoids may not become apparent for some time. Thus antihistamines and/or adrenaline may be given in conjunction with corticosteroids in such situations.

Many authors have described the clinical use of corticosteroids in the management of immunologically based diseases in the dog. A useful review is that by Schwark (1974). Amongst the more recent sources, Dodds (1977) on immune anaemias; Pedersen *et al* (1976a; 1976b) on non-infectious arthritides; and Osborne *et al* (1975) on immune conditions affecting the kidney, may be of value to the interested reader.

INFECTION

In consequence of their inhibitory actions on reticuloendothelial system activity, on inflammation, and on immunological responses corticosteroids may exacerbate infectious conditions; whilst animals subjected to extended, high dose therapy become more susceptible to infection. Nonetheless, careful glucocorticoid treatment can be of benefit in specific infectious conditions. Thus, in tetanus, a disease in which the causative organism is relatively non-invasive and principally affects the host by release of toxins, dosage with betamethasone at high levels has resulted in increased survival rates in human patients (Saunders 1970). On the other hand, a double-blind study in the effectiveness of hydrocortisone in the management of a range of severe infections was able to discern no benefit in the use of this corticosteroid (Co-operative Study Group 1963).

In certain types of infection the vigour of the host's response to the pathogen may be a greater danger to survival or future productivity than the virulence of the pathogen itself. Under such circumstances the risk of enhanced spread of the infectious agent consequent upon administration of corticosteroids becomes secondary to the more immediate benefits of corticosteroid administration in a potentially life-threatening situation. For example, inflammatory lung changes and pulmonary oedema in some forms of pneumonia may demand urgent treatment with corticosteroids, whilst the infectious organisms present may be attacked by antibiotic therapy if appropriate.

Several veterinary clinicians have reported on the usefulness of glucocorticoids in the treatment of infections (Martin 1971; Rossdale 1971; Keywood 1971; Noble 1971), and most benefit is likely to be obtained if cases are selected on the basis of whether or not exccssive inflammation, oedema or toxaemia are likely to present serious complications; if any of these factors are likely to be a problem then glucocorticoid therapy may be justifiable, but must be accompanied by suitable measures directed against the pathogen, whenever possible.

Corticosteroids may be of value in the later stages of canine distemper, in that they will reduce cerebral oedema and inhibit any immune reaction which may be involved in the production of demyelinating encephalitis, thus ameliorating central nervous system symptoms. However, use of glucocorticoids in this situation is accompanied by the risk of reactivating latent virus, and of lowering the convulsant threshold.

SHOCK

In acute circulatory failure, or 'shock', changes occur in all parts of the circulatory system, mediated in a large degree by intense and sustained catecholamine secretion and activation of the sympathetic nervous system. Blood flow is restricted in the peripheral circulation, and important capillary beds are either starved of blood or are engorged with stagnant blood. Tissue perfusion is consequently reduced; cellular dysfunction and death follow due to failure in the supply of oxygen and nutrients and due to accumulation of waste products (Table 7.1 and Fig. 7.2).

The literature on the cause, pathology, and treatment of shock is extensive, reflecting the complexity of the subject. Effective treatment

Table 7.1 Some changes in the cardiovascular system in shock

Organ	Functional change	Result
Heart	Myocardial contractility reduced Venous return reduced	Cardiac output reduced
Peripheral vasculature	Vasoconstriction	Total peripheral resistance increased
Blood	Increased viscosity Exudation	Effective blood volume reduced
Capillary red	Dilation Blood stasis	

usually requires fluid replacement regimes and, sometimes, the judicious use of compounds such as the promazine derivatives which modify the vasoconstrictor effect of excessive sympathoadrenal stimulation, and hence improve tissue blood flow. Glucocorticoids may, however, have a role to play in the treatment of this condition, and whilst extensive consideration is given to the treatment of shock in *The Physiological Basis of Small Animal Medicine* (Yoxall & Hird 1979) some discussion is relevant in the present context.

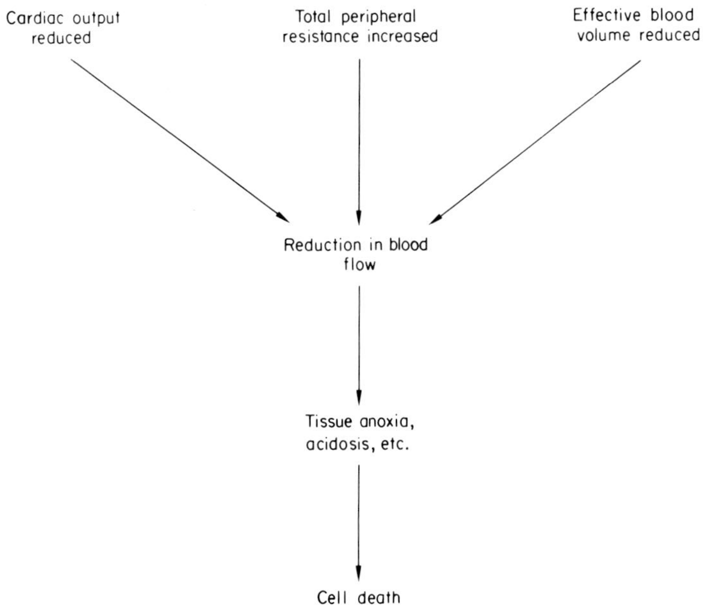

Fig. 7.2 The result of changes in the cardiovascular system in shock.

The ability of corticosteroids to ameliorate the severity of the shock syndrome has been demonstrated in various laboratory models, and clinical benefit in veterinary medicine has been reported by several authors (Keywood 1971; Martin 1971; Self 1971). In reviewing the role of glucocorticoids in shock therapy, Lefer and Verrier (1970) described the effectiveness of these steroids in many experimental models of shock when administered at high dosages before or soon after the initiation of shock-inducing procedures. Judging from laboratory experiments, the effective dose for dogs needs to be of the order 1·0 mg/kg betamethasone or equivalent. Hankes (1976) suggests that 11·0 mg/kg prednisolone sodium succinate is a minimum dose for dogs, and points out that some of the fluorinated steroids may not penetrate cells sufficiently rapidly to produce an adequate response in acute cases.

Insufficiency of corticosteroids is not a feature of shock since plasma levels of endogenous steroids are usually markedly elevated; therefore the value of glucocorticoid administration in combating acute circulatory failure presumably depends upon some pharmacological activity, rather than a correction of adrenal insufficiency. Hypotheses on the subject mostly propose that glucocorticoids either have some directly beneficial effect on the circulation, such as prevention of excessive vasoconstriction (Lillehei *et al* 1967); or stimulation of the myocardium (Tanz & Kerby 1961); or that they ameliorate the metabolic changes occurring in acute circulatory failure, perhaps by preventing the accumulation of lactic acid. Prevention of histamine or lysosomal protease release may also be important factors, as may inhibition of prostaglandin synthesis (Yoxall & Hird 1979).

Much of the substantial body of evidence, showing that animals pre-medicated with high doses of glucocorticoids resist the lethal effects of shock more successfully than non-medicated animals, has come from experimental studies on dogs and cats. Improved performance in the different compartments of the circulatory system, leading to increased blood flow during shock-inducing procedures, has been found repeatedly (Glenn 1974). Evaluation of glucocorticoids in the treatment of established shock states, in contrast to their use in preventing shock, has not progressed so far. Some reports of treatment of human patients suffering from shock suggest that survival rates are increased by glucocorticoid treatment (Lillehei *et al* 1974; James 1974; Weil 1974). Unfortunately, no reports of any thorough clinical evaluation of glucocorticoids in the treatment of shock appear to exist in the veterinary literature. Indications from experiments already referred to, however, are that dogs and cats should benefit from such treatment, provided that it is administered early in the development of the shock state.

7.5 Control of endogenous corticoid secretion

Cortisol and corticosterone are secreted by the inner regions of the adrenal cortex, namely the zona fasiculata and the zona reticularis. The rate of

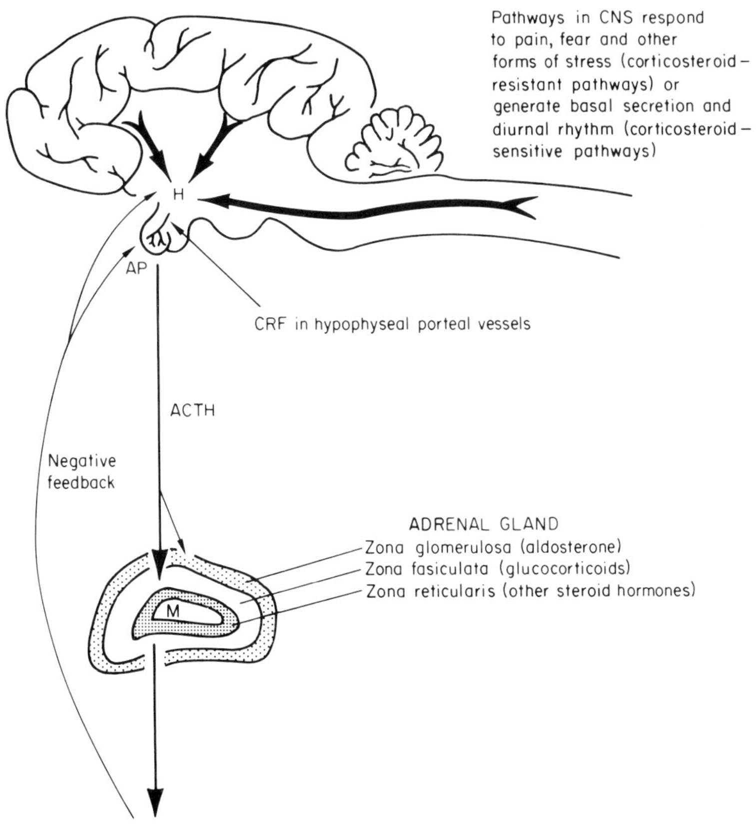

Fig. 7.3 Regulation of glucocorticoid secretion; H, hypothalamus; AP, anterior pituitary; M, adrenal medulla; CRF, corticotrophin-releasing factor.

secretion is controlled by adrenocorticotrophic hormone (ACTH), one of the anterior pituitary hormones, which stimulates the secretion of cortisol and corticosterone (Fig. 7.3). Release of ACTH is in turn influenced by a negative feedback mechanism, similar to that operating for some other hormones, so that under resting conditions rising plasma levels of corticosteroids depress the further release of ACTH. In addition, the nervous system has an important influence upon ACTH secretion, mediated through the hypothalamus; thus, in response to an appropriate stimulus, a substance called corticotrophic-releasing factor (CRF) is elaborated at neuronal endings in the median eminence of the hypothalamus and is transported in the hypophyseal-portal blood vessels to the anterior pituitary where it causes the release of ACTH. Stimuli which will initiate this pathway through the nervous system include most 'stressor' factors including pain, fright and trauma.

A circadian variation in adrenal secretion has been recognised in many mammals. Diurnal species have peak activities in the early hours with minimal secretion later in the day, whereas nocturnal animals have the reverse pattern (Bottoms *et al* 1972; Zolovick *et al* 1966; Macadam & Eberhort 1972). Even within the periods of peak activity, secretion is probably not a smooth, slowly changing process but occurs in short, episodic bursts lasting for an hour or two. In the early morning these bursts are frequent but later they occur less often or are absent; plasma corticosteroid levels are then the result of slow clearance of hormone secreted earlier (Anon 1971).

Thus the output of natural glucocorticoid hormones in undisturbed animals occurs in rhythmical daily cycles made up of short bursts of secretory activity brought about by ACTH secretion. Stress over-rides the hormonal feedback system of control by causing the hypothalamus, through nervous pathways, to modify its rate of secretion of CRF.

Aldosterone, the main natural mineralocorticoid, is secreted from a distinct region of the adrenal cortex, the zona glomerulosa. Control of its secretion is more complex than in the case of the glucocorticoids. Although ACTH does have some controlling influence, other mechanisms are much more important. The kidney contains an enzyme, renin, which is released under certain conditions into the general circulation. Renin converts a plasma globulin, angiotensinogen, to angiotensin I, which is in turn converted to angiotensin II by an enzyme in the lungs. Angiotensin II is a potent vasoconstrictor, and is believed to be responsible for stimulating secretion of aldosterone (Singer 1972).

The nature of the mechanisms controlling glucocorticoid secretion has important implications in their therapeutic use. If a dose of exogenous glucocorticoid exceeds a certain threshold level, the output of ACTH, and hence the release of cortisol and corticosterone are depressed, by interference with the negative feedback system controlling natural secretion. When such administration of exogenous steroid is prolonged, the depression of A CTH and endogenous glucocorticoid secretion becomes progressively more profound and of longer duration; effects which are often accompanied by atrophy of the zonae fasiculata and reticularis and by histological changes in the anterior pituitary. Subsequent recovery to normal hypothalamico-pituitary-adrenal (HPA) axis function may be very slow after such changes have been induced. A study of human patients showed that pituitary secretion of ACTH may take 2 months to recover, whilst the adrenal may take many more months to become responsive (Graber *et al* 1965).

Attempts have been made to devise dosage regimes which will reduce the problem of HPA axis suppression. Thus, administration of steroid therapy in the morning, the time when endogenous glucocorticoid secretion is at a peak, will ensure that there is a minimum amount of circulating exogenous steroid available to depress ACTH release when endogenous levels are at their

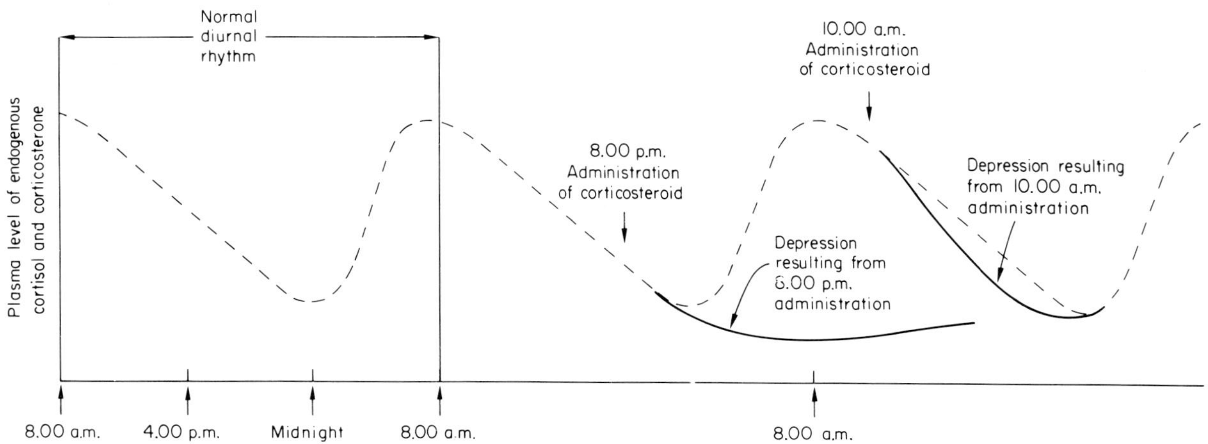

Fig. 7.4 Conceptualisation of corticosteroid suppression following morning or evening administration of exogenous corticosteroid.

lowest, in the early hours of the day. This effect is illustrated diagrammatically in Fig. 7.4.

Another possible programme is to administer steroids on alternate days only, at twice the normal daily dose. This approach should allow the HPA axis to recover on non-treatment days (Jacobson 1971).

Scott (1977) has described the use of an alternate-day dosage regime for corticosteroid administration in small animals. It is necessary to use one of the short-acting glucocorticoids, such as prednisone, prednisolone or methylprednisolone. Scott suggests that the less potent natural corticosteroids, such as hydrocortisone or cortisone, will often fail to control symptoms. The regime described by Scott is as follows:

1 Induction (5–7 days). 0·5–1·0 mg/kg prednisolone given orally, twice daily.
2 Maintenance. 2 mg/kg prednisolone orally, given on *alternate* mornings between 7 and 10 a.m. (i.e. when natural secretion is maximal).
3 The dosage is reduced by 50% each week, until the lowest maintenance dose is determined. (Usually within the range 0·5–1·0 mg/kg.)

The dose rates quoted may be rather on the high side, but in general an alternate-day regime such as this should be adopted whenever a prolonged course of glucocorticoid therapy is called for. Long-acting corticosteroid preparations produce *maximal* suppression of the HPA axis, and their use is to be discouraged. A further disadvantage of such preparations is that the amount of active steroid released over a given period of time cannot be predicted, and depends upon such factors as site of injection, as well as the physicochemical properties of the preparation used.

The effectiveness of intermittent dosage regimes depends upon the ability of glucocorticoids, in many circumstances, to produce therapeutic effects which outlast the presence of steroid in the circulation. The possibility therefore exists that pathological states may sometimes be controlled, whilst leaving the HPA axis relatively unaffected. Knowledge of the cellular events influenced by glucocorticoids helps to explain how therapeutic effects may persist after the disappearance of the steroid: once the production of the relevant messenger RNAs, enzymes and proteins influencing the pathological condition have been stimulated by the steroid, the beneficial effects obtained may well persist for longer than the presence of the steroid.

7.7 Side-effects and complications of glucocorticoid therapy

The major complications of corticosteroid therapy are iatrogenic adrenal hypofunction and iatrogenic Cushing's syndrome. Iatrogenic adrenal hypofunction may be fatal, and can arise under two sets of circumstances:

1 Following sudden withdrawal of prolonged glucocorticoid therapy. Suppression of the HPA axis may lead to withdrawal symptoms if treatment is suddenly withdrawn; a vague syndrome presenting with signs of malaise, lethargy and weakness. More often, no immediate signs present themselves, as the animal is able to meet its basal, everyday requirements for glucocorticoids. However, under conditions of stress, the depressed HPA axis may fail to respond with the increased secretion required, leading to the development of an Addisonian crisis (see above).

2 In response to acute stress during long-term corticosteroid therapy. The tissues appear to become, to some extent, acclimatised to a high circulating glucocorticoid level during long-term therapy with even fairly high doses. At the same time the HPA axis is depressed, and an Addisonian crisis may be precipitated by acute intercurrent stress, such as infection, surgery, traumatic injury, hypothermia, pregnancy, and so on.

These complications have been discussed elsewhere (Scott 1977; Rijnberk 1978). The danger of inducing overt iatrogenic Cushing's syndrome may be averted by giving a minimal dose of glucocorticoid for long-term maintenance, and by implementing an alternate-day dosage regime. Medication alternative to continuous corticosteroid should be considered whenever possible. In spite of general recognition of the problem, cases of iatrogenic Cushing's syndrome are being diagnosed with increasing frequency in the USA, and Scott (1977) ascribes this situation to the increasing use of slow-release injectable preparations.

In order to avoid secondary adrenal hypofunction consequent upon suppression of the HPA axis, an alternate-day regime may be implemented, and additional steroid may be given when periods of stress are anticipated, (e.g. elective surgery), or when stressful situations arise. Owners should be rigorously instructed in the potential dangers of suddenly withdrawing therapy, and the dose may be gradually tailed-off at the end of the required course of treatment. Consideration should also be given to reinstituting glucocorticoid therapy if an animal is subjected to severe stress in the weeks or months following a prolonged course. If such a case should require elective surgery, a soluble hydrocortisone preparation should be given as premedication at a dose rate of 5–10 mg/kg, intramuscularly. A further 1–5 mg/kg may be given intravenously if sudden hypotension or other signs of collapse occur during the course of the procedure. It may be wise to repeat the premedication dose postoperatively.

The other side-effects and complications of glucocorticoid therapy are probably less serious than the two already discussed. The nature of the side-effects produced is related to the properties of the steroid: marked sodium and water retention, with concomitant potassium loss may result from administration of compounds with significant mineralocorticoid activity, although many modern synthetic corticosteroids have relatively little mineralocorticoid activity. The most common observable changes occurring with the use of such compounds are polydipsia and polyuria. In general, these complications are no more than an inconvenience to animal owners, and do not appear to reflect any underlying damage to renal or other tissues. However, hypokalaemia can be a problem in long-term corticosteroid therapy, with consequent clinical signs of muscular weakness and lethargy. Although there are no absolute contraindications to the use of corticosteroids, the presence of pre-existing cardiac disease must be regarded as a strong relative contraindication. Hypokalaemia will have an adverse effect upon myocardial function, and will tend to exacerbate the ionic changes which occur in the myocardium in cardiac disease, whilst retention of salt and water will increase the circulatory load.

Glucocorticoids may occasionally provoke other changes. The occurrence of diabetes mellitus has been reported in dogs following corticosteroid administration (Anderson 1968; Walker 1962). It seems unlikely that glucocorticoids could initiate the diabetic state in normal dogs, but clearly they may exacerbate a pre-existing subclinical diabetic condition by their actions to decrease glucose uptake by peripheral tissues, by enhancing gluconeogenesis, and by increasing the production of free fatty acids from fat stores. In normal dogs, increased insulin secretion compensates for these effects.

Rogers and Ruebner (1977) have described hepatic lesions associated with corticosteroid administration in dogs. Hepatomegaly, with vacuolation, hypertrophy, ballooning and necrosis of hepatocytes is reported in dogs which have either been treated with corticosteroids, or which are suffering from hyperadrenocorticism (Cushing's syndrome), and these findings appear to be related to an increased serum alkaline phosphatase level. The authors point out that dogs appear to be particularly susceptible to glucocorticoid-induced hepatopathy, whilst laboratory rodents and man appear to be relatively resistant; extrapolation of toxicological data across species is therefore unwise. However, the induced hepatic pathology appears to be reversible.

The general catabolic actions of glucocorticoids can produce undesirable results after long courses of treatment. Weakness and wasting of muscle, thinning of skin, weakening of connective tissue, osteoporosis and increased susceptibility to infection are all potential problems when animals are given extended dosage. Reduction in fibroblastic proliferation and increased collagen breakdown contribute to reduced healing of wounds.

In some laboratory animals, namely mice (Fraser & Fainstat 1951) and rabbits (Fainstat 1954), it has been demonstrated that corticosteroids administered in early pregnancy can induce fetal abnormalities, the most common being cleft palate. The fetus of these species appears to be susceptible to this effect during a short critical period when the palate should be fusing. Generally, the doses used to produce these experimental effects were higher than those used in veterinary medicine, but clinical dosage does appear to be capable of causing deformities in puppies when administered to the pregnant bitch.

7.8 Conclusion

Corticosteroids therefore offer something of a challenge to the clinician. Modern, potent preparations provide tools with which the course of many diseases may be beneficially modified. This fact is acknowledged by the large amounts of these medicaments which are distributed by the pharmaceutical industry to veterinary surgeons. Yet, the potential of these substances for causing side-effects is as great as their ability to assist in treatment. Any tendency, therefore, towards their routine use will be likely to cause as much harm to patients as benefit. The key to their safe and successful application is skilled clinical management. The principles necessary for such management have been outlined in the preceding pages. As a generalisation it should be noted that single doses of glucocorticoids, even if large, are virtually without harmful effect (Haynes & Larner 1975) unless they are specifically contraindicated by pregnancy or diseases which they may exacerbate, such as diabetes mellitus. Side-effects become more serious and more common as duration of treatment and dosage increase. Therefore, to minimise side-effects when treating chronic conditions, it is best to use as infrequently as possible the smallest dose necessary to achieve the desired therapeutic effect.

References

Anderson D. C. (1968) Corticosteroid overdosage in dogs. *New Zealand Vet. J.* **16**, 18.

Anon (1971) Intermittent hormones. *Brit. Med. J.* **3**, 493.

Baxter J. D. & Forsham P. M. (1972) Tissue effects of glucocorticoids. *Amer. J. Med.* **53**, 573.

Bottoms G. D., Roesel O. F., Rausch F. D. & Akins E. L. (1972) Circadian variation in plasma cortisol and corticosterone in pigs and mares. *Amer. J. Vet. Res.* **33**, 785.

Claman H. N. (1972) Corticosteroids and lymphoid cells. *New Eng. J. Med.* **287**, 388.

Cooperative Study Group (1963) The effectiveness of hydrocortisone in the management of severe infections. *J. Amer. Med. Assoc.* **183**, 462.

Dodds W. J. (1977) Autoimmune haemolytic anaemia and other causes of immune-mediated anaemia: An overview. *J. Amer. Anim. Hosp. Assoc.* **13**, 437.

Fainstat T. (1954) Cortisone-induced congenital cleft palate in rabbits. *Endocrinology* **55**, 502.

Fraser F. C. & Fainstat T. (1951) Production of congenital defects in the offspring of pregnant mice treated with cortisone. *Pediatrics* **8**, 527.

Gabrielsen A. E. & Good R. A. (1967) Chemical suppression of adoptive immunity. *Adv. Immunol.* **6**, 91.

Gell P. G. H. & Coombs R. R. A. (1968) Classification of allergic reactions responsible for clinical hypersensitivity and disease. In *Clinical Aspects of Immunology*, eds. P. G. H. Gell, R. R. A. Coombs & P. J. Lachmann. Blackwell Scientific Publications, Oxford.

Glenn T. M. (1974) *Steroids and Shock.* University Park Press, Baltimore.

Graber A. L., Ney R. L., Nicholson W. E., Island D. P. & Liddle G. W. (1965) Natural history of pituitary-adrenal recovery following long-term suppression with corticosteroids. *J. Clin. Endoc. Metab.* **25**, 11.

Greaves M. W. & McDonald-Gibson W. (1973) Itch: Role of prostaglandins. *Brit. Med. J.* **3**, 608.

Halliwell R. E. W. (1971) The immunology of alergic skin disease. *J. Small Anim. Pract.* **12**, 431.

Hankes G. H. (1976) Therapy of shock: the corticosteroid question. *Vet. Clin. N. Amer.* **6:2**, 277.

Haynes R. C. & Larner J. (1975) Adrenocorticotrophic hormone; adrenocortical steroids and their synthetic analogs; inhibitors of adrenocortical steroid biosynthesis. In *The Pharmacological Basis of Therapeutics*, 5th edn. eds. L. S. Goodman & A. Gilman, p. 1472. Macmillan, New York.

Jacobson M. E. (1971) The rationale of alternate day corticosteroid therapy. *Postgrad. Med. J.* **49**, 181.

James P. M. (1974) Response of patients in shock to treatment with corticosteroids. In *Steroids and Shock*, ed. T. M. Glenn. University Park Press, Baltimore.

Jasani M. K. (1972) Possible modes of action of ACTH and glucocorticoids in allergic diseases. *Clinical Allergy* **2**, 1.

Keywood E. (1971) In *The Applications of Corticosteroids in Veterinary Medicine*. Glaxo Laboratories, Greenford, Middlesex.

Lefer A. M. (1974) Myocardial action of corticosteroids. In *Steroids and Shock*, ed. T. M. Glenn. University Park Press, Baltimore.

Lefer A. M. & Verrier R. L. (1970) Role of corticosteroids in the treatment of circulatory collapse. *Clin. Pharmacol. Therap.* **11**, 630.

Lillehei R. C., Dietzman R. H. & Movsas S. (1967) The visceral circulation in shock. *Gastroenterology* **52**, 468.

Lillehei R. C., Dietzman R. M., Motsay G. H., Beckman C. B., Romero L. H. & Shatney C. H. (1974) Growth of the concept of shock and review of present knowledge. In *Steroids and Shock*, ed. T. M. Glenn. University Park Press, Baltimore.

Macadam W. R. & Eberhart R. (1972) Diurnal variation in plasma corticosteroid concentration in dairy cattle. *J. Dairy Sci.* **55**.

Makinodan T., Santos F. W. & Quinn R. P. (1970) Immunosuppressive drugs. *Pharmacol. Rev.* **22**, 189.

Martin B. (1971) In *The Applications of Corticosteroids in Veterinary Medicine*. Glaxo Laboratories, Greenford, Middlesex.

Michell A. R. (1974) The metabolic consequences of trauma. *J. Small Anim. Pract.* **11**, 257.

Myles A. B. & Daly J. R. (1974) *Corticosteroid and ACTH Treatment*. Edward Arnold, London.

Noble W. A. (1971) In *The Applications of Corticosteroids in Veterinary Medicine*. Glaxo Laboratories, Greenford, Middlesex.

Osbaldiston G. W. (1971) Renal effects of long-term administration of triamcinolone acetonide. *Can. J. Comp. Med.* **35**, 28.

Osborne C. A., Finco D. R. & Low D. G. (1975) Renal failure: Diagnosis, Treatment and prognosis. In *Textbook of Veterinary Internal Medicine*, ed. S. J. Ettinger, vol. 2, p. 1465. W. B. Saunders, Philadelphia.

Pedersen N. C., Pool R. C., Castles J. J. & Weisner K. (1976a) Non-infectious canine arthritis: Rheumatoid arthritis. *J. Amer. Vet. Med. Assoc.* **169**, 295.

Pedersen N. C., Weisner K., Castles J. J., Ling G. U. & Weiser G. (1976b) Non-infectious canine arthritis: The inflammatory non-erosive arthritides. *J. Amer. Vet. Med. Assoc.* **169**, 304.

Rijnberk A. (1978) Systemic glucocorticoid therapy in dogs and its complications. *Proc. Assoc. Vet. Clin. Pharm. Therap.* **2**, 39.

Rogers W. A. & Ruebner B. H. (1977) A retrospective study of probable glucocorticoid-induced hepatopathy in dogs. *J. Amer. Vet. Med. Assoc.* **170**, 603.

Rossdale P. D. (1971) In *The Applications of Corticosteroids in Veterinary Medicine.* Glaxo Laboratories, Greenford, Middlesex.

Saunders R. K. M. (1970) Tetanus: new treatment and prophylaxis. *Lancet* i, 526.

Scott D. W.(1977) Systemic glucocorticoid therapy. In *Current Veterinary Therapy VI*, ed. R. W. Kirk, p. 1032. W. B. Saunders, Philadelphia.

Schwark W. S. (1974) Pharmacologic management of allergic diseases. *Vet. Clin. N. Amer.* **4:1**, 57.

Self A. D. (1971) Treatment and care of the road accident case. *Vet. Rec.* **88**, 96.

Singer B. (1972) Adrenal corticosteroids — physiological considerations. *Brit. Med. J.* **1**, 36.

Tanz R. D. & Kerby C. F. (1961) The inotropic activity of certain steroids upon cardiac tissue; with comments on steroidal cardiotonic structure-activity relationship. *J. Pharm. Exp. Therap.* **131**, 55.

Thomson E. B. & Lippman M. E. (1974) Mechanism of action of glucocorticoids. *Metabolism* **28**, 189.

Walker D. (1962) Diabetes mellitus following steroid therapy in a dog. *Vet. Rec.* **74**, 1543.

Weil M. H. (1974) Corticosteroid therapy in circulatory shock. In *Steroids and Shock*, ed. T. M. Glenn. University Park Press, Baltimore.

Weston W. L., Claman H. N. & Kreuger G. G. (1973) Site of action of cortisol on cellular immunity. *J. Immunol.* **110**, 80.

Yoxall A. T. & Hird J. F. R. (1979) *The Physiological Basis of Small Animal Medicine*, Blackwell Scientific Publications, Oxford.

Zolovick A., Upson D. W. & Eleftheriou B. E. (1966) Diurnal variation in plasma glucocorticosteroid levels in the horse. *J. Endoc.* **35**, 249.

8

Corticosteroids
II. Chemistry and biochemistry

K. J. THROWER & A. T. YOXALL

The previous chapter has discussed the pharmacological and physiological actions of corticosteroids, and has described the therapeutic uses of this group of compounds. This chapter will concentrate on the fundamental mechanisms of corticosteroid action, and will provide an introduction to the properties of the various corticosteroid preparations available. It is hoped that this information will enable the clinician to select the preparation most suitable for a particular purpose, and provide a basis upon which he may evaluate the products produced in the future.

8.1 Structure

Corticosteroids have 21 carbon atoms, arranged in four rings (Fig. 8.1). As with all biologically active molecules the stereochemical arrangement is important, and is shown in Fig. 8.2. If the rings are considered as a flat structure when viewed from the side, then the methyl groups at C10 and C13, the hydroxyl group at C11, and the side-chain (C20 and C21) at C17 project above the plane of the steroid, and are designated β. The hydroxyl group at C17 projects below the plane of the rings, and is designated α. The importance of these spatial arrangements will become apparent later in the chapter.

8.2 Transport, metabolism and excretion

In plasma, 90% or more of circulating corticosteroids is reversibly bound to two protein fractions. One fraction is transcortin, a glycoprotein with high affinity and low total binding capacity, but with sufficient capacity to bind most corticosteroids at normal concentrations. The second fraction is plasma albumin, which binds corticosteroids non-specifically, with a low affinity and high total binding capacity. When the rate of synthesis of corticosteroids is increased, both the free plasma concentration and the amount

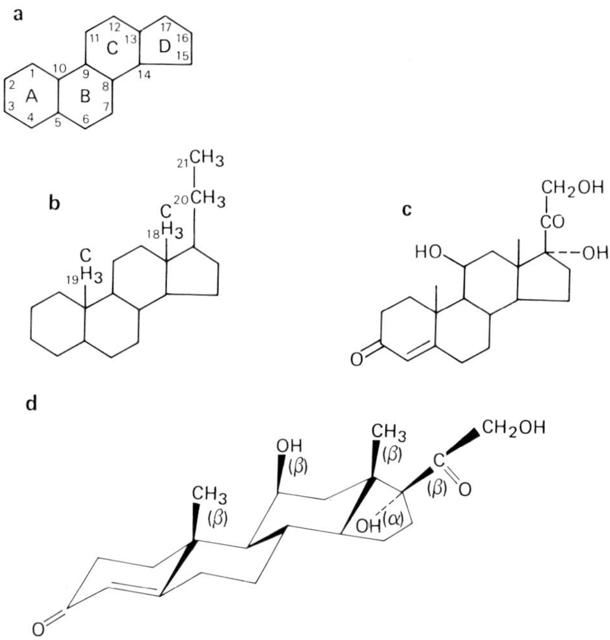

Fig. 8.1 (a) Basic steroid structure; (b) nucleus of the 21-carbon atom (pregnane series); (c) exemplified by cortisol (hydrocortisone); (d) graphical representation of stereochemical structure of cortisol as illustrated in Fig. 8.2. Bonds designated ▬ come out of the plane of the paper (β); bond designated --- goes into plane of paper (α).

bound to plasma albumin are increased, due to saturation of available transcortin-binding sites; the cortisol-binding capacity of canine transcortin being about 6·5 μg cortisol per 100 ml plasma (Seal & Doe 1965), and the resting cortisol level being about 0·9–3·7 μg/100 ml plasma (Becker *et al* 1976).

The metabolism of corticosteroids is complex, but the major pathway appears to be reduction of the 4,5 double-bond and subsequent reduction of the ketone group at C3 to hydroxyl. This hydroxyl group is then conjugated enzymatically with sulphate or glucuronic acid prior to excretion of the metabolised steroid in the urine (Siegel 1965). In the dog, only about 50–60% of endogenous corticosteroid is excreted by this route (Rijnberk *et al* 1968), the remainder being excreted in the bile (Van der Vies 1969). In man, the main route of excretion for synthetic corticosteroids is the urine (Myles & Daly 1974) and the same is probably true in the dog. The synthetic steroids appear to undergo less metabolism, being less able to bind to metabolic enzymes (see 8.6), and a much higher proportion is excreted unchanged compared with the natural steroids.

The synthetic steroids tend to have much longer plasma half-lives than natural corticosteroids, but, since the effects of administration of synthetic

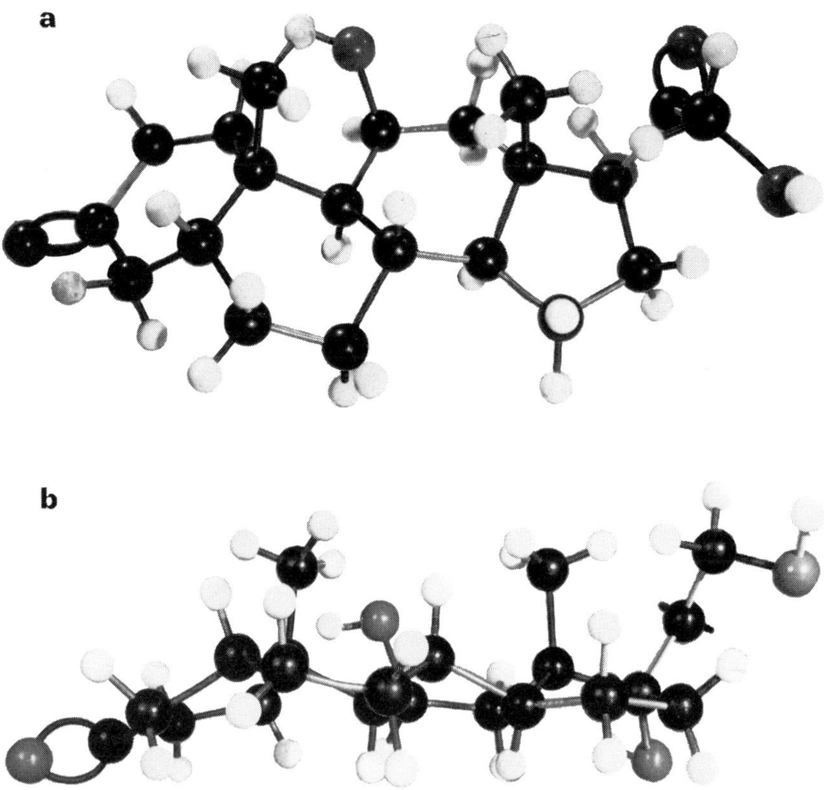

Fig. 8.2 (a) Model of structure of 17-hydroxycorticosterone (cortisol) as viewed from above to show ring structure; (b) viewed from the side to show bulk of substituent molecules protruding from the (upper) β surface of the plane of the structure.

corticosteroids continue for some long time after the steroid has been excreted (see Chapter 7) the plasma half-life is often not the major factor. Much more important are the time taken to exert an effect following administration, and the duration of the clinical and physiological effects. It has been shown that a non-fluorinated corticosteroid, methylprednisolone sodium succinate, is able to enter the intracellular compartment more rapidly than certain fluorinated steroids (Hankes 1976). Since corticosteroids probably have to enter the cell in order to exert their effects, it might be thought that this would give rise to a more rapid onset of action. However, this cannot be considered proven. Changes in the structure of synthetic steroids cause changes in the disposition of electrical charges around the molecule, so that addition of polar groups, such as hydroxyl or ketone groups, will tend to decrease lipid solubility, and hence reduce the ability of the molecule to cross cell membranes, leading to less rapid onset of action. On the other hand, the same structural changes may *enhance* the rapidity of onset of action, by decreasing plasma protein binding, by increasing the rate of metabolic activation, or by increasing the intrinsic effectiveness of the molecule. Nonetheless, as a general rule the steroids with the fewest substitutions in the molecule (hydrocortisone, cortisone, prednisolone, prednisone, methylprednisolone) appear to have the most rapid onset, but shorter duration, of action, than the more heavily substituted derivatives. These less-substituted compounds are therefore suitable for alternate-day treatment regimes, as discussed in the previous chapter (see also Scott 1977).

8.3 Function

Corticosteroids have many and varied physiological functions making them of considerable interest both pharmacologically and therapeutically. There are two main groups, the mineralocorticoids and the glucocorticoids. The former exert their greatest effect on the excretion of fluid and electrolytes, and in particular are responsible for sodium retention. The glucocorticoids exhibit primarily gluconeogenic and anti-inflammatory effects. Corticosteroids show both types of activity and the division is for convenience, emphasising the degree of each activity of the two groups. Much of the work with synthetic corticosteroids has been concerned with trying to separate the two classes of activity.

8.3.1 Mineralcorticoid activity

The most potent naturally occurring mineralocorticoid is aldosterone which is over 100 times as effective as cortisol in its sodium retaining activity. Mineralocorticoids play an important role in the regulation of sodium and potassium balance through the retention of sodium and the excretion of potassium. Phosphorus, calcium and hydrogen ion may also be excreted while chloride and water are retained.

8.3.2 Glucocorticoid activity

Glucocorticoids show an amazing diversity of effects, which are difficult to relate to any simple pattern of activity, but it may be that their major role overall is in protection against stress. While the liver has long been recognised as a primary target of glucocorticoid activity, the direct involvement of peripheral tissue with glucocorticoids also seems to be significant and receptors have been identified in many such tissues. An understanding of these effects is necessary to the good therapeutic use of corticosteroids and an appreciation of the effects they may cause.

8.4 Biochemistry of corticosteroid action

It is clear that corticosteroids exert at least part of their range of effects by stimulating the synthesis of certain proteins, and the description which follows outlines a widely accepted hypothesis as to how this synthetic action might be mediated. However, although a certain amount of evidence exists to suggest that this hypothesis might be true, it cannot be considered proven, and other mechanisms may play a part. The concept is illustrated in Fig. 8.3.

It appears that the corticosteroid first has to enter the cells; this process will be relatively easier for the more lipid-soluble steroids. The steroid then interacts with specific cytoplasmic proteins, which may be regarded as receptor proteins. These receptors have been fairly well characterised (Rousseau *et al* 1972; Ballard *et al* 1974), and appear to be proteins of molecular weight about 50 000–150 000. It also appears that it is the β surface of the steroid molecule which binds to these receptors, and that the receptors themselves have to be activated in some way before they are able to bind with steroid molecules. An equilibrium exists between the active and inactive forms, so that as more of the active form is used in binding steroid more of the inactive form is converted to the active form. There also appear to be differences between receptors in different tissues, although their binding of glucocorticoids appears to be identical, firm, and specific for glucocorticoids. Following binding of the glucocorticoid the steroid-receptor complex migrates in to the cell nucleus, where the steroid is transferred to a nuclear receptor and subsequently bound to chromatin. The nature of this binding is not clear but it is known that the nuclear binding sites can distinguish between complexes originating in different tissues.

Once inside the nucleus and bound to chromatin the steroid-receptor complex is able to regulate the synthesis of proteins, by controlling either the transcription (i.e. formation of messenger RNA from the DNA template) of m-RNA or the translation process, in which the code in the RNA is used to direct the formation of proteins. The former is thought to be more probable, in that chromatin isolated from steroid-treated tissue shows increased template activity when used to regulate RNA synthesis in cell-free preparations, and because steroid administration enhances utilisation of radioactively labelled RNA precursors into new RNA (see review by Tomkins & Gelehrter 1972). It may be that the steroid-receptor complex is able to remove a regulatory protein from its binding site on a specific gene; the binding of the protein to the gene inhibiting genetic transcription. 'Derepression' of the gene would then enhance the transcription process (Tomkins & Martin 1970).

Glucocorticoids may cause an increase or decrease in the synthesis of proteins, depending upon the tissue and protein being considered. Thus in the liver, glucocorticoids increase the quantity of those enzymes associated with

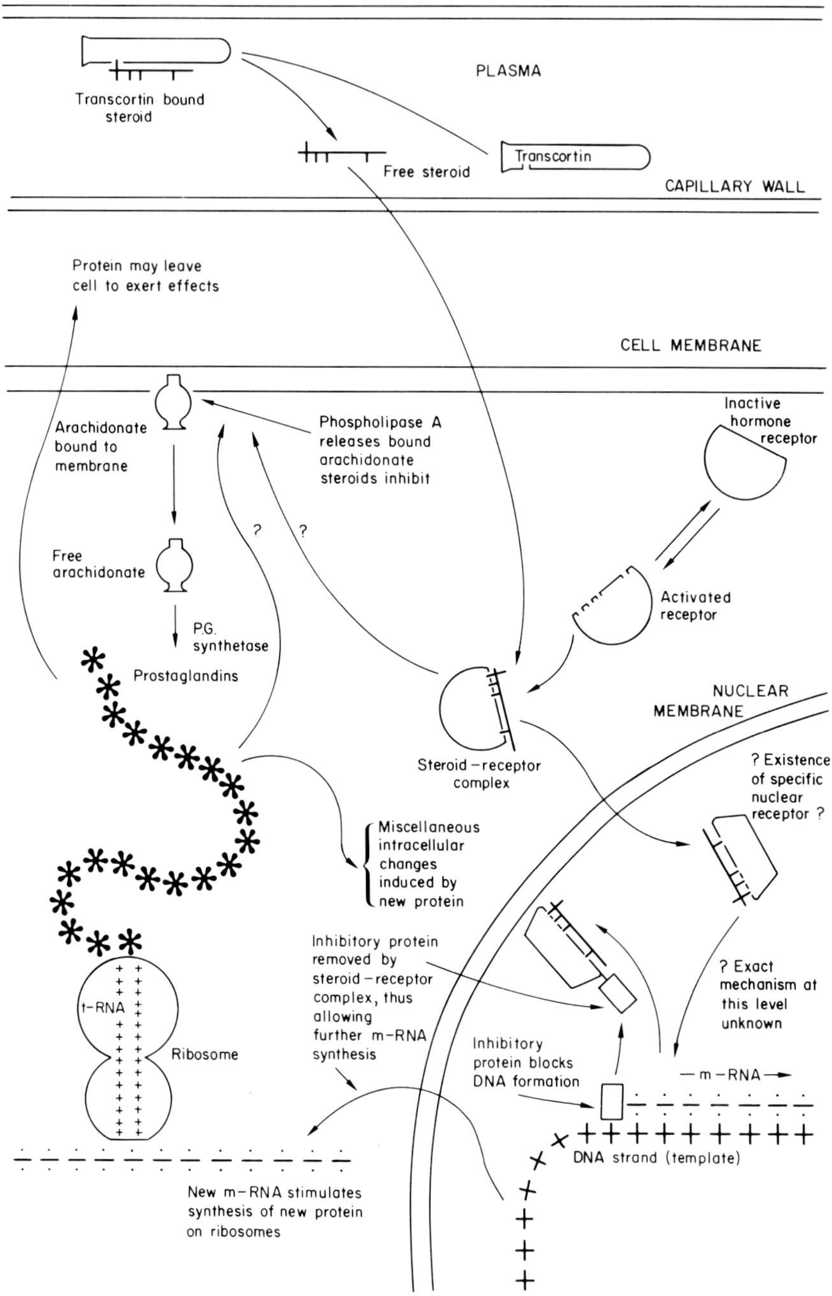

Fig. 8.3 Stylised schematic illustrations to demonstrate some of the processes, which on the basis of current evidence, may be involved in the fundamental mechanism of action of glucocorticoids.

gluconeogenesis and amino acid metabolism, whilst peripherally, many tissues suffer wastage and degeneration. A very widespread effect is the inhibition of DNA synthesis and mitosis, resulting in the cessation of growth of affected tissues, which include epidermis, brain, fibroblasts and liver. The mechanism for this inhibition is not clear but is probably one of the results of the binding of steroid-receptor complex to chromatin. Makman *et al* (1971) have suggested that some of the suppressive actions of glucocorticoids on lymphatic cells may be related to the synthesis of an inhibitory protein.

Whilst many of the actions of glucocorticoids may be explained by the effect they have on enzyme levels through binding of a steroid-receptor to chromatin, there are exceptions. Other mechanisms postulated include changes of membrane permeability, stability or binding properties, and allosteric effects on enzymes (see Cope 1972; Sayers & Travis 1970 for reviews). The effects of glucocorticoids may also be mediated to some extent through cyclic 3′5′ adenosine monophosphate (cyclic AMP). It has been suggested that glucocorticoids might inhibit the phosphodiesterase enzymes which metabolise cyclic AMP, thus allowing the cyclic nucleotide to accumulate (Myles & Daly 1974), an effect which has been demonstrated experimentally (Birnbaum & Goodman 1973), although the evidence is far from conclusive. Such an effect would, however, explain how glucocorticoids sensitise tissues to catecholamines, which depend upon cyclic AMP as an intracellular 'messenger' to exert their effects. Stabilisation of lysosomal membranes has been suggested as a mode of action for the anti-inflammatory properties of glucocorticoids (Weissmann 1969), whilst agents which are known to elevate intracellular cyclic AMP levels have also been shown to stabilise lysosomal membranes (Hoffstein & Weissmann 1975).

However, more recent studies have suggested that the anti-inflammatory actions of corticosteroids are mediated to a large extent by their ability to inhibit prostaglandin synthesis, probably by inhibiting release of the prostaglandin precursor, arachidonate, from its stores in membrane phospholipid (Nijkamp *et al* 1976). However, the means by which glucocorticoids are able to exert this effect is not clear, and it is not known whether it is related to the effects of glucocorticoids on protein synthesis.

8.5 Synthetic corticosteroids

As the glucocorticoids are of such interest and use therapeutically, much effort has been expended in synthesising molecules which are more potent than corticol, with a minimal increase in side-effects. In the synthesis of new glucocorticoid molecules, the aim has been to separate the desirable effects (chiefly anti-inflammatory action), from the undesirable effects (mineralocorticoid and catabolic activity, suppression of the HPA axis), as well as to increase potency. This approach has been partially successful in that modern glucocorticoids are more potent than their forerunners, and have little or no mineralocorticoid activity. However, it has not been possible to reduce the catabolic effects proportionately and there seems to be a close relationship between the anti-inflammatory and HPA axis suppressive effect of corticosteroids (Boss *et al* 1971). Thus, equally potent doses of hydrocortisone and its synthetic derivatives are likely to produce similar unwanted effects, apart from mineralocorticoid effects. In practice, the exact relationship between desired and undesired effects will depend also upon such factors as the dosage regime (see Chapter 7), the site of administration and, perhaps, the species. The steroids beclomethasone and clobetasone butyrate have less HPA axis suppressive effects than would be expected from their anti-inflammatory activity when applied topically; in the case of beclomethasone this is probably due to an unusually high rate of metabolic inactivation (Harris *et al* 1973).

To estimate the total number of synthetic steroids which have been produced is impossible, but from this very large number only a handful of suitable molecules have emerged. Most of the glucocorticoids used today in veterinary medicine started life, and were developed for, human therapy, although in some cases special derivatives and formulations have been made for veterinary use.

8.6 Relationship between chemical structure and activity

During research into new synthetic glucocorticoids, much has been learned about the relationship between chemical structure and biological activity. In some cases biological activity can be abolished completely, whilst in others the balance between mineralocorticoid and glucocorticoid can be markedly altered. Before discussing this further it is worthwhile remembering that cortisone (11-keto) itself is inactive; it must be converted to hydrocortisone (11-hydroxy) usually by liver enzymes, although there is some evidence that this conversion may take place in the skin for topically applied glucocorticoids. Prednisone must likewise be converted to prednisolone, but it appears, in man, that the latter conversion is much more efficient than the former (Jenkins 1967). It has been determined that the following structural features are essential to glucocorticoid activity (Fig. 8.1c):

1 Unsaturation in the Δ^4 position (i.e. a double-bond between carbons 4 and 5) in the *A* ring.

2 A 3-ketone group. Some glucocorticoids with 3-hydroxy have been reported as having reasonable activity, but it seems that such compounds are usually too rapidly excreted to be useful.

3 An 11β-hydroxy group. As stated above, cortisone and other glucocorticoids with 11-keto groups are active because of enzymatic conversion to 11-hydroxy. Substituents, such as 2α-methyl which inhibit this conversion, result in loss of activity. A change in the steric configuration from the β to the α position (i.e. from above to below the plane of the molecule) also results in loss of activity.
4 A 20-keto group.
5 A 21-hydroxy group or derivative (often acetate). Some progesterone-type molecules (i.e. with a 21-methyl) have glucocorticoid activity, especially if 9α or 6α fluoro groups are present, and one compound (clobetasol) with a 21-chloro group is very active topically.

Discussion of the relationship between structure and activity of any group of pharmacologically active substance is always difficult as the interactions between different parts of the molecule are complex and what appear to be 'golden rules' often have to be rewritten as exceptions come to light. The list given below of changes in glucocorticoid structure which result in enhanced activity is therefore very general and must be viewed as such. Structures of some of the more commonly used glucocorticoids are given below, and their relative activities compared.

In the following structural formulae, the potency of the agents is related to the potency of cortisol as having a potency of 1 in terms of each effect.

PREDNISOLONE
Anti-inflammatory potency 4.
Mineralocorticoid potency 0·8.

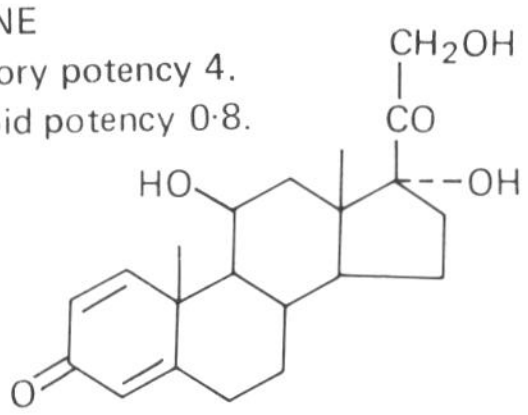

METHYLPREDNISOLONE
Anti-inflammatory potency 5.
Mineralocorticoid potency 0.

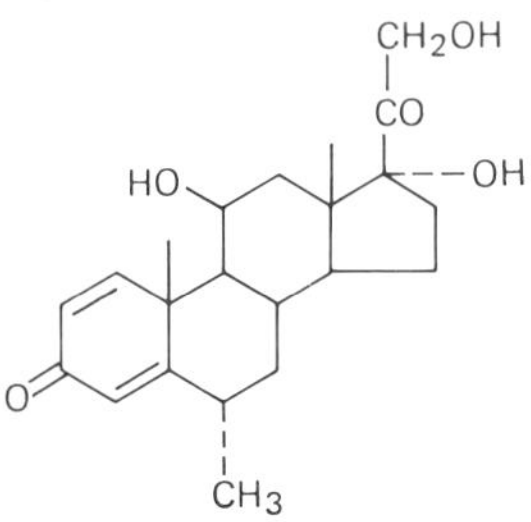

1 Introduction into the *A* ring of hydrocortisone of a 1,2 double-bond gives a fourfold enhancement of glucocorticoid activity, with no increase of mineralocorticoid activity. Most, if not all, of the synthetic glucocorticoids available have a 1,2 double-bond. Further unsaturation results in loss of activity.
2 Substitution at the 6 and 9 positions of the *B* ring generally results in considerably increased glucocorticoid activity and markedly reduce mineralocorticoid activity. Substituents at C6 include methyl (methylprednisolone, oxylone), chloro (chloroprednisolone) and fluoro groups (paramethasone, fluprednisolone, flumethasone, fluocinolone). With two exceptions substitution at C9 is with a fluoro group and the list includes fluorohydrocortisone (increased mineralocorticoid activity), betamethasone, dexamethasone, triamcinolone, fluocinolone, flumethasone, fluoroprednisolone, clobetasol and clobetasone. The exceptions are beclomethasone and flucortolone which have a 9-chloro group, but fluoro groups generally give the greatest increase in glucocorticoid activity. All substitutions at C9 are α.

9-FLUOROPREDNISOLONE
Anti-inflammatory potency 17.
Mineralocorticoid potency 0.
Has relatively high gluconeogenic potency (25)

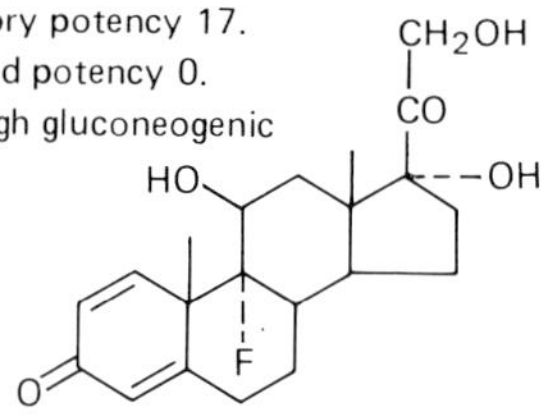

PREDNISONE

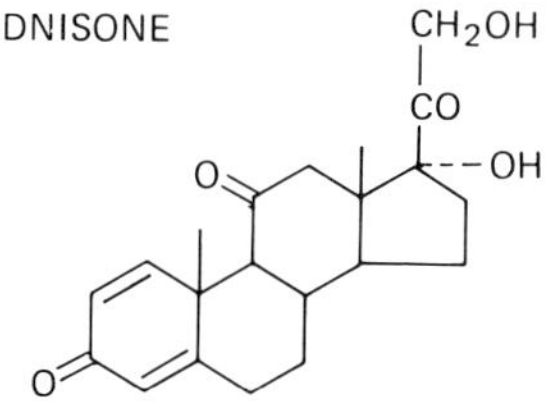

3 The *C* ring has not been very fruitful ground for derivatisation although flucortolone (11-chloro) and clobetasone (11-keto) both have good activity topically. It is the 11-keto groups on cortisone and prednisone which are converted to hydroxyl in the metabolic activation of these steroids.

4 Substitution at C16 in the *D* ring is very common and substitutents include methyl, both α (paramethasone, flumethasone, dexamethasone) and β (betamethasone, beclomethasone, clobetasol and clobetasone), and α-hydroxy groups (triamcinolone, fluocinolone). Methylation results in parturition induction during the last trimester of pregnancy, whilst hydroxylation markedly reduces sodium retention, but has little effect on glucocorticoid activity.

5 Most marketed glucocorticoids have a 17-hydroxy group although this may sometimes be derivatised to form an acetonide, propionate or acetate. An exception is flucortinbutyl in which the methyl group is absent.

	BETAMETHASONE	DEXAMETHASONE
Anti-inflammatory potency	30	29
Gluconeogenic potency	7	25
Mineralocorticoid potency	0	0

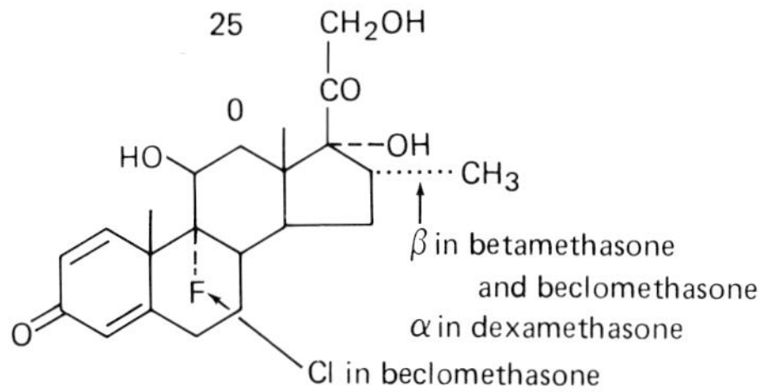

	TRIAMCINOLONE	FLUMETHASONE
Anti-inflammatory potency	3	30
Gluconeogenic potency	3	25
Mineralocorticoid potency	0	0

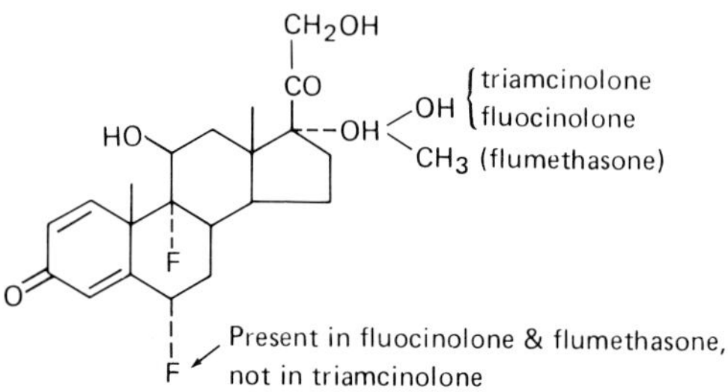

The question arises as to why these substitutions change activity, and what biochemical pathways are being affected? While our knowledge of the mechanism of corticoid activity is imperfect, the answer must be incomplete, but there would appear to be two main effects. The first is interference with enzymic metabolism. The 1,2 double-bond decreases the rate of reduction of the 4,5 double-bond and 3-keto group in the *A* ring, while the 9α-fluoro group retards oxidation of the 11β-hydroxy group and groups at 16α protect the C20-keto group from reduction. The second reason relates to the plasma protein binding, which is reduced in the synthetic glucocorticoids because of substituents on the α surface of the molecule. Thus more unbound steroid is circulating and so activity is increased. Cortisol is 95% bound to transcortin while dexamethasone and betamethasone are less than 70% bound to plasma proteins. Synthetic corticosteroids are less conjugated as the glucuronide than cortisol, and a greater proportion is usually excreted unchanged in the urine. They also have a longer plasma half-life than cortisol (80–90 minutes compared with 200 minutes from dexamethasone) and are more extensively tissue bound so that the tissue activity of dexamethasone, for example, persists up to 72 hours. One problem in quoting figures such as those given above is that most of those readily available refer to man; species differences in metabolic pathways, tissue and plasma binding mean that they should be transferred to animals with caution.

It will be noted from the above descriptions that the majority of the substitutions in the steroid structure take place in the α plane of the molecule. It is this plane as well as the 11β-hydroxy group which is believed to be chiefly involved in the binding of the molecule to transcortin. Substitutions on this surface of the molecule would, therefore, be expected to inhibit plasma protein binding (Burton & Westphal 1972). Similar considerations might apply to the interactions between steroids and metabolic enzymes. As mentioned above, binding to the cytoplasmic receptor appears to be on the β surface of the steroid molecule.

8.7 Derivatives and formulation

Many of the glucocorticoids available commercially are ester or salt derivatives of the steroid itself (e.g. betamethasone adamantoate). Generally, derivatives are not active themselves but must be converted back to the parent glucocorticoid (e.g. betamethasone). Derivatives are usually found in injectable or topical formulations and are chosen to give the glucocorticoid molecule the necessary desirable characteristics.

For intravenous use clear aqueous solutions are required so that sodium phosphate, sodium succinate or m-sulphobenzoate derivatives are made to increase the generally poor solubility of glucocorticoids. On the other hand decreased solubility, leading to slow absorption, is required for longer acting injections and this is achieved by making derivatives such as adamantoate, trioxundecanoate, phenyl propionate, acetate, trimethylacetate, acetonide or isonicotinate. Such derivatives are usually on the C21- or C17-hydroxy groups.

Topical preparations present different problems in formulation. In this case the steroid is most active when it is present as a saturated solution, but the preparation must have other suitable properties. It is particularly important that it is cosmetically acceptable and suitable for the type of lesion to which it is to be applied. Thus many glucocorticoids are offered for topical use as creams, ointments and lotions. An important ingredient of many modern topical formulations is propylene glycol, but the physical characteristics of glucocorticoid are frequently modified by making a derivative and suitable ones may be dipropionate, propionate, acetonide, acetate, butyrate or valerate. The use of suppositories in human medicine is fairly common in Europe although there is not a great acceptance in the UK. It should perhaps be considered more frequently as the reproducibility of absorption is often similar to that for oral administration although the extent of absorption may be lower.

In common with other drugs, preparations of glucocorticoids have been formulated for a particular route of administration at a particular concentration, and it is generally unwise to dilute or otherwise alter the formulation except on the manufacturer's instructions. This is especially important with topical preparations or long acting injections.

8.8 Recent trends

High doses of glucocorticoids over long periods cause wasting of tissues, reduced muscle mass, decreased mass of lymphoid tissue, osteoporosis, thinning of the skin and altered fat patterns. They may also suppress immune reactions, lead to a generally decreased resistance to infection, and delay wound healing after surgery, due to the inhibition of the formation of new collagen and the production of ground substance. Insufficient natural production results in weakness and fatigue, due to diminished work capacity of striated muscle, inadequacy of the circulation system. Psychological changes are also seen.

This has led to changes in therapeutic regimes, and especially the introduction of alternate day dosing. There has also been some alteration of views on the use of high potency fluorinated glucocorticoids in topical therapy. It has recently been recognised that systemic side-effects can occur with some topical steroids. Clobetasol propionate, which is potent and effective, has been mentioned in several reports. There is increasing interest in less potent steroids, in which the topical effect is only moderate, but the systemic effect is minimal. Modern concepts of formulation technology have also been applied to topical preparations of some older glucocorticoids, hydrocortisone in particular.

Glucocorticoids for veterinary medicine generally come into use following their introduction for human medicine. It is therefore pertinent to mention some of the more recent introductions into the latter field. Most of these have been for topical use although triamcinolone hexacetonide for intra-articular, intra- or sublesional and synovial use is an exception. The following new glucocorticoids for topical use have been introduced within the last few years: clobetasol propionate, fluprednylidene acetate, hydrocortisone butyrate, clobetasone butyrate, diflucortolone valerate, flucortin butyl, desonide and diflorasone diacetate.

Further reading

The literature on the use of glucocorticoids is voluminous, but the following general articles could prove helpful and give leads for further reading. Specific questions about particular steroids may be directed to the manufacturer or supplier who often has a considerable amount of unpublished material.

Azarnoff D. E. (ed) (1975) *Steroid Therapy*. W. B. Saunders, Philadelphia.

Leung K. & Much A. (1975) Peripheral actions of glucocorticoids. *Ann. Rev. Physiol.* **37**, 245.

Melby J. C. (1977) Clinical pharmacology of systemic corticosteroids. *Ann. Rev. Pharmacol. Toxicol.* **17**, 511.

Thompson E. B. & Lippman M. E. (1974) Mechanisms of action of glucocorticoids. *Metabolism* **23**, 159.

A Glaxo Guide to Corticosteroids (1975) Glaxo Laboratories, Greenford, Middlesex.

The Use of Corticosteroids in Veterinary Practice (1976) Glaxo Laboratories, Greenford, Middlesex.

Corticosteroids in Veterinary Medicine (1974) The Upjohn Company, Kalamazoo, Michigan.

References

Ballard P. L., Baxter J. D., Higgins S. J., Rousseau G. C. & Tomkins G. M. (1974) General presence of glucocorticoid receptors in mammalian tissues. *Endocrinology* **94**, 998.

Becker M. J., Helland D. & Becker D. N. (1976) Serum cortisol (hydrocortisone) values in normal dogs as determined by radioimmunoassay. *Amer. J. Vet. Res.* **27**, 1101.

Birnbaum R. S. & Goodman H. M. (1973) Effects of hypophysectomy on cyclic AMP accumulation and action in adipose tissue. *Fed. Proc.* **32**, 535.

Boss N., Kluge F., Müller O. A., Pickerdt C. R. & Scriba P. C. (1971) Quantitative assay of the suppressive effect of synthetic corticoids in man. *Acta Endoc.* **67**, 508.

Burton R. M. & Westphal U. (1972) Steroid hormone binding proteins in blood plasma. *Metabolism* **21**, 253.

Cope C. L. (1972) *Adrenal Steroids and Disease*. Pitman Medical, London.

Hankes G. H. (1976) Therapy of shock: the corticosteroid question. *Vet. Clin. N. Amer.* **6:2**, 277.

Harris D. M., Martin L. E., Harrison C. & Jack D. (1973) The effect of oral and inhaled beclomethasone diproprionate on adrenal function. *Clin. Allergy* **3**, 243.

Hoffstein S. & Weissmann G. (1975) Mechanisms of lysosomal enzyme release from leukocytes. IV Interaction of monosodium urate crystals with dogfish and human leukocytes. *Arthr Rheumat.* **18**, 153.

Jenkins J. S. (1967) Conversion of cortisone to cortisol and prednisone to prednisolone. *Brit. Med. J.* **2**, 205.

Makman M. H., Dvorkin B. & White A. (1971). Evidence for induction by cortisol *in vitro* of a protein inhibitor of transport and phosphorylation in rat thymocytes. *Proc. Nat. Acad. Sci. (USA)* **68**, 1269.

Myles A. B. & Daly J. R. (1974) *Corticosteroid and ACTH Treatment.* Edward Arnold, London.

Nijkamp F. P., Flower R. J., Moncada S. & Vane J. R. (1976) Partial purification of rabbit aorta contracting substance-releasing factor and inhibition of its activity by anti-inflammatory steroids. *Nature* **263**, 479.

Rijnberk A., der Kinderen P. J., & Thijssen J. H. H. (1968) Investigations on the adrenocortical function of normal dogs. *J. Endocr.* **41**, 387.

Rousseau G. C., Baxter J. D. & Tomkins G. M. (1972) Glucocorticoid receptors, relations between steroid binding and biological effects. *J. Molec. Biol.* **67**, 99.

Sayers G. & Travis R. H. (1970) Adrenocorticotrophic hormone; adrenocortical steroids and their synthetic analogs. In *The Pharmacological Basis of Therapeutics* 4th edn., eds. L. S. Goodman & A. Gilman, p. 1604 Macmillan, New York.

Scott D. W. (1977) Systemic glucocorticoid therapy. In *Current Veterinary Therapy VI*, ed. R. W. Kirk. W. B. Saunders, Philadelphia.

Seal U. S. & Doe R. P. (1956) Vertebrate distribution of corticosteroid-binding globulin and some endocrine effects on concentration. *Steroids* **5:6**, 827.

Siegel E. T. (1965) Determination of 17-hydroxycorticosteroids in canine urine. *Amer. J. Vet. Res.* **26**, 1152.

Tomkins G. M. & Gelehrter T. D. (1972) The present status of genetic regulation by hormones. In *Biochemical Actions of Hormones*, ed. G. Litwack, vol. 2. Academic Press, London.

Tomkins G. M. & Martin D. W. (1970) Hormones and gene expression. *Ann. Rev. Genet.* **4**, 91.

Van der Vies J. (1969) Personal communication, quoted in Lubberink A.A.M.E. *Diagnosis and Treatment of Canine Cushing's Syndrome.* Thesis, University of Utrecht.

Weissmann G. (1969) The effects of steroids and drugs on lysosomes. In *Lysosomes in Biology & Pathology*, eds. J. T. Dingle & H. B. Fell, vol. 1. North-Holland, Amsterdam.

9

Pain and inflammation: analgesic and anti-inflammatory agents

A. T. YOXALL

Grief for a while is blind, and so was mine.
I wish no living thing to suffer pain.
Percy Bysshe Shelley
(Prometheus Unbound)

The experience of pain is a subjective phenomenon, which involves the appreciation of painful stimuli initiated by physical or chemical means, and mediated by means of the peripheral and central nervous systems. This chapter describes the sequence of events which lead to the whole experience which we describe as 'pain', and will discuss the pharmacological instruments which may be used to diminish it.

Pain is an abstract phenomenon which we cannot describe in absolute terms, but we can usually understand something of the pain suffered by another person by referring his verbal description of his pain to our own experience. Animals are capable neither of formulating a verbal description, nor, as far as we can ascertain, of formulating an abstract concept. We therefore depend upon other clinical signs in attempting to diagnose pain in animals, and it is very likely that we underdiagnose pain in animals in consequence. The indicators of pain in animals fall into three major groups as follows:

1 Visible or audible indicators of 'distress': moaning, or other abnormal vocalisation; abnormal posture.
2 Autonomic signs: tachycardia; tachypnoea and panting; sweating and piloerection; vomiting.
3 Interference with normal function: lameness; dysphagia; dysuria and dyschezia; unwillingness to engage in normal activity; restlessness and change in demeanour.

Pain is usually diagnosed in animals by observing gross disturbance in function, which may be accompanied by visible or audible indicators. The clinician may attribute autonomic signs to pain directly, or to 'shock'. Such a diagnostic approach will reveal the presence of acute pain which is well localised, such as that associated with traumatic injury or acute inflammation, but may well fail to reveal the presence of rather unlocalised chronic pain. Equivalent syndromes in man to this latter type of pain would include headache and the 'lower back pain' syndrome. Pain in animals may be indicated by no more specific signs than a general depression and lethargy, and it may not be possible to elicit acute signs of pain from such cases, which may lead the unwary to fail to diagnose the presence of pain. For example, most tumours are associated with pain, and analgesic treatment will produce a marked improvement in the observed 'quality of life' in the canine patient. Similarly, postoperative analgesic medication will enhance recovery from painful surgical procedures, and the traumatic injury victim will often improve rapidly when an analgesic is administered. Examples of commonly undiagnosed pain are legion, and as a general rule it is probably wise for the veterinarian to be aware of the probability of the presence of pain in all circumstances where pain would be present in the human patient.

9.1 Inflammation

The inflammatory response is almost invariably associated with pain, and is, moreover, an integral part of many disease processes. It is considered here in some detail, as many of the analgesic agents to be discussed act by inhibiting some stage of the inflammatory process, and because the fundamental nature of this process render it an extremely important process in relation to medicine as a whole. One drawback to the study of inflammation in isolation is that the process is closely interlinked with other protective mechanisms, such as blood clotting, and immune mechanisms, especially the complement system. Any separation of these systems lends some degree of distortion to any approach to the problem of inflammation itself.

Many specific and non-specific stimuli may initiate the inflammatory response, either alone or in combination, for example: tissue injury due to physical, chemical or infectious factors; ischaemia; the deposition of immune complexes; the action of bacterial toxins; and activation of certain clotting factors. These stimuli all activate various chain reactions (Fig. 9.1), but it is unlikely that they all do so in the same way, or that the exact nature of the inflammatory response which is stimulated is the same in each particular case. There are marked differences, in addition, in the nature of the inflammatory response invoked in different tissues, and variations in the exact mechanisms involved between different species.

9.1.1 Role of kinins in the inflammatory reaction

Two plasma peptides, bradykinin and kallidin, appear to be important in the initiation of the inflammatory response. Many other kinins are known to

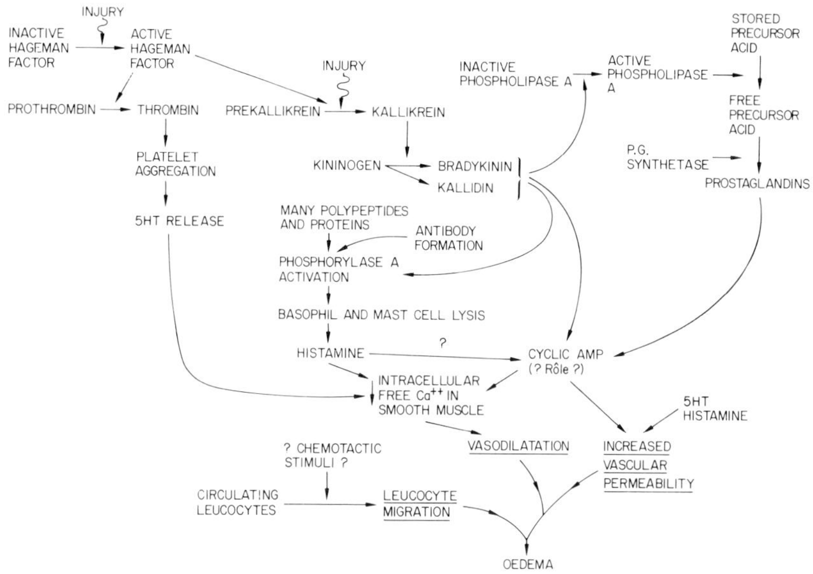

Fig. 9.1 Some of the inter-relationships between putative mediators of the inflammatory response which have been identified in various species.

exist, but their role is uncertain. Bradykinin, a nonapeptide, and kallidin, a decapeptide, are derived from certain plasma α_2-globulins, by the actions of a group of enzymes, the kininogenases, especially a group known as kallikreins, which have a particularly widespread tissue distribution. Kallikrein itself is usually present in an inactive form, prekallikrein, but conversion to the active form can be initiated by various factors, most of which are associated with tissue damage. Changes in pH or temperature, the presence of foreign materials, and some intracellular factors will stimulate activation of this enzyme, but the activation process itself is extremely complex. The factors involved in this enzyme activation process are also those which activate the blood clotting system, and the two systems appear to run closely in parallel. Clotting factor XII, Hageman factor, can activate the change from prekallikrein to kallikrein directly, and Hageman factor is itself activated by the sort of physical and chemical factors which have already been mentioned.

Bradykinin itself, once formed, is very short-lived in plasma and is rapidly hydrolysed by specific enzyme systems. Nonetheless, it is pharmacologically extremely potent and small amounts will induce changes closely resembling the inflammatory reaction when injected into tissues. It is a particularly potent vasodilator, and increases the permeability of the microcirculation, thus giving rise to hyperaemia and oedema. Kinins released from local foci of activation into the circulation may be important in the aetiology of shock and anaphylaxis, by causing widespread vasodilatation, and hence hypotension.

Bradykinin seems to be especially effective in stimulating the peripheral pain receptors (see below), but this effect can be largely inhibited by salicylates and some other anti-inflammatory agents. Such agents can inhibit the synthesis of prostaglandins from arachidonic acid, and this finding, along with other evidence, has led to the conclusion that kinins exert at least some of their physiological effects by liberation of other chemical mediators. However, it is worth noting in passing that salicylates also appear to inhibit kallikrein activation to some extent, as do glucocorticoids, so that the therapeutic action of salicylates should not be thought to be confined to the inhibition of prostaglandin synthesis (see below). The role of kinins has been comprehensively reviewed by Lewis (1968).

9.1.2 Role of prostaglandins in the inflammatory reaction

The role of the prostaglandins in initiating or maintaining the inflammatory process has yet to be fully elucidated. Different prostaglandins have different effects on different tissues, and in some cases two prostaglandins will be mutually antagonistic. Local vasodilatation is certainly an important part of the inflammatory process, and several prostaglandins are potent vasodilators. They may also cause an increase in capillary permeability, and may have a variety of effects on platelet aggregation and blood clotting. However, the effects of prostaglandins, when administered experimentally, do not exactly mimic the oedema or pain of inflammation (Ferreira 1972), and it appears that intermediate metabolites in the prostaglandin synthetic pathway may be more important mediators of the inflammatory process than true prostaglandins (Svensson *et al.* 1975). Fig. 9.2 shows the way in which the proposed mediators PGG_2, PGH_2, and thromboxane A_2 may be released. It appears that a tissue-destructive free radical, possible an hydroxy radical, is produced when PGG_2 is converted to PGH_2 (Kuehl *et al* 1977), and there is some evidence to implicate the involvement of hydroxy radicals in the inflammatory process (Oyangui 1976). A releasing factor has been isolated from the lungs of guinea-pigs with induced anaphylactic reactions, which is capable of stimulating the release of these prostaglandin-like mediators (Nijkamp *et al* 1976). Arachidonic acid appears to be an essential precursor for prostaglandin biosynthesis, although there is very little free arachidonic acid present in cells, the majority being stored in the phospholipid fraction of the cell. Nijkamp and his colleagues suggest that corticosteroids may block the response to the releasing factor by inhibiting the release of the stored acid, whilst aspirin (at rather high levels), phenylbutazone, and some other anti-inflammatory agents block the conversion of arachidonic acid to PGG_2.

It appears that prostaglandins probably play a role in the production of the more persistent aspects of inflammation (Douglas 1975), and large

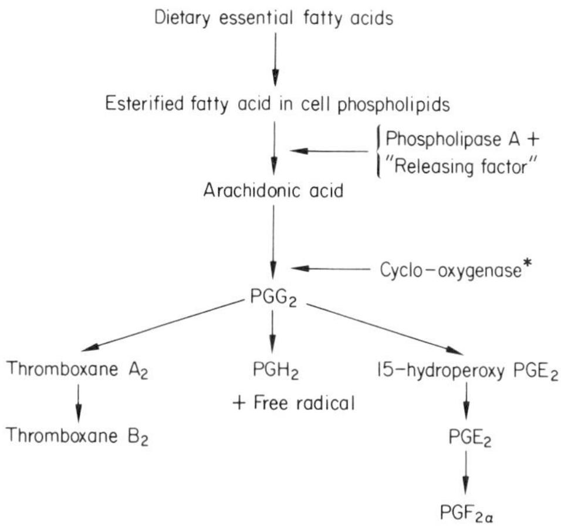

*Cyclo-oxygenase may be regarded as part of the prostaglandin synthetic enzyme system, known collectively as prostaglandin synthetase.

Fig. 9.2 Synthesis of some of the prostaglandin series of potential mediators of inflammation.

quantities of prostaglandins can be found in chronic inflammatory exudates, (from some arthritic joints, for example).

9.1.3 Role of histamine in the inflammatory reaction

Histamine is stored in some quantity in tissue mast cells, and in circulating basophils, and there is no doubt that this histamine, complexed with heparin, is actively released by these cells at the site of tissue injury. In particular, when a specific antigen binds with cell bound reaginic antibody (IgE) on the surface of a mast cell or basophil, the cell is stimulated to extrude the complexed histamine, and this process plays a considerable part in the development of some allergic reactions. It also appears that several proteins and kinins associated with tissue damage may be capable of stimulating mast cells and basophils in this way. Present evidence suggests that histamine has only a transient role in the development of inflammation when the response is not due to an immediate hypersensitivity reaction. However, the effects of histamine release in such a hypersensitivity reaction can be dramatic. There is marked capillary dilatation and an increase in capillary permeability, which is accompanied by arteriolar dilatation to the extent that a precipitate fall in blood pressure may occur, and this forms a major component of anaphylactic shock. Since several other chemical mediators are involved in the development of anaphylaxis, an antihistamine alone cannot be relied upon to reverse the whole process, but such an agent can often effect a dramatic improvement in a potentially life-threatening situation. This type of dramatic reaction is occasionally seen clinically in response to some drugs, such as penicillin, especially when these are given intravenously. In this situation, adrenaline is the drug of choice, given intravenously, and an antihistamine may be given at the same time. Many antihistamines are available, and there is little to choose between them. Chlorpheniramine is virtually painless on injection, and is preferred by some clinicians.* The inclusion of an antihistamine in multiple drug preparations has nothing to recommend it.

9.1.4 Role of 5-hydroxytryptamine in the inflammatory reaction

The chief role of 5-hydroxytryptamine in the body is as a neurotransmitter, and as a transmitter in the myenteric plexus (i.e. those cells in the intestinal wall responsible for the maintenance of peristalsis). It is found in inflammatory exudates, and although it is sometimes capable of producing some of the elements of vasodilatation and increased capillary permeability associated with the inflammatory process, this activity is not constant, and its role in inflammation is unclear.

9.1.5 Pathology of inflammation

Some of the chemical mediators which may play a part in the initiation of the inflammatory process have been discussed. Other mediators are undoubtedly also involved. The interactions of these mediators give rise to the cardinal signs of inflammation, which are:

1 Redness } due chiefly to local hyperaemia.
2 Heat }
3 Swelling: due to oedema and migration of leucocytes to the affected area.
4 Pain: due to stimulation of pain receptors.
5 Loss of function: due to the effects of factors 1–4.

OEDEMA AND HYPERAEMIA

The net effect of the various chemical mediators described above seems to be relaxation of the precapillary arterioles, with, possibly, some constriction of the larger veins in some cases. Consequently, the hydrostatic pressure within the capillary bed and postcapillary venules rises, and fluid passes out of these vessels into the tissues. The endothelial cells of the postcapillary venules become rounded so that large molecules, such as plasma proteins, can pass

*A particular use for chlorpheniramine in small animal practice is the use of an oral sustained release preparation in the treatment of cats with upper respiratory infections. Used in this context, the agent may be spectacularly successful in reducing the excessive production of mucus which is often a feature of these cases. The cat is thereby enabled to resume an oral intake of food and fluids, and recovery is then usually rapid (Tyree 1968).

through the spaces between these cells, and thence into the tissues, the basement membrane being permeable even to large molecules. A good account of this process is given by Spector and Willoughby (1968).

LEUCOCYTE MIGRATION

The mechanism whereby leucocytes are attracted into an inflammatory lesion remains obscure. The process of leucocyte migration is an active process, and it is possible to observe cells actively passing through and between the cells of the vascular endothelium by various methods (Spector & Willoughby 1968), and the bulk of evidence from *in vivo* studies suggests that there is some form of chemotactic attraction operating, although *in vitro* evidence is lacking (Keller *et al* 1975). In the cell-mediated immune response, sensitised lymphocytes have been shown to be capable of producing a factor which inhibits macrophage motility, so that macrophages tend to congregate in the area, since they cannot move away. Corticosteroids block the effect of this factor (Balow & Rosenthal, 1973), and it is likely that similar factors operate in other inflammatory situations.

Lysosomes are intracellular organelles which are present in all cells, but particularly in neutrophils. These lysosomes contain several destructive enzymes, including proteases, and rupture of lysosomes causes extensive local damage. The exact significance of the leakage of enzymes from leucocyte lysosomes in the maintenance of the inflammatory process is unclear. However, there is substantial evidence that the presence of these enzymes within the joint cavity is an important factor in inflammatory joint disease in the dog (Phelps & McCarty 1966).

Hoffstein and Weissman (1975), have shown that the release of leucocyte lysosomal enzymes can be considerably reduced *in vitro* by the use of agents which will elevate intracellular cyclic AMP levels. Amongst the agents which will exert this effect is prostaglandin E, but most anti-inflammatory agents will also stabilise lysosomal membranes to some extent. The role of anti-inflammatory agents in modifying prostaglandin synthesis has already been described, and it may be that their lysosomal stabilising properties are secondary to their effects on prostaglandin synthesis, although the relationship is not yet clear, and *in vivo* studies have not altogether confirmed the relationship between cyclic AMP levels and enzyme release (Deporter *et al* 1977).

PAIN

Many of the chemical mediators which have been implicated in the initiation of the inflammatory response are also capable of producing pain in experimental situations. Histamine, 5-hydroxytryptamine, lysosomal enzymes, and intracellular components such as K^+ ions and adenosine phosphates

(AMP, ADP, ATP), will all produce pain when applied to an exposed blister base. The pain produced by prostaglandins is slow in onset, but long-lasting, and prostaglandins will potentiate the pain caused by other agents alone. The mediator most studied, however, is bradykinin — a particularly effective algogenic agent. The importance of bradykinin in the genesis of pain in ischaemia, injury, or inflammation has been emphasised by Lim (1968), and bradykinin has been shown to induce both visceral and cutaneous pain (Lim *et al* 1967).

The skin has a rich sensory innervation, and although some free nerve-endings exist, the majority of the afferent nerve fibres terminate peripherally in specialised receptors, which may be regarded as transducers which convert physical stimuli, such as touch or temperature, into volleys of impulses in the afferent nerves. These receptors may be classified physiologically according to the type of stimulus which will produce the maximal response in the related afferent nerve fibre. A number of receptors can be identified, which show no response to stimuli of relatively low intensity, such as touch, or changes in ambient temperature, but which only start to respond to stimuli of sufficiently high intensity such that if the stimulus was continued, damage to the tissues would result. These pain receptors appear to be the peripheral units of distinct neural pathways concerned only with the sensory phenomenon of pain. However, it must not be thought that pain results simply from stimulation of these receptors, for the pain pathways within the central nervous system are extremely complex, and peripheral stimulation does not automatically result in the production of that sensory experience which we describe as pain.

Impulses from the peripheral pain receptors pass via small unmyelinated C-fibres, and unmyelinated or partially myelinated Aδ-fibres to the dorsal horn of the spinal cord. Exactly what happens within the dorsal horn remains unclear, for a complex series of neural interconnections appears to exist, such that the afferent pain input may be amplified or diminished at this level by itself, by other sensory input, and by descending spinal influences. The modulated input is transmitted upwards in spinoreticular fibres, and thence to mesencephalic and thalamic nuclei, via the brainstem reticular formation. This incoming volley of impulses stimulates not only those brain centres concerned with the integration, appreciation, and interpretation of pain, but also stimulates central analgesic centres, which modulate the afferent impulse at several levels (see Mayer & Price 1976, for a review of central mechanisms of analgesia).

The role of bradykinin in initiating stimuli which may result in stimulation of central pain nuclei has been elucidated by Besson *et al* (1974), who demonstrated that intra-arterial injection of bradykinin resulted in excitation of appropriate cells in the nucleus gigantocellularis, an area of the brain which has been especially implicated in the appreciation of pain.

On the other hand, bradykinin is not the only mediator involved and it remains uncertain whether noxious physical stimuli affect pain receptors directly, or via a chemical mediator, released from damaged tissues. Lindahl (1974) has formed a unifying hypothesis, which postulates that all pain-eliciting stimuli cause a local fall in pH about the receptors, and that it is this fall in pH which ultimately stimulates the receptors. This hypothesis is not altogether acceptable to most conventional neurophysiologists.

9.2 Treatment of pain

The treatment of pain can be approached in a variety of ways:

1 Reduction in the intensity of the exciting cause (e.g. removal of a foreign body, immobilisation of a fracture, reduction of the inflammatory process).
2 Antagonism of chemical mediators which may be responsible for stimulation of receptors.
3 Inhibition of afferent nerve transmission.
4 Inhibition of ascending spinal transmission.
5 Inhibition of central pain recognition mechanisms.
6 Stimulation of central and peripheral analgesic mechanisms.

Pharmacologically, items 1 and 2 on this list may be taken together, as the drugs which act on these stages of the pain/inflammatory reaction comprise that group of agents classified as anti-inflammatory drugs.

9.2.1 Reduction in intensity of the exciting cause

9.2.2 Antagonism of chemical mediators which may be responsible for stimulation of receptors

Fig. 9.3 summarises some of the information available on the proposed sites of action of various anti-inflammatory agents.

The classification of a drug as an anti-inflammatory agent is somewhat arbitrary. Aspirin, for example, is normally classified as analgesic, rather than an anti-inflammatory, by virtue of its centrally mediated analgesic activity, although it does have a definite anti-inflammatory action. Aspirin remains the drug of choice for treatment of rheumatoid arthritis in man (Laurence 1973), but the efficacy of the drug in the treatment of this particular form of arthritis is probably related to the peculiar pathogenesis of this disease, and other drugs are of more value in the treatment of other arthritides and inflammatory conditions. It is noteworthy that salicylate is a less effective anti-inflammatory agent than aspirin itself, and is also a less potent inhibitor of prostaglandin synthesis (Laurence 1973). This point is particularly relevant in veterinary medicine, since aspirin may cause severe vomiting in dogs, due to its effects on the gastric mucosa (see Chapter 1) and the vomiting centre. Salicylate may be used as an alternative. Both aspirin

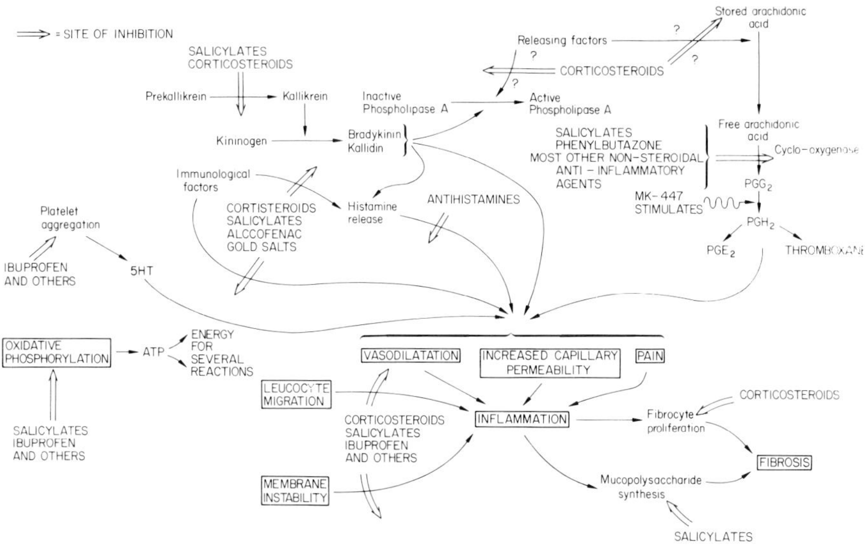

Fig. 9.3 Some of the proposed sites of action of some anti-inflammatory agents.

and salicylate are nephrotoxic in the dog, salicylate being rather worse than aspirin in this respect (Quintanilla & Kessler 1973). Aspirin can be used in the dog, if a 'protected' preparation is used, such as aloxiprin a condensation product of aspirin and aluminium hydroxide, which is stable at acid pH, so that the aspirin is not released until the preparation reaches the small intestine. However, the indications for the use of this drug are extremely limited. Better agents exist for the non-specific treatment of pain or inflammation, although aspirin is very occasionally useful to reduce fever, an effect which is mediated by its ability to inhibit synthesis of the prostaglandins responsible for the production of pyrexia in the hypothalamus (Woodbury & Fingl 1975). Other features of the salicylates are usually only manifest at toxic doses. The high degree of toxicity of the salicylates in the cat is well known, and may be related to the presence of a toxic metabolite, since the metabolism of salicylates in the cat is not fully understood (Davis & Short 1967).

The corticosteroids are, perhaps, the anti-inflammatory agents *par excellence*, and their pharmacology and use are described elsewhere (see Chapters 7 and 8).

Phenylbutazone is probably less toxic in the dog than in man. In man, agranulocytosis may be a lethal complication to the use of this drug. Phenylbutazone is much less heavily plasma protein bound in the dog than in man, with a half-life of only 6 hours, as opposed to 72 hours in man. This feature reduces the cumulative effect of the drug (so that an initial loading dose is not necessary when treating dogs), but also increases the urinary excretion of the drug, so that high renal papillary concentrations may be attained. Toxic effects of phenylbutazone may, therefore, be subtle in the dog, in that it may contribute to pre-existing renal disease, so that consequent renal signs may be attributed to chronic renal disease, rather than to the drug. Other toxic effects have been reported in the dog (Tandy & Thorpe 1967; Reid 1974) and in the cat, in which species toxicity may occur even at therapeutic doses (Wilkinson 1966; Carlisle *et al* 1968).

A serious problem with phenylbutazone is that of tachyphylaxis (i.e. the dose required to produce the desired effect increases as use of the drug is continued, so that eventually the dose required may approach the toxic level, without producing satisfactory alleviation of symptoms). This effect arises because phenylbutazone is a potent inducer of hepatic microsomal enzymes, which are responsible for its own metabolism. As described in Chapter 2, these enzymes are also responsible for the metabolism of many other drugs, the most noteworthy of which are the barbiturates. Barbiturate tolerance may thus be seen in animals which have been treated with phenylbutazone.

Phenylbutazone may also produce gastric symptoms, including vomiting and gastric ulceration. The pathogenesis of this effect is not known, but it is shared by almost all the anti-inflammatory drugs. Prostaglandins appear to exert an inhibitory or controlling effect on gastric secretion (Robert *et al* 1974), so this adverse effect of anti-inflammatory agents may be related to their ability to inhibit prostaglandin synthesis.

Since the toxicity of aspirin limits the usefulness of this drug in the treatment of rheumatoid arthritis in man, many alternative anti-inflammatory agents have been produced, most of which have only marginal advantage over aspirin or over each other, in the hope of securing a share of a large and lucrative market. A few of these preparations may be of considerable value in the treatment of chronic arthritic conditions in dogs. Those described below are a representative selection, which have been used in the treatment of dogs. Since aspirin is of less value in osteoarthritis than in rheumatoid arthritis, and in view of the undesirability of embarking on prolonged courses of corticosteroid therapy, and the probable toxicity of phenylbutazone, these agents might be considered the first line of treatment in canine osteoarthritic disease. None of these agents is, however, entirely without drawbacks, and a particular case may need to be tried on several alternative drugs in order to obtain the optimum therapeutic effect. At present these agents cannot be recommended for use in cats.

Many propionic acid derivatives have been introduced, but only ibuprofen appears to have been used in dogs to any extent. This drug is metabolised slowly in the dog (Mills *et al* 1973) and cumulation may occur if a continuous high dose is given. Uraemia has been observed in a few dogs, and this seems to occur within a few days of starting treatment (K. W. Clarke, pers. comm.), so that vomiting should be regarded as an indication for the immediate discontinuation of treatment with this agent, although this complication was not observed in earlier trials (Adams *et al* 1969). A loading dose of 30 mg/kg in divided doses, followed by 16 mg/kg, has produced beneficial results in cases which have failed to respond satisfactorily to phenylbutazone.

Alclofenac is, perhaps, the most interesting anti-inflammatory agent to have been used in the dog. It is at present the subject of a clinical trial in this species, and few side-effects have been observed so far, although vomiting may be a minor problem (R. E. Ablett, pers. comm.). The dose used in the trial is 50 mg/kg and this dose has been used by the present writer and has produced very promising results in the treatment of canine osteoarthroses. This drug has a central analgesic action equivalent to codeine, in addition to a peripheral anti-inflammatory action similar to phenylbutazone (Table 9.1).

Other anti-inflammatory agents which may be of use in the treatment of small animals have been listed elsewhere (Yoxall 1978) but all these agents suffer from some drawbacks which limit their usefulness. Certain agents, such as gold, may be associated with severe toxicity and limited efficacy.

9.2.3 Inhibition of the afferent nerve impulse

Local anaesthetic agents exert their effects by virtue of their ability to interfere with conduction of the nervous impulse. In the presence of local anaesthetics, the action potential which may be recorded in response to stimulation of the nerve is diminished, and eventually disappears altogether. There is, however, no change in the resting potential of the unstimulated nerve, which suggests that these agents exert their effect by interfering with the movement of Na^+ ions across the neuronal membrane which is responsible for the action potential, or with the enzyme systems associated with this ionic movement. A nerve fibre bathed in an electrolyte solution low in Na^+ requires

Table 9.1 Analgesic activity of alclofenac in rats. Modified from Lambelin *et al* (1970)

Order of efficacy	Hot plate test	Protection against pressure-induced pain in inflamed paw	Protection against pain induced by intraperitoneal acetic acid	Protection against pain induced by electrical stimulation
1	Codeine	Codeine	Codeine	Codeine } = 1
2	Alclofenac	Pentazocine	Alclofenac	Alclofenac } = 1
3	Propoxyphene	Propoxyphene	Propoxyphene	Phenacetin
4	Aspirin	Alclofenac } = 4	Pentazocine	Aminophenazone
5	Paracetamol	Glaphenine } = 4	Benzydamine	Phenazone
6		Benzydamine	Glaphenine	Aspirin
7		Aminophenazone	Aspirin	
8		Aspirin	Phenacetin	
9			Aminophenazone	
10			Paracetamol	

less local anaesthetic to block transmission, whilst an extracellular environment high in Na^+ requires more of the agent. Local anaesthetics have a common structure:

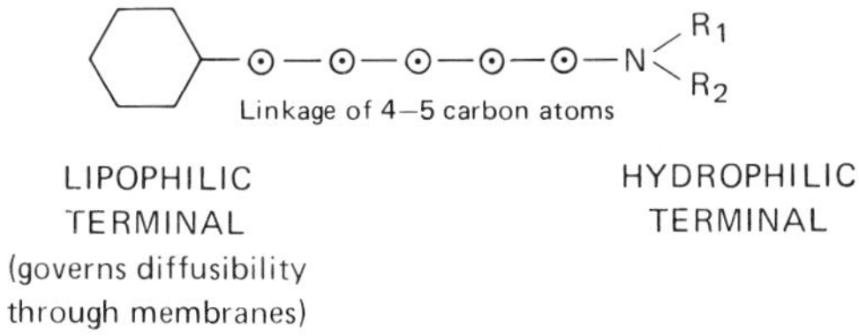

If the length of the molecule exceeds 6–9 A, activity is lost, whilst substitutions in the benzene ring will increase the duration of action of the drug, or improve its diffusibility. Side-chains on the linkage may serve to increase the activity.

The benzene ring may be joined to the chain by an ester or an amide linkage, and an amide linkage will give rise to a longer duration of action, since the drug will be resistant to cholinesterase.

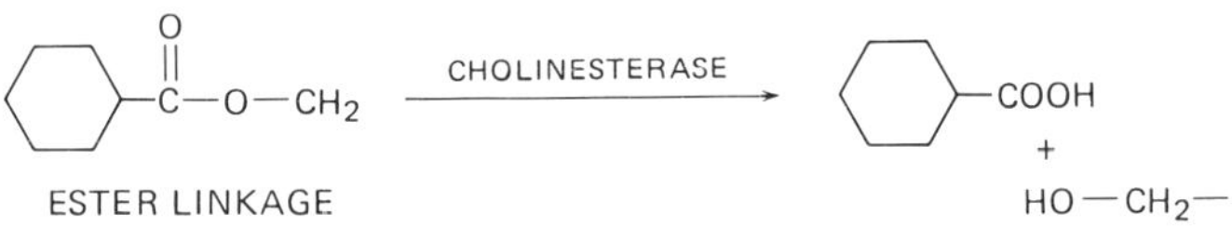

ESTER LINKAGE

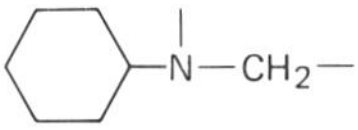

AMIDE LINKAGE

All local anaesthetics are tertiary amines, and are thus insoluble, and they are therefore produced as hydrochlorides, dissolved in water. The p*Ka* of the resulting solution is important since the ionised form of the drug is necessary for activity:

$$R{\equiv}N + HCl \rightleftharpoons R{\equiv}NH^+ + Cl^-$$

Where $R{\equiv}NH^+$ is the active form of the drug.
The p*Ka* will govern this equilibrium.

On the other hand, the unionised form is much better at penetrating the nerve sheath (Ritchie & Greengard 1966). If the local pH in the tissues is low, then the drug will tend to have a slow onset of activity, since little of the drug will be present in the unionised form:

$$R{\equiv}N + M^+ \longrightarrow R{\equiv}NM^+$$

One approach to the paradoxical situation where the drug should ideally be present in both the ionised and unionised forms has been to use carbonated solutions. The CO_2 in the solution will then diffuse rapidly inwards to the axon, leaving the pH unchanged around the nerve sheath, but causing it to fall in the region of the nerve membrane, so that the anaesthetic agent is present in an unionised form in the vicinity of the sheath, but ionised in the region of the nerve membrane.

Small nerve fibres have a relatively greater surface area than large nerve fibres, so that the small fibres are affected before the large fibres, and, as one would expect, myelinated fibres are affected only at relatively high concentration. However, the postganglionic sympathetic fibres are the smallest of all, and are blocked before the pain fibres, so that local hyperaemia, due to blocking of sympathetic vasoconstrictor fibres, is a feature of the use of local anaesthetics.

Local anaesthetic agents have significant toxicity. An anaphylactic type of response may be seen in association with some of the ester-type agents, but this is probably related to the adrenaline which is often combined with these agents to produce local vasoconstriction and thus delay absorption. This slow absorption will increase the duration of action and reduce the incidence of toxic effects on the CNS, but if an agent such as lignocaine is used, which has an inherently long duration of action and slow absorption, addition of adrenaline is unlikely to be necessary for most veterinary purposes. It is recommended, therefore, that preparations containing adrenaline should be avoided. The chief toxic effect of local anaesthetics on the CNS is the production of convulsions (although they may be anticonvulsant at low doses — phenytoin has a local anaesthetic structure and activity). Convulsions are not of themselves lethal, but the associated anoxia may be dangerous in the extreme. Treatment of such convulsions should, therefore, be aimed at establishing adequate ventilation, usually by means of endotracheal intubation or tracheostomy. Intravenous barbiturates or diazepam may be useful in controlling the convulsions of the local anaesthetic toxicity, but are not invariably effective. Local anaesthetics also have a depressant effect upon the myocardium (lignocaine, procaine derivatives and phenytoin are used clinically for their antiarrhythmic activity).

9.2.4 Inhibition of ascending spinal transmission

The general level of afferent input to the spinal cord in a segment in which there are incoming pain impulses will tend to modulate the ongoing transmission of these impulses. Therefore manoeuvres such as rubbing the affected part, or the application of heat or cold, will tend to reduce the degree of pain experienced.

9.2.5 Inhibition of central pain recognition mechanisms

The central analgesic activity of aspirin has already been mentioned (see p. 127). Paracetamol has a similar analgesic activity to asprin, that is a moderate efficacy against peripheral skeletal or muscular pain and headache, but no activity against pain or visceral origin. Paracetamol does not have the most troubling side-effects of aspirin and so may be useful for owners to administer at home, as it may be preferable not to recommend the use of aspirin. It does however, have side-effects, and may be hepatotoxic at doses not grossly in excess of those required to obtain clinical benefit, especially in the cat (Eder 1964). Nonetheless, paracetamol is probably safer than aspirin for general use.

Paracetamol is a para-aminophenol derivative and has replaced other agents of this class, such as phenacetin, in view of the fact that these other agents appear to be metabolised to paracetamol and have a greater toxicity than paracetamol, due to the production of other toxic metabolites.

9.2.6 Stimulation of peripheral and central analgesic mechanisms

Morphine has been described as 'the queen of drugs' and it is perhaps fitting that the opiates, a group of drugs which has been in clinical use since at least the third century BC and possibly since the days of the ancient Sumerians, about 4000 years BC, should provide one of the classic stories of modern pharmacology. A story which is, as yet, far from complete, but which has already produced some of the most elegant pharmacological work of recent years. A useful review for the clinician of 'the story so far' has been provided by Snyder (1977).

Briefly, consideration of the specificity of the active opiates, and of the opiate antagonists suggested that specific opiate receptors might exist within the brain. Once these receptors had been found, further studies suggested that there was a complex relationship between sodium ion concentrations and the ability of opiate agonists and antagonists to bind with the receptors. This led to the hypothesis that opiates might alter the membrane permeability of certain neurones to sodium, when bound to these specific receptors. The nature of the relationship between this change in membrane permeability to sodium, and the reduction in intracellular cyclic AMP levels and rise in cyclic GMP levels, which may be associated with the actions of opiates is unclear. It is perhaps more than coincidental that opiates depress the prostaglandin-stimulated synthesis of adenyl cyclase (the enzyme responsible for formation of cyclic AMP), whilst aspirin and paracetamol depress prostaglandin synthesis.

If specific receptors for opiates exist within the brain, it seemed likely that they would be present in association with a natural opiate-like substance in the brain, which might be a neurotransmitter. Two such substances, encephalins, have been isolated and their structures elucidated by Hughes and his colleagues (1975). These encephalins appear to be part of a whole series of specific peptide hormones, which are found especially in the pituitary (ACTH, MSH, FSH), and in various peripheral tissues (somatostatin, gastrin), whilst the encephalins themselves are found specifically in brain, and in the gastrointestinal tract. (Hence, possibly the tonic effect of opiates on the bowel and related sphincters.)

The distribution of opiate-encephalin receptors within the brain is of considerable interest. These receptors are found especially in the periaqueductal grey matter, and electrical stimulation of this region appears to be capable of producing analgesia, an effect which can be blocked by opiate antagonists, such as naloxone, which presumably bind to the receptor sites, but without producing changes within the neurone. Opiate receptors are also found in thalamic nuclei which deal with various aspects of pain sensation, and in the substantia gelatinosa of the spinal cord, an area which has long been implicated in the modulation of incoming painful impulses. Receptors are also found in various brainstem nuclei, such as that controlling the cough reflex, and in the chemoreceptor trigger zone, which activates the vomiting centre. Hence the antitussive and emetic effects of the opiates.

The encephalins are not, however, the only neurotransmitters which appear to be involved in analgesic pathways and there is good evidence that 5-hydroxytryptamine (5HT) may also be involved at some stage (Mayer & Price 1976). It seems likely that encephalin may be a transmitter at one level, whilst 5HT may be a transmitter further down the analgesic pathway, so that synaptic release of 5HT will depend upon encephalin-mediated stimulation of the presynaptic neurone, either directly or indirectly.

Morphine remains the potent analgesic of choice for small animal use. Other opiates, either natural or synthetic, are available, but none have a clear advantage over morphine in the treatment of severe pain. By and large, it has not proved possible to produce an agent with the analgesic properties of morphine, but without its side-effects, especially respiratory depression resulting from a direct depressant effect on the respiratory centre. Indeed, most synthetic opiates are rather less desirable than morphine in this respect. There has been some controversy over the use of morphine in cats, since this species appears to be especially sensitive to opiates, with excitement and mania being produced at relatively small doses. However, morphine may be safely used in cats at doses not exceeding 0·1 mg/kg, whilst up to 16 mg may be given to dogs by intramuscular or subcutaneous injection. Clinical experience suggests that morphine is more effective than pethidine in producing analgesia in small animals, when given in doses which produce equivalent levels of respiratory depression.

Certain contraindications to the use of opiates exist. They tend to cause a rise in intracranial pressure and so should not be used in cases of head injury. Neither should they be used to relieve the pain of acute pancreatitis, since they produce spasm of the pancreatic ducts. Where respiratory embarrassment results solely from chest-wall pain, opiates may produce a striking improvement in ventilation, but in all other cases of respiratory depression opiates should be used only with the greatest circumspection. Opiates are, perhaps, of most value in dealing with road traffic accident cases, or other traumatic injuries, and as premedicants in cases in which postoperative pain is likely to be significant. In the latter type of case, postoperative morbidity may be considerably reduced by the judicious use of opiates.

For less severe pain, codeine may be extremely useful. This drug has about a quarter of the analgesic activity of morphine, but only a tenth of the side-effects of the more potent drug. It may be given orally, as may the more potent derivative dihydrocodeine. 'Codeine', as bought across the chemist's counter is usually in fact a compound preparation, containing other analgesics, whilst many veterinary clinicians will use codeine itself as the phosphate, as a non-specific antidiarrhoeal. The constipating effect of codeine is its chief drawback, and dextropropoxyphene may be preferred by virtue of the absence of this side-effect, as well as its reduced tendency to cause respiratory depression (Brown Robbins 1955). Dextropropoxyphene is available in combination with paracetamol as 'Distalgestic', and this combination may be recommended as the most suitable oral analgesic for use in small animal practice. Clinical experience suggests that up to 32·5 mg per os dextropropoxyphene may be given three times daily to large dogs, whilst Davis and Donnelly (1968) suggest that a total daily dose of 32·0 mg per os, or 2·2 mg/kg by intramuscular injection, should be safe in cats.

References

Adams S. S., McCullough K. F. & Nicholson J. S. (1969) The pharmacological properties of ibuprofen, an anti-inflammatory, analgesic, and antipyretic agent. *Arch. Int. Pharmac. Ther.* **178**, 115.

Balow J. E. & Rosenthal A. S. (1973) Glucocorticoid suppression of macrophage migration inhibitory factor. *J. Exp. Med.* **137**, 1031.

Besson J.M., Guilbaud G. & Lombard M. C. (1974) Effects of bradykinin intra-arterial injection into the limbs upon bulbar and mesencephalic reticular unit activity. In *Advances in Neurology* ed. J. J. Bonica, vol. 4, p. 207. Raven Press, New York.

Brown Robbins E. (1955) The pharmacologic effects of a new analgesic α-4-dimethylamino-1,2-diphenyl-3-methyl-4-propionyloxybutane. *J. Amer. Pharm. Ass.* **44**, 497.

Carlisle C. H., Penny R. H. C., Prescott C. W. & Davidson H. A. (1968) Toxic Effects of phenylbutazone on the cat. *Brit. Vet. J.* **124**, 560.

Davis L. E. & Short C. R. (1967) Species differences in biotransformation and excretion of salicylate. *Fed. Proc.* **26**, 619.

Davis L. E. & Donnelly E. J. (1968) Analgesic drugs in the cat. *J. Amer. Vet. Med. Ass.* **153**, 1161.

Deporter D. A., Dieppe P. A., Glatt M. & Willoughby D. A. (1977) The relation of cyclic AMP levels to phagocytosis and enzyme release in acute inflammation *in vivo*. *J. Path.* **121**, 129.

Douglas W. W. (1975) Polypeptides and prostaglandins. In *The Pharmacological Basis of Therapeutics*, eds. L. S. Goodman & A. Gilman 5th edn., p. 646. Macmillan, New York.

Eder H. (1964) Chronic toxicity studies on phenacetin, *N*-acetyl-p-aminophenol, and acetylsalicylic acid on cats. *Acta pharmacol. et toxicol.* **21**, 197.

Ferreira S. H. (1972) Prostaglandins, aspirin-like drugs, and analgesia. *Nature New Biol.* **240**, 200.

Ferreira S. H. & Vane J. R. (1974) New aspects of the mode of action of non-steroid anti-inflammatory drugs. *Ann. Rev. Pharmacol.* **14**, 57.

Hoffstein S. & Weissman G. (1975) Mechanisms of lysosomal enzyme release from leukocytes (IV). *Arthr. Rheum.* **18**, 153.

Hughes J., Smith T. W., Kosterlitz H. W., Fothergill L. A., Morgan B. A., & Morris H. R. (1975) Identification of two related pentopeptides from the brain with potent opiate agonist activity. *Nature* **258**, 577.

Keller H. U., Hess M. W. & Cottier H. (1975) Physiology of chemotaxis and random mobility. *Seminars in Haematology* **12**, 27.

Kuehl F. A., Humes J. L., Egan R. W., Ham E. A., Beveridge G. C. & Van Arman C. G. (1977) Role of prostaglandin endoperoxide PGG_2 in inflammatory processes. *Nature* **265**, 170.

Lambelin G., Roba J., Gillet C. & Buu-Hoi N. (1970) Pharmacology of a new analgesic, antipyretic and anti-inflammatory agent 4-allyloxy-3-chloro-phenylacetic acid. *Arzneimittel Forschung* **20**, 610.

Laurence D. R. (1973) *Clinical Pharmacology*, 4th edn. Churchill Livingstone, Edinburgh.

Lewis G. P. (1968) Pharmacologically active polypeptides. In *Recent Advances in Pharmacology*, eds. J. M. Robson & R. S. Stacey, p. 213 Churchill, London.

Lim R. K. S. (1968) *Pharmacology of Pain.* P. 169. Pergamon Press, Oxford.

Lim R. K. S., Miller D. G., Guzman F., Rodgers D. W., Rodgers R. W., Wang S. K., Shao P. Y. & Shih T. Y. (1967) Pain and analgesia evaluated by the intra-peritoneal bradykinin-evoked pain method in man. *Clin. Pharm. Ther.* **8**, 521.

Lindahl O. (1974) Pain — a general chemical explanation. In *Advances in Neurology*, ed. J. J. Bonica, vol. 4, p. 45. Raven Press, New York.

Mayer D. J. & Price D. D. (1976) Central nervous system mechanisms of analgesia. *Pain* **2**, 379.

Mills R. F. N., Adams S. S., Cliffe E. E., Dickinson W. & Nicholson J. S. (1973) The metabolism of ibuprofen. *Xenobiotica* **3**, 589.

Nijkamp F. P., Flower R. J., Moncada S. & Vane J. R. (1976) Partial purification of rabbit aorta contracting substance-releasing factor and inhibition of its activity by anti-inflammatory steroids. *Nature* **263**, 479.

Oyangui Y. (1976) Participation of superoxide anions at the prostaglandin phase of carrageenan foot oedema. *Biochem. Pharmac.* **25**, 1465.

Phelps P. & McCarty D. J. (1966) Crystal-induced inflammation in canine joints. II Importance of polymorphonuclear leukocytes. *J. Exp. Med.* **124**, 115.

Quintanilla A. & Kessler R. H. (1973) Direct effects of salicylate on renal function in the dog. *J. Clin. Invest.* **52**, 3143.

Reid, J. S. (1974) Osteoarthritis. In *Current Veterinary Therapy*, ed. R. W. Kirk, p. 707. W. B. Saunders, Philadelphia.

Ritchie J. M. & Greengard P. (1966) On the mode of action of local anaesthetics. *Ann. Rev. Pharmac.* **6**, 405.

Robert A., Nylander B. & Andersson S. (1974) Marked inhibition of gastric secretion by two prostaglandin analogs given orally to man. *Life Sci.* **14**, 533.

Snyder S. H. (1977) Opiate receptors in the brain. *New Eng. J. Med.* **296**, 266.

Spector W. G. & Willoughby D. A. (1968) *The Pharmacology of Inflammation.* English Universities Press, London.

Svensson J., Hamberg M. & Samuelsson B. (1975) Prostaglandin endoperoxides, IX characterisation of rabbit aorta contracting substance (RCS) from guinea pig lung and human platelets. *Acta Physiol. Scand.* **94**, 222.

Tandy J. & Thorpe E. (1967) A fatal syndrome in the dog following administration of phenylbutazone. *Vet. Rec.* **81**, 398.

Tyree R. C. (1968) *Vet. Med. Small Anim. Clin.* **63**, 144.

Wilkinson G. T. (1966) *Diseases of the cat.* Pergamon Press, Oxford.

Williams D. M. & Johnson N. W. (1976) Alterations in peripheral blood leucocyte distribution in response to local inflammatory stimuli in the rat. *J. Path.* **118**, 129.

Woodbury D. M. & Fingl E. (1975) Analgesic-antipyretics, anti-inflammatory agents, and drugs employed in the therapy of gout. In *The Pharmacological Basis of Therapeutics* 5th edn., eds. L. S. Goodman & A. Gilman, p. 325. Macmillan, New York.

Yoxall A. T. (1977) Pain in small animals — its recognition and control. *J. Small Anim. Pract.* **19**, 423.

10

Agents acting on the cardiovascular system I. Modes of action

H. M. SNOW and A. T. YOXALL

The management of cardiac disease is perhaps the example *par excellence* for the demonstration of the necessity for the clinician to have some comprehension of the fundamental mode of action of the therapeutic agents at his disposal in order to produce the optimal clinical response. The treatment of cardiac disorder leans heavily upon the use of particularly powerful drugs, and is one of the relatively few conditions in veterinary practice which calls for the judicious use of combinations of two or more interacting drugs in many cases, and if these agents are to be used to the best advantage it is important that the clinician should be able to relate the expected and observed effects of these agents to the pathological and physiological processes taking place in the patient.

This chapter will deal with the relevant aspects of cardiac physiology and pathophysiology, and the ways in which therapeutic agents may modify the processes involved, whilst the following chapter will deal with the more practical aspects of the clinical use of such agents.

10.1 Cardiac function

The heart has only one function; to subserve the requirements of tissue respiration by supplying oxygenated blood to the tissues, and by removing deoxygenated blood and passing it to the lungs for the removal of carbon dioxide and uptake of oxygen. In order to carry out this function, the heart has to keep a certain volume of blood moving round the circulation (i.e. it has to maintain a certain flow). Since the resistance offered to this flow will vary mainly with the degree of vasomotor tone in the peripheral circulation, the heart must be capable of developing sufficient pressure to maintain flow in the face of such peripheral resistance as may be present.

The heart is said to be in failure when it is unable to maintain an adequate output (i.e. adequate tissue blood flow). The heart may be regarded as a pump which accepts what comes back to it at a low pressure — the venous return — and pumps this out on the arterial side of the circulation at a higher pressure. The input filling pressure is a major determinant of the output of the heart. In heart failure the relationship between input or filling pressure and output breaks down because of a loss of contractility of the heart muscle. In order to maintain an adequate output the heart has to work at higher filling pressures.

In order to maintain adequate cardiac function, the myocardium has five particular properties.

1 Excitability. The ability to respond to an (electrical) stimulus.
2 Conductivity. The ability to conduct such a stimulus from any point in the myocardium to any other.
3 Automaticity. The ability to maintain spontaneous electrical activity.
4 Contractility. The ability to respond to an electrical stimulus by mechanical (muscular) contraction.
5 Refractoriness. Failure to respond to a further stimulus in the period immediately following the response to a stimulus.

These properties are related to the fundamental properties of the myocardial cells, which are related in turn to the movement of ions across the myocardial cell membranes, and the ability of these cells to actively transport ions against concentration gradients. Thus, as shown in Fig. 10.1 the active extrusion of Na^+ in exchange for K^+ results in a concentration gradient of about 50:1 for Na^+ ions outside:inside, with a concentration gradient of about 1:35 for K^+ ions outside:inside. The mechanism by which Na^+ is extruded against its concentration gradient is an active, energy-consuming process, known as the Na^+/K^+ pump (Skou 1965). The activity of this pump means that the resting cell membrane is effectively impermeable to Na^+ ions. When the distribution of ions across the cell membrane is at equilibrium the chemical potential (concentration gradient) of the K^+ ions is balanced by an equal and opposite electrical potential and thus the resting potential of the myocardial cell is largely determined by the permeability of the membrane to K^+ and the K^+ ion concentration gradient.

When the cell is stimulated either electrically, mechanically or chemically, changes in membrane permeability (conductance) take place. The initial change is the opening of sodium 'gates', which allow Na^+ ions to enter the cell (phase 0), whilst K^+ ions move outwards. Ca^{++} ions enter the cell less rapidly (phase 2), and the resting potential is eventually restored as Na^+ is removed from the cell, which returns to the K^+ equilibrium potential (phase 3). Fig. 10.2 illustrates these changes in a cell of the specialised conducting system (Purkinje cells) of the sheep heart, and is taken from Noble (1975), where a fuller account of the mechanisms involved may be found. These particular cells show automaticity or spontaneous (pacemaker) activity, and the potential across the membrane never actually becomes stable. The membrane remains slightly permeable to Na^+ ions, and the influx of these ions causes the potential to rise gradually above the resting potential to a

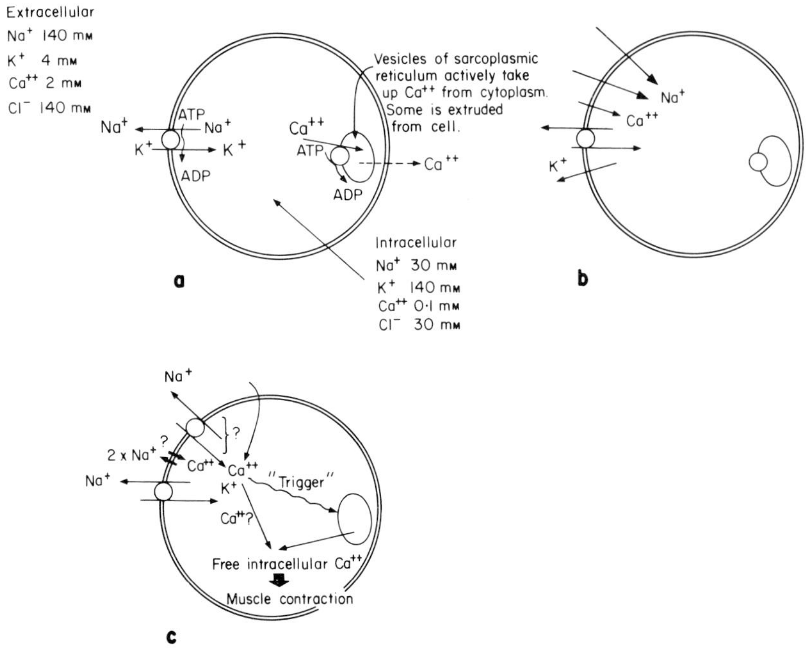

Fig. 10.1 (a) Resting cardiac cell. Ionic pump in cell membrane keeps intracellular $[Na^+]$ low and $[K^+]$ high. Since a chemical gradient exists of K^+ the difference in concentration of K^+ inside the cell and out will cause a potential difference to exist due to the charges on the K^+ ions. Charges on Na^+ ions balanced by Cl^-. (b) Early phase of action potential. Cell becomes permeable to Na^+ ions which rush in down their concentration gradient. A certain amount of Ca^+ also enters — but slightly later, and for a longer period. K^+ leaves the cell. (c) Excitation-contraction coupling. Resting potential is gradually restored as Na^+ is pumped out, whilst Ca^{++} enters in exchange, thus causing no change in potential difference across membrane. The mechanism by which Ca^{++} enters is uncertain. Three possibilities are illustrated: the active pump may exchange Na^+ for Ca^{++}, the normal membrane pump may include Ca^{++} as well as K^+ inward pumping — possibly at separate sites; transmembranal exchange of Na^+ for Ca^{++}. The presence of high intracellular free Ca^{++} level may then 'trigger' release of more Ca^{++} from sarcoplasmic reticulum by inhibiting Ca^{++} pump. Free intracellular Ca^{++} activates contractile process.

threshold level, above which the 'sodium gates' open widely, and the process described above follows spontaneously. In other cells which do not normally show automaticity, the slight increase above resting potential required to reach the threshold level is provided by an electrical stimulus from adjacent cells.

Under normal circumstances, the cells of the sinoatrial node show the most rapid rate of spontaneous discharge (automaticity), and the electrical impulse thus generated is distributed through the myocardium. Other cardiac tissues show automaticity, but at a slower rate than the sinoatrial node, so that the nodal discharges normally predominate, and thus determine the heart rate. If the sinoatrial node fails, or if its rate of spontaneous discharge

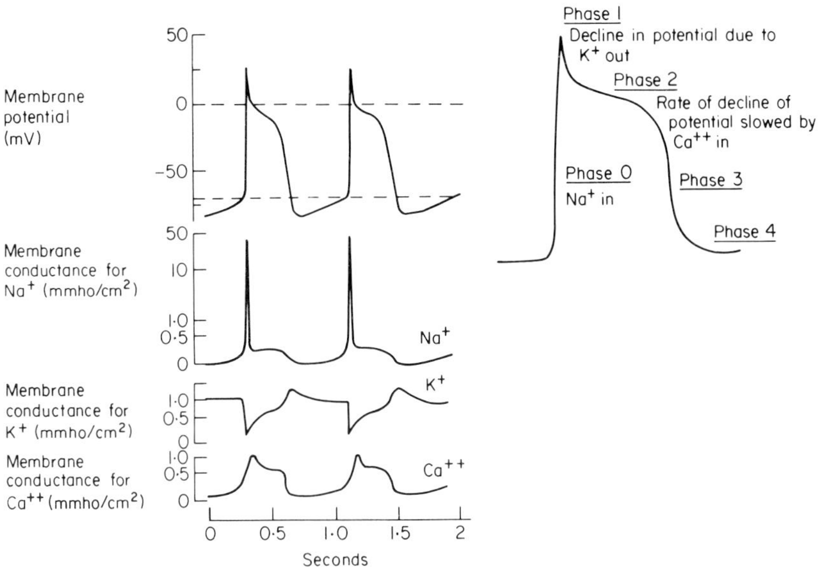

Fig. 10.2 Action potential in isolated Purkinje cell of the sheep heart. The changes in potential across the cell membrane which occur during the action potential are shown. The upper trace shows the changes in potential which occur whilst the lower three show the accompanying changes in membrane conductance of Na^+, K^+, Ca^{++}. Note the very large increase in sodium conductance (ordinate is logarithmic scale) relative to changes in K^+ and Ca^{++} conductance. Also shown is a representation of the action potential of a contractile fibre with the ion movements annotated. Modified from Noble (1975).

falls, then the next most rapidly spontaneously discharging tissue will take over the role of pacemaker. Under certain circumstances, pacemaker activity from the Purkinje system or other cells may give rise to ectopic beats.

The discussion so far has shown, very briefly, how the electrical properties of the myocardial cells confer the properties of excitability, conductivity and automaticity upon the heart. Refractoriness follows because a high level of K^+ permeability exists for a short period after a discharge. The next section will deal with the contractile properties of heart muscle, and show how myocardial contraction is linked to electrical excitation of the cells.

10.2 Myocardial contractility

The contractile element of muscle consists of a complex of the two proteins actin and myosin. Actin is associated with the transverse Z-membranes of the muscle fibrils, from which it extends longitudinally into the fibrils (Fig. 10.3). Myosin is a complex protein, made up of fragments of light and heavy meromyosin. Under suitable physiochemical conditions, myosin aggregates

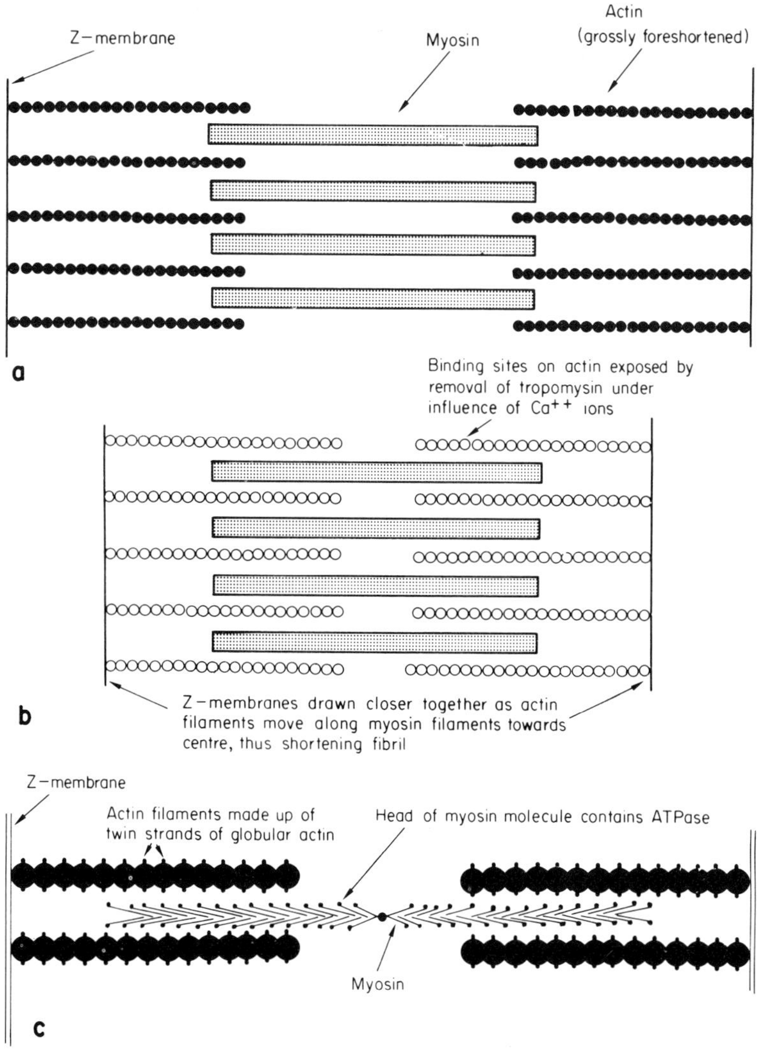

Fig. 10.3 Schematic representation of a few contractile proteins with a muscle fibril. (a) When the muscle is relaxed; (b) when the muscle is partially contracted; (c) To show myosin structure. Filaments greatly foreshortened, since in life they contain several thousand molecules, rather than the small number shown here.

to form a molecule shaped rather like a golf club, with a head and a long tail. The molecules so formed aggregate further to form a filament, the body of which is composed of the tails of the molecules, with the heads protruding along the surface (Fig. 10.3). The myosin filaments are orientated parallel to the actin filaments, but are disposed at the centre of the fibrils, so that they partially overlap the actin filaments, the degree of overlap being greater when the fibril is relaxed, and less when the fibril is overstretched, but being maximal when the fibril is slightly stretched. Where the actin and myosin fibres overlap, cross-bridges can be formed between individual molecules of the actin filament and the protruding heads of the myosin filaments. During diastole the formation of such bridges is inhibited by the presence of a protein complex, consisting of troponin and tropomyosin, which appears to block the myosin binding sites on the actin molecules. Muscle contraction occurs when the blocking tropomyosin molecules are removed, apparently under the influence of calcium ions, and cross-bridges between adjacent actin and myosin filaments are formed (Katz 1970). The cross-bridges are broken down and re-established on adjacent molecules, so that the actin filaments move along the myosin filaments, and, being attached to the transverse Z-membranes, thus cause the muscle fibril to be shortened. The movement of the actin filaments by means of the cross-bridges may be likened to the movement of a centipede, the cross-bridges being analogous to the legs. This process requires energy, which is provided by the breakdown of adenosine triphosphate (ATP). The head of the myosin molecule contains the enzyme ATPase, which, in the presence of Ca^{++} ions, is capable of hydrolysing ATP to ADP (adenosine diphosphate) and inorganic phosphate, with the release of energy from the high energy phosphate bond lysed in the process. (For further details of the mechanisms outlined above the reader is referred to reviews by Braunwald *et al* 1967; Huxley 1969; and Katz 1970.)

It will be apparent from the foregoing remarks that muscular contraction will occur in the presence of Ca^{++} and ATP, and in order to prevent a state of tetany developing, the intracellular Ca^{++} concentration is normally maintained at a low level (about 10^{-7}M), when the muscle is at rest. Ca^{++} ions are stored chiefly in the vesicles of the sarcoplasmic reticulum, and an 'ionic pump' exists, which is capable of extracting Ca^{++} ions from the cytoplasm and transferring them to the sarcoplasmic reticulum against their concentration gradient (Hasselbach & Makinose 1961). If this system is responsible for the increase in free intracellular Ca^{++} to about 10^{-5}M which occurs during systole, then it is necessary to propose some mechanism by which the Ca^{++} pump is 'turned off' during systole, thus allowing rapid release of Ca^{++} into the cytoplasm (i.e. some excitation–contraction mechanism must be proposed, by means of which ionic movements across the cell membrane may be related to the activation of actin–myosin contraction by Ca^{++} ions). Unfortunately, there is no satisfactory explanation for the mechanism of this process in cardiac muscle, although a good explanation has been presented for the process in striated muscle (Nakagima & Endo 1973).

When the myocardial cell membrane is depolarised during the action potential, Na^+ enters the cell and K^+ leaves. During the plateau phase, Ca^{++} enters, but probably insufficient to cause the whole increase in the intracellular Ca^{++} concentration observed during contraction (Bassingthwaight &

Reuter 1972). On the other hand, the activity of the sarcoplasmic reticulum Ca^{++} pump does not seem to depend upon Na^{+} or K^{+} levels (Martonosi & Feretos 1963). It has therefore been postulated that the influx of a small amount of Ca^{++} across the cell membrane triggers the release of more Ca^{++} from the sarcoplasmic reticulum (Fabiato & Fabiato 1975). A further hypothesis suggests that the sarcoplasmic reticulum plays little or no part in excitation-contraction coupling, and that it is only important in sequestering Ca^{++} ions and thus ending contraction. The accumulated Ca^{++} would then be passed directly from the sarcoplasmic reticulum to the extracellular fluid. In this scheme, sufficient Ca^{++} to activate actin-myosin contraction enters the cell across the cell membrane, in exchange for Na , which is removed from the cell following its entry in the early stages of the action potential. It is suggested that this exchange takes place either via a specific membrane carrier (Langer 1971), or via the Na^{+}/K^{+} pump (Lindenmayer & Schwartz 1975). According to the Langer hypothesis, one Ca^{++} ion would be exchanged for two Na^{+} ions so that the exchange would be electrically neutral, and thus not detectable by normal electrophysiological methods. According to the Lindenmayer–Schwartz hypothesis, one Ca^{++} ion plus one K^{+} ion would enter the cell in exchange for three Na^{+} ions — again an electroneutral transfer.

Whatever the details of excitation-contraction coupling, it is apparent that in the case of cardiac muscle extracellular Ca^{++} is of some importance, and that binding of Ca^{++} to the external surface of the cell membrane may also be important (Sanborn & Langer 1970). The role of intracellular mediators in the context remains uncertain. Cyclic 3′ 5′ adenosine monophosphate (cyclic AMP) may well play an important role, since it is known to influence not only events at the cell surface (Roberts *et al* 1973), but also to have significant interactions with the Ca^{++} ion in a variety of situations (Rasmussen 1970). When the intracellular concentration of cyclic AMP is elevated by drugs, increased myocardial contractility and excitability are seen (see below). For a general review of the biochemistry of myocardial contraction in relation to small animal therapeutics, the reader is referred to Parker and Adams (1977).

Further consideration will be given to the biochemical events involved in myocardial contraction in the later parts of this chapter devoted to the discussion of the modes of action of some cardioactive compounds. First, however, it is worth considering how the observable clinical parameters of cardiac function may be related to the biochemical events discussed.

10.3 Mechanical properties of cardiac muscle

The rate at which muscle fibres contract when myosin bound ATPase is activated depends upon the load applied, and in this process, chemical energy released by the hydrolysis of the high energy bonds in ATP, is converted to physical energy. This physical energy appears in two forms — heat and mechanical work. The factors which determine both the total amount of physical energy released and the partition of this energy into heat and work may be divided into two classes:

1 Physical factors (e.g. length of fibres; load applied).
2 Chemical factors (e.g. concentration of Ca^{++} ions; intracellular cyclic AMP level).

The most important of the physical factors is the relationship between the initial or resting length of the muscle and the energy produced during a contraction, known as Starling's law of the heart. The curve shown in Fig. 10.4 demonstrates this law in operation in the dog heart. As the size of the heart at the beginning of each beat (end-diastolic volume) is increased, muscle fibres are stretched, and the resultant work obtained from each beat (stroke work) is also increased.

At least two cellular mechanisms are thought to contribute to the operation of Starling's law:

1 The degree of overlap of the actin and myosin filaments; the greater the overlap the more active sites on filaments are available for the development of tension.
2 As the muscle is stretched, its radius decreases, and it is thought that this decrease in radius leads to a more complete and rapid activation of the mechanisms whereby Ca^{++} is released from the sarcoplasmic reticulum by the diffusion of Ca^{++} across the cell membrane during the action potential.

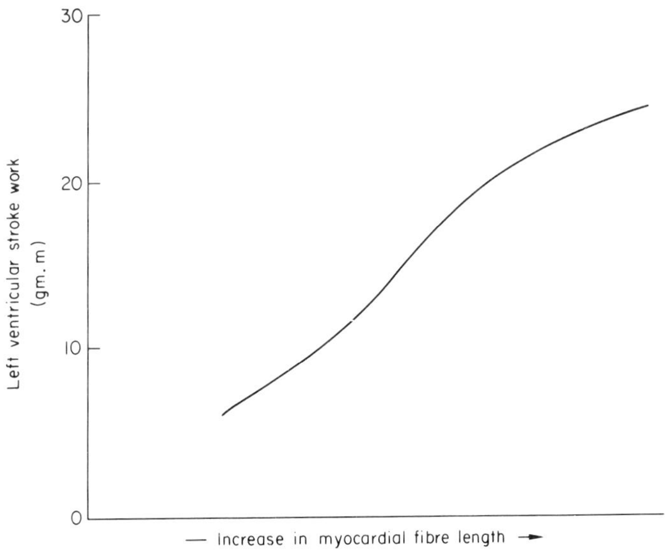

Fig. 10.4 Relationship between the left ventricular myocardial fibre length and stroke work (hypothetical curve derived from several sources).

A further way in which physical, or more properly geometrical, factors affect the work of the heart is through the law of La Place. The tension in the wall of the heart is proportional to the radius of curvature and to the pressure within. Thus, the tension in the wall of a large dilated heart is much higher than that in a small heart when the pressure in the ventricles is the same. However, in the dilated heart in which compensatory hypertrophy has not taken place to a sufficient degree (e.g. when the heart is in failure), then the fibres in the dilated heart have to contract against a much higher wall tension if systolic blood pressure is to be maintained.

The above considerations have important consequences with respect to the partitioning of the total energy produced by the heart into heat and work.

It is known that, for the same amount of mechanical work produced, the heart working at high fibre tension produces much more heat than the heart working at normal or low fibre tension (Gibbs & Mommaerts 1967). Thus, the higher the fibre tension, the more inefficient the heart becomes. This latter point is demonstrated in Fig. 10.5, where it may be seen that, for the same amount of work done, the oxygen cost when the blood pressure is high and the stroke volume low is much greater than when the pressure and stroke volume are within normal limits. If the heart's requirement for oxygen exceeds that which is available from the cardiac circulation then the heart will not be able to produce the work required to maintain an adequate cardiac

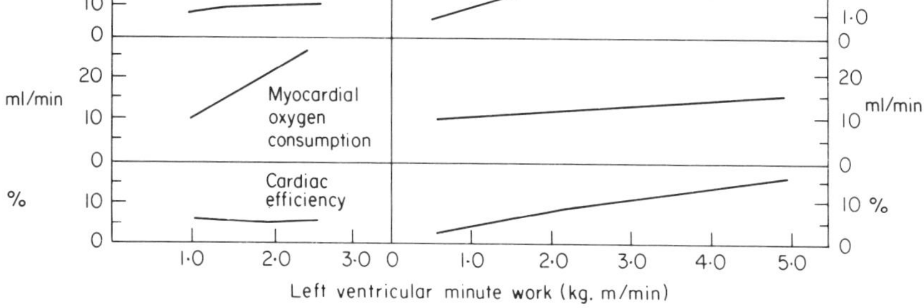

Fig. 10.5 Effect of increasing cardiac work by raising aortic pressure (left), or by augmenting cardiac output (right) on myocardial oxygen consumption and cardiac efficiency. Note that heart is much better able to produce an efficient response to volume increase than to pressure increase — 69·6% increase in work for only 53% increase in oxygen consumption. For increased pressure, increased oxygen consumption = increased work. From Sarnoff *et al* (1958) with permission.

output, and some degree of circulatory failure will follow. Therapeutic measures are therefore aimed at reducing cardiac size and at reducing any elevation of blood pressure, as well as improving cardiac efficiency (usually by improving contractility) so that more useful work is produced.

Of the chemical factors involved in the production of cardiac energy, and its partition into mechanical work and heat, the role of Ca^{++} ions will be apparent from previous sections. The catecholamines also have an important role. Catecholamines have an inotropic effect; they are capable of producing changes in the force of contraction, without any change in initial fibre length.

They also have a chronotropic effect (i.e. they increase the heart rate).

The catecholamines appear to exert their effects on the myocardium by stimulating the membrane bound enzyme adenylate cyclase, which catalyses the formation of cyclic AMP from ATP. This in turn appears to accelerate the entry of Ca^{++} into the cell (Daniel *et al* 1970), and the increased inward current so produced increases the amplitude of the action potential (Noble 1975). It would be expected that this increased inward Ca^{++} current would also increase the duration of the action potential, but increased movement of K^{+} into the cell in fact shortens the duration of the action potential, so reducing the refractory period, and allowing the heart rate to rise — an effect which is amplified by an increased rate of rise of the pacemaker potential. Despite the reduced duration of the action potential, the increase in the magnitude of the Ca^{++} current is sufficient to cause an increase in intracellular Ca^{++} concentration. The overall effect of catecholamines may thus be summarised by saying that they enhance the movement of ions across the cell membrane. For further details, the reader is referred to Noble (1975).

The chief disadvantage of the catecholamines is that by reducing the refractory period and increasing the rate of rise of the pacemaker potential, they tend to induce various dysrhythmias, including, at worst, ventricular fibrillation. This tendency limits their clinical usefulness (see below). For the same reason, sympathetic dominance of the heart is associated with the spontaneous incidence and persistence of dysrhythmias. The other problem associated with catecholamines is that they reduce cardiac efficiency. Although they increase the amount of work done by the myocardium, they increase the myocardial oxygen requirement to a greater extent. Since myocardial hypoxia is likely to be a significant problem in the failing heart, this effect must be regarded as a potentially serious drawback to their use.

Several other cardioactive agents appear to exert their effects by activation of adenyl cyclase. An example is provided by the polypeptide hypoglycaemic hormone, glucagon. This hormone has similar metabolic effects to the catecholamines, and exerts inotropic and chronotropic effects on the heart similar to those of noradrenaline (Levey *et al* 1970) and has been used clinically in man. It does not, however, have the arrhythmogenic properties of noradrenaline, and Jenkins and Clark (1977) state that its cardiostimulatory properties are greater in the dog than in man.

The methylxanthines also give rise to an increase in the intracellular 'messenger' cyclic AMP, but act by inhibiting the enzyme phosphodiesterase, which metabolises cyclic 3′5′AMP to cyclic 5′AMP (Fig. 10.6), rather than by stimulating cyclic AMP production by stimulating adenyl cyclase (Butcher & Sutherland 1962). There is evidence that the increased levels of cyclic 3′5′AMP following methylxanthine administration give rise to an increased concentration of free intracellular Ca^{++} (Bianchi 1975), which may account for the inotropic and chronotropic effects of this class of compounds. Since the rate of cyclic 3′5′AMP synthesis is normally low, the methylxanthines do not produce a very spectacular effect when given alone, but markedly potentiate the actions of catecholamines, when the rate of cyclic AMP synthesis is accelerated by activation of adenyl cyclase (Rall & West 1963). The methylxanthines — caffeine, aminophylline, theophylline, theobromine, etamiphylline, and other derivatives — are widely used clinically for their cardiotonic effects, which are accompanied by respiratory stimulation and the induction of diuresis.

10.4 Autonomic control of the heart and circulation

The foregoing discussion has been concerned with a description of the electrical and mechanical properties of heart and smooth muscle and of how these properties may be modified. In this section, an attempt will be made to give an integrated description of the autonomic control of the heart.

The two naturally occurring hormones, noradrenaline and adrenaline, have a stimulant action on the heart, as already shown, with both heart rate and force of contraction being increased. Noradrenaline is released from sympathetic nerve endings in the heart and a mixture of adrenaline and noradrenaline is released into the blood from the adrenal medulla. There is now available a wide variety of drugs which mimic some of the actions of noradrenaline and adrenaline, and a list of some of these sympathomimetic drugs is given in Table 10.1.

The existence of at least three types of receptor site in the cardiovascular system have been proposed, namely α, β_1, and β_2. In general, the experimental evidence suggests that the heart contains β_2-type receptors and that the smooth muscle of the arteries and veins contains α and β_2 receptors (Ahlquist 1948). Thus, stimulation of β_1 receptors results in an increase in heart rate and force of contraction; stimulation of β_2 receptors results in a relaxation of smooth muscles, and stimulation of α receptors results in a contraction of smooth muscle.

10.4.1 Noradrenaline (Norepinephrine, levarterenol)

Noradrenaline is a short-acting stimulant of both α and β_2 receptors. When given intravenously, its most obvious action is an increase in blood pressure.

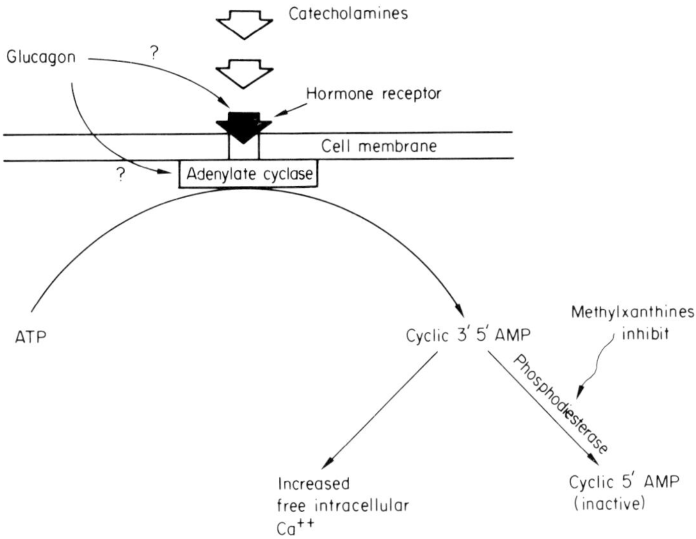

Fig. 10.6 Modes of action of agents which increase intracellular cyclic 3′5′ AMP levels.

This increase occurs because of the α stimulating effects of noradrenaline upon the smooth muscle of the resistance vessels of the arterial circulation. Although noradrenaline is physiologically very important, its clinical use in veterinary practice is limited because, in the animal with heart failure, noradrenaline may well reduce cardiac output by increasing the load against which the heart has to pump, thus masking the cardiac effects.

10.4.2 Adrenaline (Epinephrine)

Adrenaline is released into the bloodstream along with noradrenaline from the adrenal medulla. It is not released from sympathetic nerve endings. In terms of the profile of activity of adrenaline on the heart and circulation, it differs from noradrenaline in that it has a higher affinity for the β_2 receptor site. As might be expected, low doses of adrenaline dilate peripheral blood vessels (β_2 action), whereas at high doses the profile of activity is similar to that of noradrenaline (α action). At low doses, the combination of both cardiac stimulation and peripheral vasodilatation results in an increase in systolic blood pressure, either a small fall or no change in diastolic blood pressure and an increase in heart rate. Cardiac output is increased, the extra output being mostly to skin and skeletal muscle. As the dose of adrenaline is increased, the α stimulating activity becomes apparent, and vasoconstriction occurs; the overall picture is then similar to that obtained with noradrenaline.

Adrenaline is used clinically in small animals in cases of anaphylactic

Table 10.1 Some of the more important agents acting on the autonomic nervous system. The compounds listed are representative of each group only, and this list should not be regarded as being in any way comprehensive.

Mode of action	Agents available	Mode of action	Agents available
Mixed α and β adrenergic agonists	Adrenaline (ephedrine) Amphetamine Ephedrine Phenylpropanolamine	Adrenergic neurone blocking agents	Guanethidine Bretylium Reserpine
		Mixed α and β blocking agent	Labetolol
Mainly α agonist, some β agonist action	Noradrenaline (norepinephrine, levarterenol) Metaraminol	Mainly α adrenergic blocking action	Phenoxybenzamine, dibenamine Tolazoline, phentol-amine Phenothiazines Butyrophenones
Almost entirely α agonist action	Phenylephrine Methoxamine		
Mixed α and β agonist, but also some specific receptors	Dopamine	Mainly β adrenergic blocking action	Propranolol Sotalol Tolamol Metopralol Pindolol Atenolol Oxyprenolol
Mainly β agonist, limited α agonist action	Isoprenaline (isoproterenol) Dobutamine Mephentermine Nylidrin Isoxuprine	Cholinergic agents	Carbachol Bethanechol Methacholine Pilocarpine Opiates Suxamethonium
Selective β agonist action	Orciprenaline (metaproterenol) Salbutamol Terbutaline Fenoterol Ritodrine Isoetharine Quinterenol	Anticholinergic agents	Atropine Hyoscine Propantheline Emepronium Dicyclomine Most antihistamines

shock and in cardiac arrest, in which case it may be given intravenously or by the intracardiac route. The use of catecholamines in this circumstance is not without problems. They tend to give rise to tachyarrhythmias, and even ventricular fibrillation, especially when the myocardium is sensitised (e.g. by anaesthetic agents). The clinician must ensure that the heart is in asystole, rather than in ventricular fibrillation, lest adrenaline should make the situation worse. The recommended dose is up to 5 ml of 1:10 000 adrenaline hydrochloride for large dogs, given into the left ventricle. The dose may be repeated (Hall 1971), and external cardiac massage should be given to expel the drug into the coronary circulation. Clark (1977) recommends that lignocaine (1–2 mg/kg body weight) should be given prior to adrenaline, by the same route, to reduce the incidence of dysrhythmias.

10.4.3 Isoprenaline (Isoproterenol)

Isoprenaline is a short-acting synthetic catecholamine. In contrast to noradrenaline and adrenaline it has no α stimulating activity. The affinity of isoprenaline for the β_2 receptor site is about three times that of its affinity for the β_1 receptor site. At low doses, the predominant effect is dilatation of the blood vessels of the skin and skeletal muscles. There is a marked fall in diastolic blood pressure as a result of the decrease in peripheral vascular resistance. Heart rate and force of contraction increase partly as a direct action of the drug on β_1 receptors in the heart, and partly as a result of reflex activity brought about by the fall in blood pressure. The increase in cardiac output is greater than that obtained with adrenaline and noradrenaline. At high doses of isoprenaline, the combination of a very low resistance to blood flow and a large increase in heart rate and force of contraction results in a decrease in the size of the heart to such a degree that compression of the endocardium occurs, resulting in both mechanical damage and impairment of blood flow (Ferrans *et al* 1964). Thus, overstimulation of the heart with isoprenaline or any other drug which combines cardiac and vasodilating stimulant properties, whilst providing a transient increase in the output from the heart may result in damage to the myocardium of a permanent or long-lasting nature. Because its vasodilator action should enhance tissue perfusion, in addition to its effects on the heart, isoprenaline has been used in the treatment of acute circulatory failure ('shock'). Ogburn (1976) discusses its value in this respect. In severe acute cardiac failure, isoprenaline may be given in an intravenous infusion, but there is considerable danger of producing excessive tachycardia and of increasing the myocardial oxygen requirement beyond the limits of the available oxygen supply. Rapid intravenous digitalisation is preferable in all but the most peracute of cases.

10.4.4 Dobutamine

It will be apparent from the foregoing discussion that none of the three catecholamines so far considered have the ideal properties required to support the heart which is unable to maintain an adequate cardiac output. Dobutamine is now used in man to support the heart in low output failure. Its main action is on the cardiac β_1 receptors, although it also has some α

constrictor effects on blood vessels. In the normal dog, cardiac output and blood pressure are increased, with only a small associated increase in heart rate (Snow, unpubl. obs.). Whether or not dobutamine specifically stimulates particular β_1 receptors concerned with the force of contraction of the heart, rather than those concerned with heart rate is controversial (Bolter & Ledsome 1976) It is likely that the small increase in heart rate, relative to the larger increase in force of contraction, observed in the normal animal with intact cardiovascular reflexes, is the result of vagal slowing of the heart in response to the increase in blood pressure.

Dobutamine is short-acting and has to be given by intravenous injection. It is capable of producing the same maximum effects on the heart as isoprenaline, but the above two features of dobutamine make it unsatisfactory for the long-term treatment of heart failure.

A large number of non-catecholamine sympathomimetic and adrenergic receptor blocking drugs are available, but, at present they appear to have very few indications in veterinary medicine, being used in man chiefly in the treatment of hypertension (α blocking agents, β blocking agents), in the treatment of angina (β blocking agents), and in the treatment of bronchial asthma (β_1 mimetic agents). It is worth noting, in passing, that β_1 mimetic agents, such as orciprenaline, are not suitable for the treatment of bronchial asthma in dogs, since even small doses have significant cardiovascular effects. The reason for this is not clear. However, the β blocking agent propranolol has been used in small animal practice, in the treatment of hypertension in the dog and in feline hypertrophic cardiomyopathy (see Chapter 11).

Amphetamine has a potent α and β sympathomimetic activity, and can produce a spectacular response in neonatal animals suffering from severe circulatory and respiratory depression following prolonged parturition or arising from other causes (W. D. Roberts, pers. comm.). In this situation it is given by intracardiac injection and massaged into the circulation. Its benefit here arises from its ability not only to stimulate the heart, but also from its potent stimulatory effect on the medullary respiratory centre.

Injudicious administration of several agents used in general anaesthesia may cause profound hypotension, by virtue of their α adrenergic blocking properties, causing peripheral vasodilatation. Use of sympathomimetic agents is rarely called for in this situation, but a specific α mimetic, with minimal cardiac activity, such as methoxamine, may be used to arrest profound and progressive hypotension, if conservative treatment fails. Any agent with β activity should always be avoided during anaesthesia if possible, as many anaesthetic agents sensitise the myocardium to the actions of catecholamines, and severe arrhythmias may be set up.

The discussion so far has dealt with the sympathetic aspects of the autonomic control of the heart. The parasympathetic system has rather the opposite effects, so that acetylcholine or parasympathetic stimulation cause slowing of the heart and a decrease in the force of contraction. If vagal stimulation is intense, slowing may progress even to complete asystole. Under normal circumstances, the heart appears to be under continuous sympathetic and parasympathetic discharges, its performance being a function of the balance of the effects of the degree of discharge from each system at any moment. In animals which are physically fit and accustomed to undertaking vigorous exercise (such as racing greyhounds), and which require to have a considerable degree of reserve cardiac capacity for their vigorous exertions, the degree of parasympathetic tone at rest is greater than in normal animals. Such animals are therefore at greater risk of developing a dangerous degree of bradycardia consequent upon vagal stimulation. However, the vagus has little direct effect upon the force of contraction of the ventricle (Furnival *et al* 1973).

Acetylcholine acts by increasing the permeability of the cell membrane to K^+, leading to a hyperpolarisation of the membrane by as much as 10 mV. Also the rate of rise of the pacemaker potential in sinoatrial node cells is reduced (Hutter & Trautwein 1956). In this way the heart rate is reduced. The amplitude and duration of the action potential is also reduced, and thus the amount of Ca^{++} entering the cell during the plateau phase of the action potential is decreased (Noble 1975). The reduction in the amplitude of the action potential (i.e. the magnitude of the initial Na^+ current plus the Ca^{++} current), effectively slows transmission of the potential from one cell to another. This is particularly so at the cells of the atrioventricular node, where release of sufficient acetylcholine may cause complete block of transmission from the atrial muscle to the specialised conducting tissue of the ventricles.

Cholinergic drugs, such as methacholine, or reversible cholinesterase inhibitors, such as neostigmine, have been used in the treatment of states characterised by excessive atrial activity, such as paroxysmal atrial tachycardia (Jenkins & Clark 1977).

10.4.5 Atropine

Atropine combines with the postsynaptic acetylcholine receptors, and so prevents acetylcholine from exerting its effects. It thus abolishes or reduces vagal tone on the heart. It may therefore be of value in the treatment of heart block, and following cardiac arrest. It is also of considerable importance in general anaesthesia. Normal cardiac activity is maintained by a balance of sympathetic and parasympathetic activities, and abolition of vagal tone will produce:

1 An increase in heart rate (due to sympathetic dominance).

2 Increased conductivity, especially in the specialised conducting tissues of the heart.

Clinically, atropine is used for anaesthetic premedication (there are very few anaesthetics which are not improved by atropine premedication) in order to improve cardiac stability. Atropine premedication is obligatory when anaesthetic agents which are potent myocardial depressants are to be used (e.g. etorphine, halothane, barbiturates). Atropine may also be used to treat bradycardia, sinus arrest or atrioventricular block occurring under anaesthesia. Whilst these conditions may occur as a result of undue vagal stimulation (by the effects of irritant vapours on the upper respiratory tract; by surgery involving parts of the head and neck; or by traction on anterior abdominal viscers), some drugs with cholinergic properties may also play a significant part (e.g. suxamethonium, opiates, anticholinesterase agents).

10.5 Cardiac glycosides

The cardiac glycosides are a most important group of drugs. They are widely used because of their ability to improve cardiac contractility without producing a corresponding increase in myocardial oxygen consumption (Lee & Klaus 1971).

The measurable effects of the cardiac glycosides on the failing heart are as follows:

1 Inotropic action — improved contractility.
2 Slowing of heart rate (negative chronotropic effect) due to:
  a Reduced excitability.
  b Slowed conduction.
  c Increased atrioventricular refractory period.
  d Reduced sensitivity of myocardium to catecholamines.
  e Increased sensitivity to acetylcholine.

In the normal animal these effects tend to be masked by reflex homeostatic mechanisms.

Although these effects are well documented in standard texts, and although a great deal of work has been done on the mechanism of action of this group of agents, much remains unclear as to their mode of action at a biochemical level. Nonetheless, it is possible to draw a general picture, which can explain the effects described above.

It has long been apparent that the cardiac glycosides were capable of causing potassium loss from contractile tissues (Calhoun & Harrison 1931), and it subsequently became clear that this effect was mediated by inhibition of the active Na^+/K^+ membrane pump (Schatzmann 1953). Much of the work on the cardiac glycosides has been done on red cells, since they appear to have similar effects on transmembranal ion movements in the red cell, and studies using this model revealed no evidence that inhibition of the cation pump was related to impairment of the energy supply required to run the pump (Scnatzmann 1953; Kuntz & Sulser 1957). However, it subsequently appeared that digitalis not only affected the active pumping of K^+ into the cell, but also

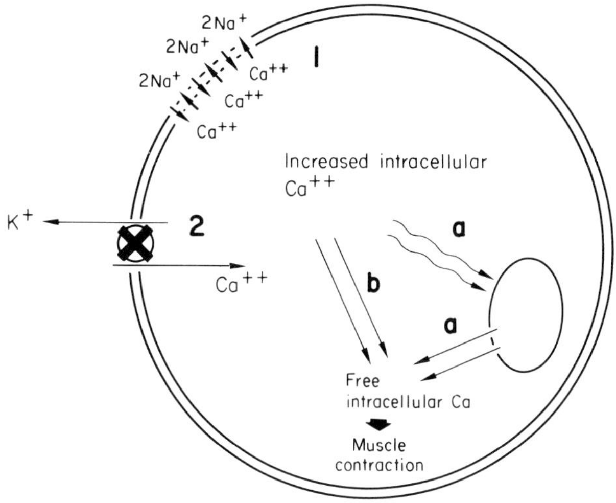

Fig. 10.7 Modes of action of cardiac glycosides (cf. Fig. 10.1c). Cardiac glycosides inhibit the membrane ionic pump, so Na^+ which enters during action potential less easily removed from the cell. There are two theories as to how this might lead to an increased intracellular free Ca^{++}, (1) increased transmembranal exchange — $2 \times Na^+$ for each $1 \times Ca^{++}$ to maintain electrical neutrality; (2) Ca^{++} influx and K^+ efflux exchange through glycoside inhibited pump. Increased free intracellular Ca^{++} from sarcoplasmic reticulum, (a) or itself is sufficient; (b) to produce enhanced contraction of actinomyosin.

the passive efflux of K^+ from the cell (Grupp 1963). The Na^+/K^+ pump is fuelled by ATP, which is broken down by membrane bound ATPase, the released energy is in some way transferred to a 'sodium carrier'. Some authors (Post *et al* 1960) have considered that the cardiac glycosides compete with sodium for this carrier, whilst others (Repke 1964) have suggested that they inhibit the membrane bound ATPase itself. This discussion, however, begs the question of how, by inhibiting the Na^+/K^+ pump, the cardiac glycosides are able to improve cardiac contractility. This effect is almost certainly mediated through an increase in free intracellular Ca^{++} during the action potential, which in turn will encourage the activation of myosin bound ATPase. In a series of papers, Langer (1971, 1974) has suggested that inhibition of the Na^+/K^+ pump allows intracellular Na^+ to accumulate, which is then available for transmembranal exchange for Ca^{++} (Fig. 10.7). It will be recalled from the discussion earlier in this chapter that the transmembranal influx of Ca^{++} appears to trigger the release of Ca^{++} from the sarcoplasmic reticulum, so it may be that the proposed enhancement of transmembranal entry of Ca^{++} would encourage some augmentation of Ca^{++} release from the sarcoplasmic reticulum. Lindenmayer and Schwartz (1975) have suggested a further refinement, which is that the Na^+ pump may, in effect, pump both K^+ *and* Ca^{++} into the cell in exchange for Na^+, and that when the pump is inhibited by cardiac glycosides it may switch to pumping Ca^{++} into the cell and K^+ out. This hypothesis is particularly attractive in that it suggests an explanation for the 'force-frequency effect'. This term describes the phenomenon whereby cardiac contractility is increased as the heart rate increases, up to a certain maximal value (about 180 beats/minute in the dog). If there is indeed some Ca^{++} influx coupled to Na^{+} efflux, then the more rapid rate of depolarisation associated with a faster heart rate would call for increased Na^{+} efflux to compensate for the increased Na^{+} influx during repeated depolarisations, and increased Ca^{++} influx, and hence greater contractility, would be coupled with the increased Na^{+} efflux. It should be stated, however, that the force-frequency relationship is normally explained in terms of optimal filling of the cardiac chambers and the operation of Starling's law during more rapid rates of contraction.

Whatever the biochemical basis of glycoside action may be, it is clear that the duration of the cardiac action potential is increased following administration of these agents (see Fig. 10.2). Reduced conductivity will follow, because the prolonged period of contraction is associated with an increased length of refractory period, and so the cells will remain in an unexcitable state for a longer period.

Although the cardiac glycosides are the most important agents acting upon cardiac calcium metabolism, other agents also have significant effects. Nifedepine is a calcium antagonist, which causes a reduction of myocardial work and oxygen demand, and is used in the treatment of angina in man. Many general anaesthetic agents, such as the barbiturates and halothane interfere with intracellular calcium disposition (Nayler & Szeto 1972; Price 1974), and thus reduce myocardial contractility, and action which may be reversed by cardiac glycosides or β adrenergic agents (Harvey 1975). Verapamil is a relatively new antidysrhythmic agent, which appears to act by reducing Ca^{++} entry to myocardial cells (Singh & Vaughan Williams 1972). This observation brings the whole argument round full circle, for it is apparent that the Ca^{++} ion has a modulating activity on the Na^{+}/K^{+} pump, as well as having its own disposition modified by the action of the pump.

10.6 Antidysrhythmic agent

The mode of action of the antidysrhythmic agents has been fairly well worked-out, notably by Vaughan Williams (1975), who classifies them as follows:

Class 1. Quinidine, procainamide, lignocaine. These agents are thought to block certain of the sodium 'gates' in the cell membrane, thus reducing the rate of rise of the action potential. When the action potential rises rapidly, it is possible for a cell to become depolarised very shortly after a previous depolarisation; if the cell depolarises slowly (as would occur if the 'gates' were partially blocked) it requires to be more fully repolarised before it will discharge again. In other words, reducing the rate of rise of the action potential prolongs the effective refractory period. However, quinidine also has other effects, such as raising the threshold for depolarisation (West & Amory 1960), and reducing the rate of conduction in the specialised conducting tissues (Wallace *et al* 1966), and producing some degree of vagal block (Moe & Abildskov 1975). All the agents in this class have some degree of local anaesthetic activity, and probably act by interfering with the lipid structure of the cell membrane, thereby closing the pores through which ions may pass (Ritchie 1971).

Class 2. Dysrhythmias occur more commonly when there is excessive sympathetic drive to the heart, and therefore agents which lower the normal sympathetic drive to the heart, or which are capable of reducing increased sympathetic activity, will tend to have an antidysrhythmic action (Vaughan Williams 1975).

Class 3. Certain agents appear to be able to selectively prolong the phase of repolarisation (e.g. amiodarone) (Vaughan Williams 1975).

Class 4. Verapamil (see above).

10.7 Electrolytes

It is hoped that this chapter will have provided an integrated review of some important aspects of cardiac electrophysiology, and the modes of action of some of the therapeutic agents which are of importance in small animal medicine. Because cardiac function is intimately dependent upon the movement of certain cations, the role of these cations has been discussed at some length. An important cation, magnesium, has been omitted from this discussion, not because it is considered to be of minor significance, but because its exact role is unclear at present. There is no reason to suppose that it will not transpire to be of considerable importance, as further studies elucidate its role.

The importance of the myocardial intracellular-extracellular ion balance will be apparent from the points raised throughout the chapter. Wide variations in the normal balance are inconsistent with normal myocardial function, and if maintenance of a normal balance is important in the healthy animal, it is of yet greater importance in the animal whose cardiac function is impaired. Diseased or damaged cells tend to lose the ability to maintain adequate transmembranal electrolyte gradients, and this is especially true of cells in which optimal conditions for the biochemical processes required for the synthesis of high energy fuels, such as ATP, are no longer present. The prime example is the cell which is hypoxic. In cardiovascular disorders, the primary lesion may well involve myocardial cell damage or disease, but the resulting circulatory changes are likely to require the heart to do an increased amount of work in order to maintain an adequate output, and, as discussed earlier in this chapter, this will place an increased demand upon the availability of oxygen to the myocardial cells especially if there is cardiac dilation. At the same time, however, the efficiency of both the pulmonary and systemic circulations may be so compromised that adequate tissue oxygenation will be impossible to maintain. The situation then arises that the heart cannot function adequately unless the circulation is improved, to enhance myocardial oxygenation, whilst the circulation cannot be improved until the myocardium functions more efficiently.

As if this situation was not sufficiently alarming, it is made worse by the inability of the failing circulation to maintain adequate renal perfusion, so that further problems of electrolyte imbalance occur. The somewhat hypoxic cells of the myocardium, whose ability to maintain adequate transmembranal electrolyte gradients is already compromised by the presence of hypoxia, are then faced with the added problem of having to function in the face of gross disturbances in the composition of the extracellular fluid.

Acidosis usually goes hand in hand with hypoxia, and the hydrogen ion is a potent inhibitor of myocardial function (Safer & Davies 1973). Acidosis and hypoxia together probably account for the decreased energy production in mitochondria isolated from the failing heart, and possibly also for the serious problem of reduced intracellular Ca^{++} transport which can also be demonstrated in *in vitro*, using preparations from the failing heart (Detweiler & Knight 1977).

It is apparent, therefore, that support for the failing myocardium should include careful attention to the patient's respiratory status and electrolyte balance. The following therapeutic manoeuvres may be of value.

10.7.1 Oxygen

In the acute case, oxygen should be administered by mask, endotracheal or nasotracheal intubation. An oxygen-rich environment, such as might be provided by an improvised oxygen-tent, is of value in the management of the less acute case. Many dogs with failing hearts will seek out cool and airy environments, and this tendency may be encouraged.

10.7.2 Diuretics

The mechanisms leading to the retention of salt and water and the consequent expansion of the extracellular fluid volume in cardiac failure are complex (see reviews by Cannon 1977; Detweiler & Knight 1977), but appear to be mediated via the kidney and the renin-angiotensin system. The adverse results of fluid retention include increased circulating blood volume, ascites, oedema and hydrothorax. Retention of Na^+ leads to a rise in the concentration of this ion in the extracellular fluid, making it more difficult for the sodium pump to keep the intracellular Na^+ level sufficiently low. The retention of water adds to the circulating blood volume, so that the heart has to do more work to maintain blood flow. Whilst both the cardiac glycosides and the methylxanthines have a diuretic action, this is not generally sufficient to restore normal fluid balance, and it is usual to supplement treatment with a saluretic/diuretic agent. On the other hand, it is important to avoid undue loss of K^+ from the body, as any depletion in the K^+ concentration in the extracellular fluid will be made good by loss of K^+ from the intracellular compartment. The potassium-sparing diuretics, such as triamterene and amiloride may therefore be preferred. Ethacrynic acid and frusemide are less expensive, and frusemide seems to be less likely to cause hypokalaemia in the dog than in man, although it is potentially ototoxic (Jenkins & Clark 1977).

10.7.3 Low salt diet

A low salt diet will also help to reduce the extracellular Na^+ level, and thus reduce the amount of work necessary to maintain a low intracellular Na^+ level. Mild cases of chronic cardiac failure may respond well to little more than curtailment of exercise (to reduce the demands made on the myocardium), a low salt diet, and judicious use of suitable diuretics.

10.7.4 Potassium

Control of potassium levels is difficult in the extreme, since the important factor is the intracellular potassium level, and its relationship to the extracellular level. If the extracellular potassium level falls, the contractility of the myocardium will be initially increased, as the efflux of K^+ during the action potential will be facilitated, and according to the Lindenmayer–Schwartz hypothesis (see above), influx of Ca^{++} might be enhanced, as Ca^{++} might substitute for K^+ in the ionic pump. If the ability of the ionic pump is compromised, intracellular K^+ will rapidly be lost to the extracellular compartment. This has been postulated as the cause of failure of some cases of cardiac failure to respond to treatment, and it may be possible to restore the intracellular K^+ level by giving potassium-glucose-insulin mixtures (Julian *et al* 1974). However, care must be taken, if potassium is administered, with or without glucose and insulin, to prevent the development of hyperkalaemia. In this case, the differential between intracellular and extracellular K^+ levels is reduced, and contractility is reduced, with cardiac arrest occurring early. Hypokalaemia enhances the toxicity of the cardiac glycosides — presumably because glycoside-induced inhibition of the ion pump, coupled with a large intracellular-extracellular K^+ differential increases excitability, and allows ectopic foci to develop. It is therefore especially important to maintain normal K^+ levels in the digitalised patient, and this may best be achieved by dietary control and the avoidance of K^+-depleting diuretics.

10.7.5 Calcium

To some extent calcium and potassium antagonise the actions of each other on the myocardium, and so calcium salts may be the best line of treatment for myocardial depression associated with hyperkalaemia. A large increase in extracellular Ca^{++} causes dysrhythmias if not cardiac arrest, and a vagal mechanism has been postulated for the mediation of this effect (Littledike *et al* 1976), although a direct effect on the myocardium, such as competition for Mg^{++} binding sites, is probably responsible in part. Moderate hypercalcaemia, however, improves cardiac contractility — presumably by making more Ca^{++} ions available for entry into myocardial cells (Toda 1969). Conversely, hypocalacaemia leads to a reduction in contractility. Calcium chloride may be of value in the treatment of cardiac arrest, and Hall (1971) has recommended that up to 3 ml 10% calcium chloride may be given into the left ventricle by cardiac puncture, and that this dose may be repeated if required. Calcium chloride is, however, irritant in concentrations greater than 5%, and Clark (1977) recommends the use of calcium gluconate, although a much larger dose is required, as it is less fully ionised (10–20 ml 10% solution at 10-minute intervals for dogs of average size).

It will be noted that all the therapeutic manoeuvres so far described for the treatment of the failing heart, are intended to increase the amount of mechanical work done by the heart, hopefully with relatively less increase in myocardial oxygen consumption. An alternative, but as yet relatively unproven method, is to reduce the amount of work done. This approach has been described in relation to the dog by Hamlin (1977), and rests upon the assumption that 'failure' of the heart is, in fact, a homeostatic mechanism, whereby the mismatching of cardiac oxygen requirement and supply can be reduced to a minimum, thereby preventing the further deterioration of myocardial function. If the contractility and work of the heart decrease in cardiac failure, it may be that oxygen demand by the myocardium decreases to an even greater extent. Suggested methods of treatment include the lowering of peripheral resistance by β blocking agents or ganglion blockers, and the use of β blocking agents, such as propranolol, which reduce cardiac contractility and heart rate, but which also reduce myocardial oxygen demand, and protect against dysrhthmias. Diuretics are not used in this scheme, reduction of pulmonary oedema following the reduction in pulmonary venous pressure which follows the general reduction in blood pressure. Although it is difficult to reconcile this approach with the suggestion that myocardial oxygen utilisation is greater in the dilated heart, due to the operation of La Place's law, it is equally true that a reduction in systolic pressure will reduce the myocardial oxygen requirement in the failing heart, although this effect might be cancelled out by the increase which would follow any increase in the systolic period (Sarnoff *et al* 1958).

A great deal of work remains to be done to assess the validity of the hypotheses underlying this approach, and its application to small animal cardiology.

References

Ahlquist R. P. (1948) A study of adrenotropic receptors. *Amer. J. Physiol.* **153**, 586.

Bassingthwaighte J. B. & Reuter H. (1972) Calcium movements and excitation-contraction coupling in cardiac cells. In *Electrical Phenomena of the Heart*, ed. W. C. De Mello, p. 353. Academic Press, New York.

Bianchi C. P. (1975) Cellular pharmacology of contraction of skeletal muscle. In *Cellular Pharmacology of Excitable Tissue*, ed. T. Narahashi. C. C. Thomas, Springfield, Ill.

Bolter C. P. & Ledsome J. R. (1976) Inotropic and chronotropic responses of the *in vivo* denervated dog myocardium to dobutamine. *Can. J. Physiol. Pharmacol.* **54**, 618.

Braunwald E., Ross J. Jr. & Sonnenblick E. H. (1967) Mechanisms of contraction of the normal and failing heart. *New Eng. J. Med.* **277**, 794, 1012.

Butcher R. W. & Sutherland E. W. (1962) Adenosine 3′,5′-phosphate in biological materials. *J. Biol. Chem.* **237**, 1244.

Calhoun J. A. & Harrison T. R. (1931) Studies in congestive heart failure: IX The effect of digitalis on the potassium content of cardiac muscle in dogs. *J. Clin. Invest.* **10**, 139.

Cannon P. J. (1977) The kidney in heart failure. *New Eng. J. Med.* **296**, 26.

Clark D. R. (1977) Recognition and treatment of cardiac emergencies. *J. Amer. Vet. Med. Ass.* **171**, 98.

Daniel E. E., Paton D. M., Taylor G. S. & Hodgson B. J. (1970) Adrenergic receptors for catecholamine effects on tissue electrolytes. *Fed. Proc.* **29**, 1410.

Detweiler D. K. & Knight D. H. (1977) Congestive heart failure in dogs: Therapeutic concepts. *J. Amer. Vet. Med. Ass.* **171**, 106.

Fabiato A. & Fabiato F. (1975) Contractions induced by a calcium-triggered release of calcium from the sarcoplasmic reticulum of single-skinned cardiac cells. *J. Physiol.* **249**, 469.

Ferrans V. J., Hibbs R. G., Black W. C. & Weelbaicher D. G. (1964) Isoproterenol induced myocardial necrosis: A histochemical and electron microscope study. *Amer. Heart J.* **68**, 71.

Furnival C. M., Linden R. J. & Snow H. M. (1973) The ionotropic effect on the heart of stimulating the vagus in dog, duck and toad. *J. Physiol.* **230**, 155.

Gibbs C. L. & Mommaerts W. F. H. M. (1967) Energetics of cardiac muscle. *J. Physiol.* **191**, 16.

Grupp G. (1963) The effect of ouabain on potassium fluxes of the dog heart in situ. *Fed. Proc.* **22**, 184.

Hall L. W. (1971) *Wright's Veterinary Anaesthesia and Analgesia*, 7th edn. Baillière, Tindall, London.

Hamlin R. L. (1977) New ideas in the management of heart failure in dogs. *J. Amer. Vet. Med. Ass.* **171**, 114.

Harvey S. C. (1975) The barbiturates. In *The Pharmacological Basis of Therapeutics*. 5th. edn., eds. L. S. Goodman & A. Gilman, p. 102. Macmillan, New York.

Hasselbach W. & Makinose M. (1961) Die Calciumpompe der 'Erschlaffungsgrana' des Muskels und ihre Abhängigkeit von der ATP-Altung. *Biochem. Zschr.* **333**, 518.

Hutter O. F. & Trautwein W. (1956) Vagal and sympathetic effects on the pacemaker fibers in the sinus venosus of the heart. *J. Gen. Physiol.* **39**, 715.

Huxley H. E. (1969) The mechanism of muscular contraction. *Science* **164**, 1356.

Jenkins W. L. & Clark D. R. (1977) A review of drugs affecting the heart. *J. Amer. Vet. Med. Assoc.* **171**, 85.

Julian D. G., Kitchin A. H., Montgomery G. L. & Bouch D. C. (1974) Diseases of the heart. In *A Companion to Medical Studies*, eds. R. Passmore & J. S. Robson, vol. 3, part 1. chapt. 16. Blackwell Scientific Publications, Oxford.

Katz A. (1970) Contractile proteins of the heart. *Physiol. Rev.* **50**, 63.

Kuntz H. A. & Sulser F. (1957) Über die Hemmung des Aktiven Kationentransportes durch Herzglykosid. *Experientia* **13**, 365.

Langer G. A. (1971) The intrinsic control of myocardial contraction: ionic factors. *New Eng. J. Med.* **285**, 1065.

Langer G. A. (1974) Calcium in mammalian myocardium; localisation and movement of contractile-dependent calcium. *Circ. Res.* **34**, 1191.

Lee K. S. & Klaus W. (1971) The subcellular basis for the mechanism of inotropic action of the cardiac glycosides. *Pharmac. Rev.* **23**, 193.

Levey G. S., Prindle K. H., & Epstein S. E. (1970) Effects of glucagon on adenyl cyclase activity in the left and right ventricle and liver in experimentally-produced isolated right ventricular failure. *J. Mol. Cell. Cardiol.* **1**, 403.

Lindenmayer G. E. & Schwartz A. (1975) A kinetic characterisation of calcium on ($Na^+ + K^+$)-ATPase and its potential role as a link between extracellular and intracellular events: hypothesis for digitalis-induced inotropism. *J. Mol. Cell. Cardiol.* **7**, 591.

Littledike E. T., Glazier D. & Cook H. M. (1976) Electrocardiographic changes after induced hypercalcaemia and hypocalcaemia in cattle: reversal of the induced arrhythmia with atropine. *Amer. J. Vet. Res.* **37**, 383.

Martonosi A. & Feretos R. (1963) Observations on the calcium uptake by fragmented sarcoplasmic reticulum. *Fed. Proc.* **22**, 352.

Moe G. K. & Abildskov J. A. (1975) Antiarrhythmic drugs. In *The Pharmacological Basis of Therapeutics*, eds. L. S. Goodman & A. Gilman. Macmillan, New York.

Nakagima Y. & Endo M. (1973) Release of calcium induced by depolarisation of the sarcoplasmic reticulum membrane. *Nature New Biol.* **246**, 216.

Nayler W. G. & Szefo J. (1972) Effect of sodium pentobarbital on calcium in mammalian heart muscle. *Amer. J. Physiol.* **222**, 339.

Noble D. (1975) *The Initiation of the Heart Beat.* Clarendon Press, Oxford.

Ogburn P. (1967) Vasoactive agents in the treatment of shock. *Vet. Clin. N. Amer.* **6:2**, 121.

Parker J. L. & Adams R. (1977) Drugs and the heart muscle. *J. Amer. Vet. Med. Ass.* **171**, 78.

Post R. L., Merritt C. R., Kinsolving C. R. & Albright C. D. (1960) Membrane adenosine triphosphatase as a participate in the active transport of calcium and potassium in the human erythrocyte. *J. Biol. Chem.* **235**, 1796.

Price H. L. (1974) Calcium reversed myocardial depression caused by halothane. *Anaesthesiology* **41**, 576.

Rall T. W. & West T. C. (1963) The potentialities of cardiac inotropic responses to norepinephrine by theophylline. *J. Pharmac. Exper. Therap.* **139**, 269.

Rasmussen H. (1970) Cell communication, calcium ion, and cyclic adenosine monophosphate. *Science* **170**, 404.

Repke K. (1964) Überden biochemischen Wirkungsmodus von Digitalis. *Klin. Wschr.* **42**, 157.

Ritchie J. M. (1971) The mechanism of action of local anaesthetic agents. In *International Encyclopaedia of Pharmacology & Therapeutics*, ed. P. Lechat, vol. 1, sect. 8. Pergammon Press, Oxford.

Roberts R. M., Walker A. & Cetorelli J. J. (1973) Fucose-containing glycopeptides from the cell surface of Chinese Hamster ovary cells grown in the presence or absence of cyclic AMP. *Nature New Biol.* **244**, 86.

Safer B. & Davies R. E. (1973) Effects of H^+ on physiological and biochemical function of the heart. *Fed. Proc.* **32**, 449.

Sanborn W. A. & Langer G. A. (1970) Specific uncoupling of excitation and contraction in mammalian cardiac muscle by lanthanum. *J. Gen. Physiol.* **56**, 191.

Sarnoff S. J., Braunwald E., Welch G. H. Jnr., Case R. B., Stainsby W. N. & Macruz R. (1958) Haemodynamic determinants of oxygen consumption of the heart with special reference to the tension-time index. *Amer. J. Physiol.* **192**, 148.

Schatzmann H. J. (1953) Herzglycoside als Hemmstaffe für den Aktiven Kalium-und Natrium transport durch die Erythrocytenmembran. *Helv. Physiol. Pharmacol. Act.* **11**, 346.

Singh B. N. & Vaughan Williams E. M. (1972) A fourth class of antidysrhythmic action? Effect of verapamil on ouabain toxicity, on atrial and ventricular intracellular potentials, and on other features of cardiac function. *Cardiovasc. Res.* **6**, 109.

Skou J. C. (1965) Enzymic basis for active transport of sodium and potassium across cell membranes. *Physiol. Rev.* **45**, 596.

Toda N. (1969) Effects of Ca^{++}, Na^{+}, and K^{+} ions on contractility of isolated atria and their response to noradrenaline. *Brit. J. Pharmacol.* **36**, 350.

Vaughan Williams E. M. (1975) Antidysrhythmic drugs — their mode of action. In *Contraction and Relaxation in the Myocardium*, ed. W. G. Naylor. Academic Press, London.

Wallace A. G., Cline R. E., Sealy W. C., Young W. G. & Troyer W. G. (1966) Electrophysiological effects of quinidine: studies using chronically implanted electrodes in awake dogs. *Circulation Res.* **19**, 960.

West T. C. & Amory D. W. (1960) Single fibre recording of the effect of quinidine on atrial pacemaker sites in the isolated right atrium of the rabbit. *J. Pharmac. Exper. Therap.* **130**, 183.

11

Agents acting on the cardiovascular system II. Clinical use in small animals

M. G. DEAR

In this chapter the practical clinical use of agents acting on the cardiovascular system will be discussed. Although an individual patient may present with a number of inter-related problems, it is usually possible to distinguish an underlying cardiological problem if it is present, even if it is not possible to make a conclusive diagnosis of the exact nature of this problem. Furthermore, in many cases the underlying problem will not be amenable to curative therapy. It is therefore useful to consider cardiovascular pharmacotherapeutics in a manner which will allow it to be applied to the problem at varying stages of diagnostic resolution; and with this approach it is possible to distinguish two broad categories of drug usage:

1 Prophylactic therapy.
2 Curative (ameliorative) therapy.
  a Specific.
  b Symptomatic.
  c Supportive.

This chapter will be mainly confined to a discussion of methods of curative therapy.

11.1 Specific curative therapy

An aetiological diagnosis allows therapy to be directed at removal of the cause of the disease process in many cases. These causes may be classified as follows:

Infectious causes. Viral (e.g. canine distemper); bacterial (e.g. bacterial endocarditis) — antibiotics; protozoan (e.g. toxoplasmosis); metazoal (e.g. filariasis) — filaricides, microfilaricides.

Physical causes. Trauma, heat stroke.

Chemical causes. Heavy metals, anaesthetics — chemical antidotes.

Metabolic causes. Endocrinological: diabetes mellitus and thyroid disorders — corrective treatment; nutritional — corrective measures; immunological — possibly immunosuppression.

Neoplastic causes. Primary or secondary — surgery, if possible.

Developmental. Congenital disorders — surgery; degenerative disorders — enzymes.

Psychogenic. Systolic pump failure, tachyarrhythmias — removal of stressors.

11.2 Symptomatic and supportive pharmacotherapy

Since the heart is primarily a pump the clinical manifestations of cardiac failure, regardless of the underlying cause, are principally congestive signs precipitated by inadequate cardiac contractility. Even when the aetiology is obscure or difficult to manage, it is possible to ameliorate the signs of congestive heart failure by treating the myocardial asthenia and the fluid congestion which accompanies it. For this purpose the cardiac glycosides and diuretics provide the basis of pharmacotherapy.

11.2.1 Therapy for myocardial asthenia

CARDIAC GLYCOSIDES

Digitalis glycosides are used for the treatment of congestive heart failure arising from valvular degenerations, congenital anomalies and from cardiomyopathies, together with their resultant arrhythmias. This approach, using plant extracts containing cardiac glycosides, was employed as long ago as 1500 BC by the Egyptians, and subsequently by the Romans as diuretics and heart tonics. In 1785, William Withering used an extract of the foxglove plant, digitalis, in the treatment of dropsy. A similar application of the use of the drug was made in veterinary medicine in 1841 (Blaine).

The natural glycosides in the plant (lanatosides or digilanids) can be hydrolysed to produce pharmacologically active glycosides (digitoxin and gitoxin from the leaves of *Digitalis purpurea*; digitoxin, gitoxin and digoxin from *D. lanata* leaves). These active glycosides are further hydrolysed in the body into an aglycone (genin) which is basically a steroid nucleus and a sugar. The latter affects the solubility and hence the bioavailability of the aglycone. Digitoxin and digoxin (and rarely ouabain) are used in veterinary medicine (Fig. 11.1). The unpurified digitalis preparations are unreliable and now obsolete.

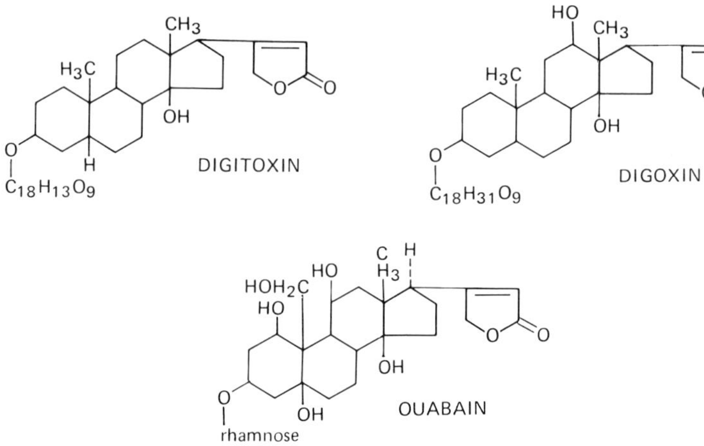

Fig. 11.1 Structural formula of the most important cardiac glycosides. Note that addition of –OH at carbon-12 position alters digitoxin to digoxin, but this small change significantly alters the degree of plasma protein binding, whilst increased polarity of molecule reduces absorption through lipid cell membranes as in gastro-intestinal tract. Highly polar ouabain with several –OH groups is not absorbed from gastro-intestinal tract and can only be given intravenously.

The kinetics of cardiac glycosides

The bioavailability and kinetics of the cardiac glycosides are dependent upon several factors:

Gastrointestinal absorption. Digitoxin powder is absorbed almost completely although only slowly from the intestinal tract of dogs, whereas the elixir form is absorbed much more readily. In both tablet and elixir form, digoxin is 60–90% absorbed, and reaches its peak plasma level within 1 hour.

Hepatic circulation and metabolism. Both digoxin and digitoxin are taken up by the liver, and undergo hepatic metabolisation. The metabolites are excreted in the bile, and reabsorbed to a certain extent — although probably to a smaller extent than in man (Jenkins & Clark 1977). Digoxin undergoes renal excretion, whilst digitoxin is chiefly excreted in the bile after hepatic metabolism.

Plasma concentration. The amount of glycoside entering the myocardial cell is dependent upon the plasma concentration of free drug. The plasma concentration of free drug depends, in turn, upon the rate of absorption from the site of administration, the rate of excretion, and degree of plasma protein binding. Plasma protein binding is itself dependent upon the glycoside concentration, and the glycoside in question. Digitoxin is 70–90% bound in the plasma concentration range 10–50 μg/ml, whereas digoxin is about 25–30% bound at therapeutic concentrations in the dog, and about 20% bound in the cat (Baggot & Davies 1973).

Since the absorption of both digoxin and digitoxin is rapid, the plasma concentration of either glycoside at any moment will depend upon the rates of metabolism and excretion for that glycoside. Estimates of the half-lives of digoxin and digitoxin in the dog have varied, but figures which may be quoted are 40–50 hours for digoxin (Hamlin *et al* 1971), and about 8 hours for digitoxin (Hamlin 1978).

The elimination kinetics of the glycosides may be altered by the presence of hepatic disease (tending to increase the half-life); impaired renal function, especially when glomerular filtration is reduced (probably most significant for digoxin); and by the stimulation of the hepatic microsomal enzyme system by agents such as the barbiturates, phenylbutazone, and diphenylhydantoin. Surprisingly, according to Hamlin (1978), the half-life of digoxin is reduced following pretreatment with barbiturates, but not that of digitoxin (see also Breznock 1975). Hamlin (1978) has observed that the plasma half-life of digitoxin in the dog is unaffected by the presence of nephritis, or by pretreatment with barbiturates, whilst the half-life of digoxin is prolonged considerably (up to 5 days) by the presence of nephritis, and is reduced after barbiturate administration. One might conclude, from these observations, that digitoxin would have some advantage over digoxin in clinical usage, in that the kinetic behaviour of the former appears to be less susceptible to interference by extraneous factors. In the same paper Hamlin has produced some evidence from clinical studies which reinforces this view. This work also emphasises the value of carrying out glycoside blood level estimations in clinical practice. At present, such estimations are routinely available from only a limited number of veterinary laboratories, but are widely available in human laboratories, and in kit form for the larger veterinary laboratory. It is to be hoped that the cost will diminish with wider use of this facility, since the relatively high cost of each individual estimation is probably the most significant bar to the wider use of this most important technique in small animal medicine. In Hamlin's study, the glycoside levels of dogs digitalised for the treatment of heart disease were measured, and classified as being within or below the therapeutic range, or within the toxic range, which extends from the upper level of the therapeutic range. It will be appreciated that some dogs will show symptoms of toxicity whilst their blood glycoside levels remain within the therapeutic range, and that in some cases adequate clinical response will not be seen at subtoxic doses. The results of Hamlin's study are shown in Table 11.1. It will be seen that an appropriate blood glycoside level was found in the great majority of cases treated with digitoxin, whilst 50% of the dogs treated with digoxin showed toxic blood glycoside levels, which were sometimes accompanied by clinical signs of digitalis toxicity.

Table 11.1 Blood levels of digitoxin and digoxin in a sample of dogs digitalised for heart failure. Modified from Hamlin 1978.

	Digitoxin treated	Digoxin treated
Total no. of cases	40	76
Therapeutic blood level	15 – 25 ng/ml	1·0 – 1·8 ng/ml
No. of cases found to have therapeutic blood level	36 (90%)	11 (14%)
No. of cases found to have subtherapeutic blood level	3 (8%)	27 (36%)
No. of cases found to have toxic blood level	1 (2%)	38 (50%)

Nonetheless, digoxin has been the glycoside of choice for most veterinary cardiologists, and much more experience has been accumulated in the use of this glycoside than in the use of digitoxin. Part of the reason for this may be that the short half-life of digitoxin calls for this drug to be given twice daily, whereas once-daily dosing is sufficient for digoxin. Another problem is that digitoxin is available in only a limited number of different preparations, which may pose problems in administration.

Action of cardiac glycosides on the heart

This topic has been dealt with more fully in the preceding chapter, but may be summarised by stating that the digitalis glycosides give rise to an increase in myocardial contractility, a reduction in heart rate, and delayed conduction through the specialised conducting tissues and the atrioventricular node.

In heart failure, these glycosides increase the contractile force of ventricular systole (i.e. the rate of rise of ventricular pressure is increased), and increase ventricular diastolic time. Filling of the coronary circulation takes place chiefly during diastole, so this effect should aid myocardial oxygenation. Myocardial oxygenation is also improved by the reduction in diastolic heart size, which, by the operation of the La Place law, will allow the heart to increase the amount of useful work done for the same oxygen consumption (see Chapter 10). A third way in which digitalis may improve myocardial oxygenation is by improving the circulation in general and by raising the arterial blood pressure, thus improving coronary perfusion.

In addition to improving myocardial contractility and oxygenation, the cardiac glycosides cause a reduction in the heart rate in the failing heart. This slowing arises partly due to prolonged intracardiac conduction times resulting from the direct effects of the glycosides on the myocardial and pace-maker cells, and partly from the ability of the glycosides to sensitise the heart to acetylcholine, and reduce sensitivity to catecholamines. However, a large part of the cardiac slowing effect of the cardiac glycosides is due to the improvement in the circulation, resulting from the increased cardiac output and elevated blood pressure which follows their administration. Improvement of the circulation enables the failing heart, which may be exhibiting tachycardia, to resume a normal rate. For this reason, tachycardia *per se* is not necessarily an indication for the use of cardiac glycosides, although a reduction of tachycardia in the failing heart can be used as indication of an improved circulation.

If cardiac conductivity is generally slowed throughout the conducting tissues of the heart, and cardiac contractility is generally increased, the effect on excitability varies in different cardiac tissues. Excitability is in general decreased, but this effect is less marked in the ventricles than in the atria (Hoffman & Singer 1964). Conversely, automaticity is increased in the ventricles to a greater extent than in the atria, and this may account for the arrhythmias seen in digitalis intoxication.

The cardiac glycosides have some extracardiac effects. They sensitise the carotid baroreceptors, but overall tend to cause an increase in blood pressure by causing some degree of peripheral vasoconstriction (Mason & Braunwald 1964), and by a central action on the vasomotor centre. The other important extra cardiac action of the cardiac glycosides is the induction of diuresis which follows improved renal perfusion.

Overall, the actions of the cardiac glycosides on the heart may be summarised in terms of increased myocardial contractility, this being the chief effect of these agents, producing an increase in cardiac output in spite of a reduction in heart rate, if this has been elevated.

Certain factors modify the effects of the cardiac glycosides upon the heart:

1 Potassium concentration. A reduced extracellular potassium concentration will sensitise the myocardium to the cardiac glycosides.
2 Magnesium and calcium. Hypomagnesaemia and hypercalcaemia increase sensitivity.
3 Thyroid function. Hypothyroid human patients require lower levels of digitalis for maintenance than euthyroid individuals. The same appears to be true in dogs.
4 Drug interactions. The following interactions are noted by Jenkins and Clark (1977): digitalis + catecholamines — arrhythmias; digitalis + propranolol — bradycardia; digitalis + succinylcholine — potentiation of digitalis effects on contractility and excitability; digitalis + ketamine or droperidol — increased tolerance to digitalis.
5 Unknown factors. There is considerable variation in individual response of the myocardium to the cardiac glycosides, necessitating individual evaluation of the glycoside dosage.

Indications for the use of cardiac glycosides

Digitalis compounds are primarily indicated for the treatment of congestive heart failure caused by mild or severe failure of one or both ventricles.

Cardiac glycosides are most beneficial in treating failure resulting from ventricular overload (e.g. aortic or mitral insufficiency). However, it is important to treat the primary disease (e.g. infection, anaemia, etc.) when heart failure is secondary.

Arrhythmias also constitute an indication for the use of cardiac glycosides. In atrial fibrillation, digitalis improves myocardial efficiency reducing the ventricular rate, increasing cardiac output, reducing venous pressure and the pulse deficit. The dose of the glycoside is increased until the heart rate falls to less than 160 beats/minute. The value of digitalis in this situation depends upon its ability to delay conduction in the atrioventricular node, so that the ventricle only responds to a limited number of the atrial impulses.

Atrial and atrioventricular functional tachycardias may be treated with digitalis. Reflex vagal stimulation and increased atrioventricular nodal refractoriness mediate the action of digitalis in these cases.

Supraventricular tachycardia may result from digitalis intoxication and generally digitalis is contraindicated for the treatment of ventricular tachycardia and premature ventricular beats since ventricular fibrillation may be induced. Cardiac glycosides have also been used for the treatment of cardiac failure resulting from complete atrioventricular block. The myocardial performance is improved even though atrioventricular conduction may be further slowed and the arrhythmia exacerbated.

Contraindications

Digitalis intoxication is the primary contraindication to the use of digitalis glycosides (see below).

Partial or complete heart block of non-digitalis origin is not necessarily a contraindication to the use of digitalis, where the drug may be helpful in alleviating congestive heart failure. Similarly, ventricular premature contractions and ventricular tachycardias of non-digitalis origin may result from myocardial irritability, and may be improved by the judicious use of digitalis to improve myocardial function and reduce myocardial hypoxia, since hypoxic areas may act as stimulus points for ectopic foci.

Treatment with calcium salts or sympathomimetic agents should be regarded as relative contraindications for the use of cardiac glycosides (see above). Similarly dogs which have prolonged vomiting, diarrhoea or diuresis, and which may be hypokalaemic will be more sensitive to the actions of the cardiac glycosides and to their toxicity.

Prophylaxis

The prophylactic use of digitalis has been discussed by Detweiler and Knight (1977). They point out that the prophylactic use of digitalis has yet to be proven to be of value in controlled studies, but that there may be some rationale in using digitalis prophylaxis in certain circumstances:

1 Prior to surgery. Digitalis protects the heart against the myocardial depressant effects of most anaesthetics, and may prevent the development of anaesthetic-induced arrhythmias. Preoperative digitalisation has been advocated for aged dogs with any evidence of compromised cardiac function, even in the absence of cardiac failure.

2 Haemorrhagic shock. Prophylactic digitalisation may prolong survival in dogs subjected to experimental haemorrhagic shock.

3 Idiopathic hypertrophic aortic stenosis. Detweiler and Knight quote the results obtained by Williams and Braunwald (1965) showing that early administration of digitalis prevented the development of cardiac hypertrophy in rats in which the aorta was experimentally constricted.

However, the prophylactic use of digitalis is definitely not indicated in constrictive pericarditis or cardiac tamponade, in which it will not reduce the heart rate, nor in sinus arrhythmia, sinoatrial block or ventricular escape beats, unless heart failure is present. In general, in view of the potential toxicity of the cardiac glycosides, the cost-benefit relationship of digitalis prophylaxis is likely to be unfavourable, and extensive use of digitalis prophylaxis cannot be generally recommended at present, except in special circumstances.

Dosage

Determination of the dosage of digitalis glycosides is dictated by the fact that there is no fixed dose suitable for every individual animal. This is exemplified by the fact that animals with heart disease frequently have accompanying degenerative conditions of other organs which affect the uptake, utilisation and excretion of these glycosides.

This author is of the opinion that in the current socioeconomic climate establishing the optimum dose of digitalis is generally best achieved in the animals's home environment except where there is acute heart failure. The latter environment contains the dietary, exertional and emotional milieu in which the dog is to be maintained. This approach is used in conjunction with slow oral digitalisation. The dosages for the main cardiac glycosides may be summarised as follows:

1 Ouabain which is used by the intravenous route for emergencies: 0·04 mg/kg i.v. 25–50% initially then 25% every hour until the desired effect is achieved.

2 Digoxin.

a 0·05 mg/kg i.v. 25–50% initially then 25% every hour until the desired effect is achieved.

b 0·025 mg/kg/day orally, divided into two equal doses for the dog, and about half this dose rate for the cat.

3 Digitoxin: 0·05–0·1 mg/kg/day orally, divided into two equal doses.

Digoxin is the preferred glycoside because it can be used intravenously or orally, it has a fairly short duration of action orally which is helpful in reducing toxicity and has a greater efficacy in relieving congestive heart failure than does digitoxin (Ettinger 1966; Detweiler 1965).

Digitoxin is probably less inclined to cause vomiting than digoxin, and may be used as an alternative if excessive vomiting limits the use of digoxin.

In general, young patients are likely to require a relatively larger dose of glycoside either because their renal clearance rate is greater or because there is increased uptake of glycosides into erythrocytes. The actual formulation of the glycoside used is very important, and whilst a particular proprietary brand should remain reasonably consistent there may be significant variations between brands.

Slow oral digitalisation. The maintenance dose of digoxin is calculated on the basis of 0·25 mg/kg/day, and the owner is instructed to give half the dose twice daily. Since the half-life of digoxin is about 40–50 hours, it will require about 7–10 days for a steady state level to be obtained (Fig. 11.2). Significant therapeutic and/or toxic signs are likely to be seen towards the end of this period, and if no response is seen, the daily dosage may be increased. This approach is suitable formild cases, in which concurrent diuretic therapy is not required. A satisfactory response is determined by the amelioration of clinical signs. The

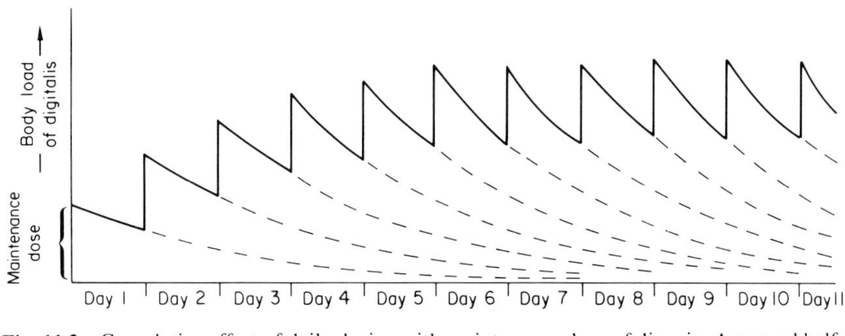

Fig. 11.2 Cumulative effect of daily dosing with maintenance dose of digoxin. A normal half-life of about 45 hours for digoxin in the dog is assumed which may not be correct for an animal in cardiac failure with impaired renal and hepatic function. Note the slow accumulation of digoxin over about 7 days (4 half-lives) after which daily dosing simply maintains total body load of digoxin without adding to it. For simplicity this Fig. shows the effect of once-daily dosing. Twice-daily dosing would produce less fluctuation in body load over each 24-hour period. ——— indicates total body load of digoxin at any given time; ---------- indicates exponential decrease in level which would occur if next dose was not given.

patient should clearly be examined at suitable intervals, in order to assess whether any alteration in dosage is called for. The dose may need to be reduced as the patient improves, as the general improvement in the circulation will lead to enhanced absorption of the glycoside. Where possible the blood glycoside levels should be monitored. Dosage errors are otherwise probably inevitable.

Rapid oral digitalisation. This method may be utilised when a more rapid response is called for in more severe cases of cardiac failure. However, this method is accompanied by a much greater risk of inducing digitalis toxicity.

A loading dose of 0·066 mg/kg is given on the first day, in divided doses. This is followed by administration of the maintenance dose, calculated as above, on day 2 and thereafter (Fig. 11.3).

Rapid parenteral digitalisation. Rapid parenteral digitalisation is reserved for cases in acute cardiac failure, especially where there is severe pulmonary oedema and cyanosis. The cardiac glycosides should be given intravenously, as intramuscular injection is painful.

The dosage regimes described above are used, and the procedure should be monitored electrocardiographically. Large intravenous doses of a suitable diuretic should also be given (e.g. frusemide 5–10 mg/kg 2-hourly), whilst morphine will reduce dyspnoea and provide sedation, as well as promoting the pooling of blood in splanchnic vessels and thus reducing pulmonary capillary pressure (Pyle 1977).

The doses quoted above should be reduced if factors enhancing bioavailability or myocardial sensitivity are thought to be present (see above). Cats are sensitive to digitalis glycosides, and rapid digitalisation should not be attempted in this species (Tilley & Weitz 1977).

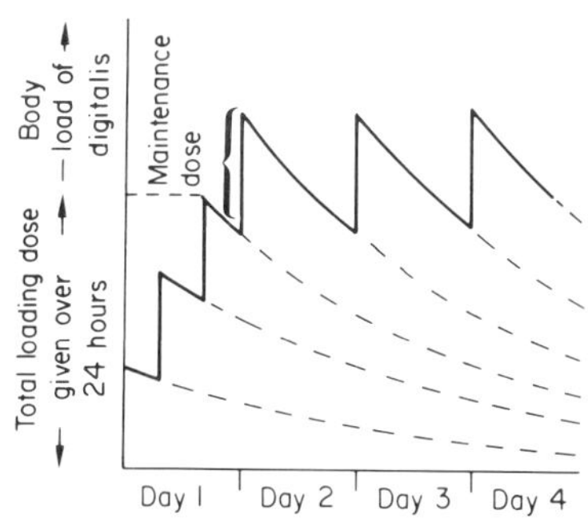

Fig. 11.3 Effect of rapid oral digitalisation on body load of digoxin. The same assumptions are made concerning half-life as in Fig. 11.2. In this case the loading dose is given in three doses over the first 24 hours, followed by daily maintenance dose. Loading dose ≏ 2.7 × maintenance dose. Constant body load is attained in 1–2 days.

Toxicity and its treatment

Clinically, the administration of an oral overdose of digitalis produces gastrointestinal signs such as anorexia, salivation and later vomiting and diarrhoea. Subsequently neurotoxic effects such as lethargy, weakness and even seizures may develop.

Electrocardiographically, cardiac glycosides produce prolongation of the P-R interval, S-T segment changes, and T-wave changes. At toxic levels, atrioventricular block proceeds to junctional arrhythmia, ventricular premature beats and ventricular tachycardia. The latter more serious arrhythmias usually follow intravenous digitialisation.

Factors promoting digitalis toxicity include patient sensitivity, renal or hepatic disease, acidosis, hypoxia and electrolyte imbalance.

Therapy for digitalis intoxication primarily involves cessation of treatment. Vomiting may be controlled with low doses of mild tranquillisers, and hypokalaemia may be rectified using potassium chloride in the food or by slow intravenous infusion. The electrocardiogram is monitored for peaking of the T wave indicating hyperkalaemia. Persistent ventricular arrhythmias may be treated with lidocaine (lignocaine) or a β adrenergic blocking agent, such as propranolol.

METHYLXANTHINES

Drugs included in this group are caffeine, theophylline, theobromine, aminophylline and etamiphylline.

The chief use of the methylxanthines in human cardiology is in acute cardiac failure, especially when accompanied by paroxysmal dyspnoea, when slow intravenous or intramuscular injection of aminophylline may produce a significant improvement in the patient rather more rapidly than intravenous digitalisation, the latter treatment being used after the aminophylline, so that the effects of the digitalis become apparent as those of the aminophylline disappear (Ritchie 1975).

As discussed in Chapter 10, the methylxanthines have powerful inotropic and chronotropic actions, and relax and bronchial smooth musculature. They also have a general stimulatory action on the central nervous system, producing a useful increase in the depth and rate of respiration by their action on the respiratory centre. They produce peripheral vasodilatation, which may be especially relevant in the coronary circulation, but this activity is offset to some extent by centrally mediated vasoconstriction resulting from stimulation of the vasomotor centre. The increased cardiac rate and contractility result in an increased cardiac output, leading to an increased glomerular filtration rate and a mild diuresis. Aminophylline may also inhibit the tubular resorption of sodium (Rubin *et al* 1968). However, Jenkins and Clark (1977) state that refractoriness develops within 1–2 days.

Indications

The methylxanthines have been used in veterinary practice when a mild diuretic action is required to augment cardiac glycoside therapy. Aminophylline, which is theophylline plus ethylenediamine, is used as an adjunct to digitalis when an adequate response to the glycoside cannot be obtained without producing toxic effects, and may be most useful in this respect, allowing satisfactory control of an otherwise intractable case to be obtained. Lack of pharmacokinetic data makes it difficult to recommend suitable dose rates for these agents in small animals, except in the case of etamiphylline camsylate (Bogan 1977). This agent has been extensively used in the UK as a mild cardiostimulatory drug in dogs believed to be suffering from some form of cardiac disorder. Bogan has shown that the plasma half-life of etamiphylline is extremely short in the dog (about 60 minutes) following oral or intramuscular injection, but that satisfactory plasma levels should be maintained provided that the camsylate were to be given orally at intervals of 4–8 hours, and in adequate dosage. In contrast to theophylline, etamiphylline does not increase heart rate, and produces a net fall in blood pressure when injected intravenously.

Toxicity

Etamiphylline camsylate was given by Bogan at doses up to 28 mg/kg, and at this dose rate there appears to be little danger of excessive stimulation of the nervous system, which is the chief toxic feature of the methylxanthines, whilst excessive tachycardia is a sign of overdosage with those members of the group which accelerate the heart rate. At high doses the methylxanthines may be arrhythmogenic, which might potentially limit their usefulness in augmenting the actions of the cardiac glycosides.

11.2.2 Antiarrhythmic therapy

The basic mechanisms which are treated are those of ectopic beats and re-entry beats. These involve the electrophysiological alterations of changes in automaticity and changes in conduction together with combinations thereof (Table 11.2).

QUINIDINE

Quinidine (the dextroisomer of quinine) exerts its effects through:

1 Depression of myocardial contractility.
2 Depression of conduction.
3 Depression of automaticity.

Table 11.2 Classification of cardiac arrhythmias

Escape rhythms

1 Sinoatrial block: digitalis intoxication; chronic degenerative myocardial disease occasionally present in healthy hearts.
2 Wandering pacemaker: usually benign; occasional A/V junctional escape beats.
3 Ventricular escape rhythm: complete A/V block.

Extrasystoles

1 Ventricular extrasystoles: usually associated with some degree of myocardial disease, but may be benign.
2 Atrial extrasystoles.
3 Junctional and sinus extrasystoles.
4 Return extrasystoles (reciprocal rhythm).

Parasystole

Ectopic beats at constant intervals due to presence of independent pacemaker.

Tachycardias

(Defined as 'runs' of more than three extrasystoles together)

Arrhythmia	Causes
1 Atrial tachycardia *2* Atrial flutter *3* Atrial fibrillation	Mitral valve disease Hypertension Ischaemia Thyrotoxicosis Thoracotomy Digitalis intoxication
4 A/V junctional tachycardia	
5 Ventricular tachycardia *6* Ventricular flutter *7* Ventricular fibrillation	Ischaemia Digitalis intoxication Hypothermia Complete heart block

4 Prolongation of the effective refractory period of hear muscle and conductive tissue.
5 Vagolytic effects and anticholinergic effects (peripheral vasodilation).

These features reduce ectopic activity but collectively result in an increased cardiac rate at therapeutic dosages and a decreased arterial blood pressure.

Indications

Atrial and junctional arrhythmias. Quinidine has long been used for converting atrial fibrillation, to sinus rhythm and for maintaining it in man. However, in dogs quinidine has proved of very limited value in this respect (Detweiler 1957; Pyle, 1967). The objective has been to lower the ventricular rate using digitalis prior to conversion with quinidine. Similarly, quinidine may be used to convert atrial flutter and is sometimes effective for treating supraventricular paroxysmal tachycardia where digitalis therapy has failed.

Ventricular premature contractions and tachycardia. Premature ventricular beats are usually a sign of serious heart disease and in an undigitalised dog quinidine may be used to convert the ectopic beats together with digitalis to improve the performance of the failing myocardium.

Persistent unifocal and multifocal ventricular tachycardia is a life-threatening arrhythmia and is controlled with lignocaine, procainamide or direct current conversion. Quinidine which takes 30–90 minutes to act following intramuscular administration may then be used for 4–6 weeks to achieve long-term control.

Contraindications

Basically, the use of quinidine is contraindicated in the following.

1 Idiosyncratic hypersensitivity.
2 Sinoatrial, atrioventricular and intraventricular block.
3 Poor myocardial function.

None of the antiarrhythmic agents in this section is safe for use in cats (Tilley & Weitz 1977).

Dosage

There is no fixed dosage for quinidine preparations. By the oral route, quinidine reaches its maximal effect in 1–3 hours and lasts for 6–8 hours. Intramuscularly, the drug reaches its peak effect in 30–90 minutes and is excreted in the urine within 24 hours in man (Moe & Abildskov 1965).

The oral range is 8–20 mg/kg, starting at the lower end of the range and being repeated every 2 hours in acute cases and every 6–8 hours in established cases until conversion is achieved or toxicity intervenes. The dosage for acute cases is used when the intramuscular route is employed. For maintenance therapy, the long-acting quinidine preparations may be given every 8–12 hours.

Toxicity (cinchonism) and its treatment

The following are features of quinidine intoxication:

1 Anorexia, vomiting, diarrhoea, inco-ordination.
2 Hypotension and decreased myocardial contractility.

3 Thrombocytopaenia.
4 Electrocardiographically, there is prolongation of the P wave, the P-R and Q-T intervals and of the QRS duration with atrioventricular block, ventricular tachycardia or ventricular fibrillation.

There is no specific antidote although combinations of quinidine with procainamide reduce the chance of toxicity.

PROCAINAMIDE

The amide of procaine was developed to prolong the action of procaine.

Mechanism of action

Procainamide acts like quinidine. It depresses automaticity and conduction in the atria and ventricles. The effective refractory period is lengthened and there is a slight vagolytic and anticholinergic effect which may increase the heart rate. Cardiac contractility is depressed less than with quinidine at therapeutic levels and there is little effect on blood pressure except when procainamide is given intravenously. The electrocardiogram shows prolongation of the QRS complex and P-R and Q-T intervals.

Indications

Procainamide is used primarily to treat ventricular arrhythmias such as ventricular premature contractions and unifocal and multifocal ventricullar tachycardia. Procainamide is preferred to quinidine for treating these arrhythmias but lignocaine or β adrenergic blocking agents are preferable when the arrhythmias are induced by digitalis. Procainamide is only of limited value for treating atrial tachycardia.

Contraindications

Procainamide is contraindicated where there is sinoatrial, atrioventricular and intraventricular block. Similarly, the drug is discontinued when nausea, vomiting and anorexia develop.

Dosage

Procainamide may be administered orally, intramuscularly or intravenously. It is absorbed completely from the gastrointestinal tract, reaching peak plasma concentration in 1 hour. The suggested total daily dosage is not to exceed 50 mg/kg divided into four equal doses daily. Intravenously, the drug is effective within minutes and should be maintained by oral administration. The safety factor is less than that by the oral route, and the animal should be monitored for signs of hypotension together with electrocardiographic monitoring. The dose rate is a 100 mg intravenous bolus which may be repeated if necessary and 10–40 mg/kg/minute via intravenous infusion. Noradrenaline may be used to maintain the blood pressure. Procainamide is excreted primarily by the kidneys in dogs and care should be used where there is impairment of renal function.

Toxicity and its treatment

Signs of toxicity include hypotension, decreased cardiac contractility, anorexia, vomiting, diarrhoea, central nervous system depression and ventricular tachycardia and asystole. Chronic administration may produce agranulocytosis. Cessation of procainamide therapy and the commencement of supportive therapy are indicated in this situation.

LIGNOCAINE

Mechanism of action

Lignocaine (diethylaminoacet 2, 6 xylidide) does not affect the systemic arterial blood pressure or myocardial contractility significantly in therapeutic dosages (Harrison *et al* 1963) but it does decrease ventricular excitability and automaticity. In normal tissue it depresses conduction but improves it in depressed tissue. The absolute refractory period is not affected significantly by lignocaine but the effective refractory period is lengthened relative to the action potential duration. Lignocaine has been widely used for the treatment of ventricular arrhythmias.

Indications

Lignocaine must be used without adrenaline and its primary indication is for the management of acute ventricular arrhythmias resulting from cardiac catheterisation, cardiac surgery, cardiac diseases and digitalis intoxication. Specifically lignocaine is used for treating R or T ventricular premature contractions, multifocal ventricular premature contractions paroxysmal unifocal ventricular tachycardia and prophylactically after ventricular fibrillation.

Contraindications

Sinoatrial, atrioventricular and intraventricular block or any time when there is excessive prolongation of the P-R interval or QRS complex form contraindications for the use of this drug.

Dosage

Lignocaine is mainly metabolised by the liver and is excreted through the kidneys. The dosage varies from 1 to 2 mg/kg as an acute bolus intravenously or from 4 to 8 mg/kg over a few minutes. The duration of effect is from 10 to 20 minutes with repeated doses at 20-minute intervals. A constant intravenous infusion of 50 μg/kg/min (12·5 ml of 2% lignocaine in 500 ml of 5% dextrose produces a 500 μg/kg/ml solution) may be used, but quinidine or other antiarrhythmic agents administered orally are preferable for prolonged therapy. For digitalis-induced ventricular tachycardia, procainamide and quinidine are not used because of the possibility of combined intoxication.

Toxicity and its treatment

Central nervous system excitement progressing to convulsions may occur with an overdose of lignocaine and is treated with diazepam or ultrashort-acting barbiturates intravenously. Hypotension and bradycardia are other signs consistent with excessive lignocaine therapy.

PHENYTOIN SODIUM (diphenylhydantoin sodium)

Mechanism of action

Diphenylhydantoin sodium depresses automaticity and improves conduction in normal and diseased tissue. Again as with lignocaine, the effective refractory period is lengthened relative to the action potential duration but in addition there is decreased efferent sympathetic activity in cardiac nerves.

Indications

This drug is most useful for the treatment of digitalis-induced arrhythmias in man. In addition, diphenylhydantoin may be used in combination with other antiarrhythmic drugs to treat supraventricular and ventricular arrhythmias.

Contraindications

There are none of major significance.

Dosage

The oral route is recommended, at a dose rate of 24 mg/kg initially, followed by 15–25 mg/kg, in 3–4 divided doses daily (Muir 1976).

Toxicity

Hypotension, sinus bradycardia and ventricular arrest may result from unduly high doses of this drug.

Of the remaining drugs that act as antiarrhythmic agents, it is helpful for the clinician to view them in the light of their pharmacological classification. Included in this category are drugs which are important in cardiovascular pharmacotherapy for their antitussive and bronchodilator effects.

DRUGS ACTING AT THE ADRENERGIC RECEPTOR SITES

1 SYMPATHOMIMETIC AGENTS

The general properties and mode of action of the sympathomimetic agents are described in Chapter 10. Adrenaline and noradrenaline have few indications other than for stimulation of the asystolic heart. Isoprenaline has an almost pure β action, and thus produces increased heart rate and contractility, relaxation of bronchial smooth muscle and peripheral vasodilatation. It is the drug of choice for the treatment of complete heart block when clinical signs such as Stokes–Adams seizures are present, as well as its use in the treatment of cardiac standstill. Heart block may be treated with isoprenaline 5 μg/ ml in 5% dextrose as an intravenous infusion, the rate of administration being adjusted until a ventricular rate of 100–120 beats/minute is achieved (Ettinger 1969), or with a single bolus of 0·05 mg/ml intravenously (Buchanan *et al* 1968). Sustained release isoprenaline tablets may be used 4–6 times daily. Elixir and sublingual preparations are not recommended.

2 ADRENERGIC BLOCKING AGENTS

The α adrenergic blocking agents phenoxybenzamine and phentolamine hydrochloride have been used in dogs in the treatment of shock (Ogburn, 1976), and in digitalis-induced arrhythmias. The object is to improve cardiac activity and increase peripheral blood flow. Fluid therapy for volume replacement is important if hypotension is to be avoided.

The most widely used β blocking agent is propranolol. Since cardiac β_1 receptors are blocked by the agent, cardiac automaticity and conductivity are decreased and there is a lengthening of the effective refractory period of cardiac cells. It is clear, therefore, that this agent will be of value in the treatment of cardiac arrhthmias.

Indications

Propranolol is used primarily for atrial arrhythmias, and, when necessary, for arrhythmias induced by digitalis glycosides. The drug is also helpful in slowing the ventricular rate in atrial fibrillation when digitalis is ineffective. When arrhythmias are thought to arise in association with excessive sympathetic activity, propranolol is clearly indicated, and also in the treatment of anaesthetic-induced arrhythmias, insofar as these have a sympathetic component. However, both propranolol and the cardiotoxic anaesthetics depress the myocardium, so propranolol should be used with great care in this situation. Tilley and Weitz (1977) suggest that propranolol is the only antiarrhythmic agent which is safe for use in the cat, and the same authors recommend its use in the treatment of both hypertrophic and congestive forms of feline idiopathic cardiomyopathy.

Contraindications

1 Severe and intractable heart failure.
2 Sinus bradycardia.
3 Restrictive and obstructive lung disease.

Dosage

1 One to three mg by slow intravenous infusion, stopping when the desired effect has been reached. Great care is required when administering this agent to animals with heart failure.
2 Five to sixty mg orally 6-hourly for maintenance.

Toxicity

Toxicity from propranolol is manifested by cardiac depression, bradycardia, hypotension and bronchospasm. During heart failure, retention of sodium and water is enhanced as a result of diminished cardiac output and altered renal haemodynamics.

11.2.3 Diuretic therapy

The primary functions of the kidney are to excrete waste material and to maintain water, electrolyte and acid-base balances. These last three functions are achieved through mechanisms which affect sodium reabsorption.

1 Active transport of sodium chloride from the glomerular filtrate throughout the tubules and collecting ducts, except in the descending limb of the loop of Henle.
2 Exchange of sodium ions for hydrogen ions, facilitated by carbonic anhydrase.
3 Exchange of sodium ions for potassium ions through the mediation of the angiotensin-aldosterone system.

Antidiuretic hormone acts chiefly in the collecting ducts to effect further resorption of water.

During heart failure, sodium and water retention are enhanced as a result of diminished cardiac output and altered renal haemodynamics, which in turn cause increased secretion of both aldosterone and antidiuretic hormone. Cardiac glycosides, and to a lesser extent the methylxanthines, tend to improve the cardiac output and renal blood flow, thus alleviating the fluid retention. In more severe cases, and when cardiac glycosides alone are ineffective, diuretics are of considerable use in relieving the sodium and water load. The following groups of diuretics are of interest to the veterinary clinician.

THIAZIDES

The thiazide diuretics act primarily as saluretics. Most evidence suggests that they inhibit sodium and chloride resorption in the proximal tubules. They are also weak carbonic anhydrase inhibitors.

Indications

Thiazides are useful diuretics, possessing high efficacy, low toxicity, high acceptability and a reasonable potency. By inhibiting proximal tubular sodium reabsorption, thiazides reduce or prevent the accumulation of both sodium and water, and are useful in the treatment or prophylaxis of ascites and pulmonary oedema. There is very little tendency to drug refractoriness with agents of this group.

Contraindications

1 Severe electrolyte imbalance.
2 Marked renal and hepatic impairment.
3 Acute circulatory failure ('shock').

Administration

Following oral administration, thiazides are well-absorbed and diuresis commences in 1 hour, and persists for 12–24 hours. Initially they may be given twice daily, but maintenance is usually achieved with a diminished dose given once daily. Several different thiazide diuretics are available: chlorothiazide, hydrochlorthiazide, benzhydroflumethiazide, and cyclopenthiazide are examples in common use. The dose range varies widely with the compound used.

Toxicity

Hypokalaemia tends to develop with protracted use, and this may be dangerous if the diuretic is given together with a cardiac glycoside. The liklihood of hypokalaemia developing may be reduced by using the medication on alternate days only. Another approach is to give potassium-rich foods, or by administering a suitable potassium preparation. If such is to be used, the slow-release preparations are very much better tolerated than potassium chloride.

FRUSEMIDE (furosemide)

Mechanism of action

Frusemide is an anthranilic acid derivative which inhibits the tubular reabsorption of sodium in the proximal and distal convoluted tubules and in the ascending loop of Henle. It does not interfere with the action of aldosterone or carbonic anhydrase inhibitors and may be used concurrently with compounds of the latter type. It is especially effective in the cat (Tilley & Weitz 1977).

Indications

The use of frusemide is indicated in almost any situation where fluid overload is to be treated. It is indicated when other diuretics have failed and when the haemodynamic state grossly reduces the glomerular filtration rate and leads to sodium overload in the body.

Contraindications

1 Severe electrolyte imbalance.
2 Shock.

Both frusemide and ethacrynic acid are potentially ototoxic, and should not be administered with the aminoglycoside antibiotics for this reason.

Dosage

1 Intravenously, frusemide is given at a rate of 5–40 mg (depending on the dog's size) initially and this may be repeated in 2 hours (Ettinger & Suter 1970). Much higher doses have been recommended (Muir 1976), but these have generally been tried in normal dogs. The diuresis starts within 5 minutes, peaks within 30 minutes and persists for 2 hours.

2 Orally, frusemide is administered at 2–4 mg/kg/day divided twice daily with an upper limit of 120 mg per dose. After oral administration diuresis begins within 1 hour, peaks at 2 hours and is complete within 6–8 hours. Intermittent rather than continuous therapy is recommended because of the high potency of frusemide.

ETHACRYNIC ACID

Ethacrynic acid is methylene butyryl phenoxyacetic acid. Although it is chemically different from fursemide its mechanism of action, indications, contraindications and toxicity are all similar to those of furosemide. Hypokalaemia, hypochloraemia and alkalosis are serious side-effects.

Dosage

1 Intravenously, 3–4 mg/kg/day is recommended.
2 Orally, 50–100 mg/day is the suggested dose rate (Muir 1976).

POTASSIUM SPARING AGENTS

1 SPIRONOLACTONE

Spironolactone is a synthetic steroid which competes with aldosterone and thereby inhibits sodium reabsorption in the distal renal tubules. Additionally, spironolactone prevents potassium loss from this portion of the nephron.

Use of the drug is indicated not only for treating the oedema of congestive heart failure but also that resulting from primary hyperaldosteronism.

The diuretic effects of spironolactone are limited and take 2–3 days to exert their effect. Spironolactone is also expensive and as a result of these properties the drug is used in combination with thiazides.

2 TRIAMTERENE

Triamterene interferes with distal tubular transport of sodium. There is an excretion of sodium and chlorine and a retention of potassium which may lead, in overdose, to hyperkalaemia. Triamterene is used in combination with other diuretics and for cases of refractory oedema. The dosage is 2–4 mg/kg/day and is available in combination with both hydrochlorothiazide and with benzthiazide.

3 AMILORIDE

Amiloride hydrochloride is another potassium sparing diuretic available either in 5 mg tablets or in combination with hydrochlorothiazide.

11.2.4 Antitussives and bronchodilators

One of the classic signs associated with left heart failure is the presence of a 'cardiac cough' which may be associated with several factors other than circulatory failure alone. Some of these factors result from the presence of a persistent cough and some exacerbate the cough, the primary cause of which is heart failure. These factors include tonsillitis, laryngitis tracheitis, bronchitis, bronchiolitis, bronchiectasis, emphysema, pulmonary fibrosis, pulmonary congestion and tracheal collapse.

Therapy of these secondary factors which may become of primary importance is as follows:

1 Antitussives.
2 Brochodilators.
3 Antibiotics.
4 Diuretics.
5 Steroids.

In treating these conditions it is important to remember that the drugs employed may have significant effect on cardiac performance. Broncho-constriction is a major component of the cough reflex and brochodilation is an important characteristic of antitussive agents. Table 11.3 lists some of the antitussive and bronchodilator agents in current use.

Table 11.3 Antitussive and bronchodilator agents

Cough suppressants
Opiates: codeine, pholcodine, methadone, dextromethorphan, noscapine (non-narcotic opiate alkaloid).
Non-opiate agents: dimethoxanate, pipazathate (phenothiazine esters), chlophedianol, carbetapentane, benzonatate, and several others. Agents in this group are of dubious efficacy in general.
Phenobarbitone, amylobarbitone.
Bronchodilators
Methylxanthines: theophylline, proxyphylline, aminophylline, choline theophyllinate, acepifylline, etamiphylline, diprophylline, bamifylline.
β adrenergic agents: isoprenaline, orciprenaline, terbutaline, adrenaline, isoetharine, methoxyphenamine, ephedrine, salbutamol.
Corticosteroids.
Anticholinergic agents.
Mixtures
Numerous mixtures of the agents listed above are available, whilst other proprietary mixtures contain both expectorants and cough suppressants.

11.2.5 Low sodium diets

A diet that is low in sodium may form an important adjunct to cardiac therapy. Normal dogs can tolerate fairly large quantities of ingested salt but a dog that is compensating for heart disease can easily be driven into heart failure in this way. Several mechanisms may be involved in the sodium retention that is associated with heart failure all of which are dependent on the diminished cardiac output (Friedberg 1966).

Because dogs with heart failure have this diminished ability to excrete ingested salt, the clinician may wish to introduce a low sodium diet. However, low sodium diets are contraindicated in chronic nephritis, adrenal cortical conditions and general debilitation, dehydration and chronic diarrhoea. In addition, a low sodium diet has generally not been recommended as a preventative or precautionary measure (Rubin 1975) although in humans, diets designed for improved longevity do restrict sodium intake (Leonard *et al* 1974). Many owners are also reluctant to adopt the use of these diets and face their inconvenience. Commercially prepared low sodium diets help to overcome this inconvenience but such diets are frequently of low palatibility. As with any dietary regime, it must be strictly adhered to without supplementation. A high caloric intake, 60–80 cal/kg in the active older dog, and high quality protein is required.

Tables for such diets are well documented in veterinary literature (Ettinger & Suter 1970; Schuchman 1974) together with guidance in making the food palatable and easy to prepare.

References

Baggott J. D. & Davis L. E. (1973) Plasma protein binding of digitoxin and digoxin in several mammalian species. *Res. Vet. Sci.* **15**, 81.

Blaine D. (1841) *Canine Pathology. A Description of the Diseases of Dogs.* 4th edn. Longmans, Orme & Co., London.

Bogan J. A. (1977) *Kinetics of etamiphylline camsylate in the dog, horse and bovine.* Unpublished report.

Braunwald E. & Pool P. E. (1968) Mechanism of action of digitalis glycosides (I and II). *Mod. Concepts Cardiovasc. Dis.* **37**, 129.

Breznock E. M. (1975) Effects of phenobarbital on digitoxin and digoxin elimination in the dog. *Amer. J. Vet. Res.* **36**, 371.

Buchanan J., Dear M. G., Pyle R. L. & Berg P. (1968) Medical and pacemaker therapy of complete heart block and congestive heart failure in a dog. *J. Amer. Vet. Med. Ass.* **152**, 1099.

Detweiler D. K. (1957) Electrocardiographic and clinical features of spontaneous auricular fibrillation and flutter (tachycardia) in dogs. *Zbl. Veterinarmed.* **6**, 509.

Detweiler D. K. (1965) Cardiac glycosides in the treatment of congestive heart failure in dogs. *Anim. Hosp.* **1**, 29.

Detweiler D. K. & Knight D. H. (1977) Congestive heart failure in dogs: Therapeutic concepts. *J. Amer. Vet. Med. Ass.* **171**, 106.

Ettinger S. J. (1966) Therapeutic digitalisation of the dog in congestive heart failure. *J. Amer. Vet. Med. Ass.* **148**, 525.

Ettinger S. J. (1969) Isoproterenol treatment of atrioventricular block in the dog. *J. Amer. Vet. Med. Ass.* **154**, 398.

Ettinger S. J. & Suter P. F. (1970) *Canine Cardiology*. 1st edn. p. 254. W. B. Saunders, Philadelphia.

Friedberg C. (1966) *Diseases of the Heart*. 3rd edn. W. B. Saunders, Philadelphia.

Hamlin R. L. (1978) Personal communication.

Hamlin R. L., Dutta S. & Smith C. R. (1971) Effects of digoxin and digitoxin on ventricular function in normal dogs and dogs with heart failure. *Amer. J. Vet. Res.* **32**, 1391.

Harrison D. C., Sprouse J. M. & Morrow A. G. (1963) The antiarrhythmic properties of lidocaine and procainamide. *Circulation* **28**, 486.

Hoffman B. F. & Singer D. H. (1964) Effects of digitalis on electrical activity of cardiac fibres. *Prog. Cardiovasc. Dis.* **7**, 226.

Jenkins W. L. & Clark D. R. (1977) A review of drugs affecting the heart. *J. Amer. Vet. Med. Ass.* **171**, 85.

Leonard Hofer & Pritikin (1974) *Live Longer Now*. Grosset & Dunop, New York.

Mason D. T. & Braunwald E. (1964) Studies on digitalis. X. Effects of ouabain on forearm vascular resistance and venous tone in normal subjects and in patients in heart failure. *J. Clin. Invest.* **43**, 532.

Moe G. K. & Adildskov J. A. (1965) Antiarrhythmic drugs. In *The Pharmacological Basis of Therapeutics* 3rd edn., eds. L. S. Goodman p. 699. Macmillan, New York.

Muir W. W. (1976) Pharmacotherapy of cardiac drugs. In *Sci. Proc. 43rd Ann. Meeting A.A.H.A.*, Anaheim, California, p. 89.

Ogburn P. (1976) The role of vasoactive agents in shock therapy. *Vet. Clin. N. Amer.* **6:2**, 287.

Pyle R. L. (1967) Conversion of atrial fibrillation with quinidine sulphate in a dog. *J. Amer. Vet. Med. Ass.* **151**, 582.

Pyle R. L. (1977) The clinical management of congestive heart failure in the dog. *Clin. Pharmacol. Newsletter* (Colorado State Univ.) **2:5**.

Ritchie J. M. (1975) The xanthines. In *The Pharmacological Basis of Therapeutics*. 5th. edn., eds. L. S. Goodman & A. Gilman, p. 367. Macmillan, New York.

Rubin G. J. (1975) Cardiovascular pharmacology. In *Sci. Proc. 42nd. Ann. Meeting A.A.H.A.* Cincinnati, Ohio. p. 58.

Rubin I. L., Gross H. & Arbeit S. R. (1968) *The Treatment of Heart Disease in the Adult*. Lea & Febiger, Philadelphia.

Schuchman S. M. (1974) Low sodium diet. In *Current Veterinary Therapy*, ed. R. W. Kirk. p. 325 W. B. Saunders, Philadelphia.

Tilley L. P. & Weitz J. (1977) Pharmacologic and other forms of medical therapy in feline cardiac disease. *Vet. Clin. N. Amer.* **7:2**, 415.

Williams J. F. & Braunwald E. (1965) Studies on digitalis. Effects of digoxin on the development of cardiac hypertrophy in the rat subjected to aortic construction. *Amer. J. Cardiol.* **16**, 534.

Withering W. (1785) An account of the foxglove and some of its medical uses. Reprinted in part in *Classics of Cardiology: A Collection of Classic Works on the Heart and Circulation*, eds. F. Willus & T. E. Keys, vol. 1. Dover Pub., New York.

12
The use of anthelmintics in dogs and cats

R. M. CONNAN

The helminths of the dog and cat which are more or less common in Britain are listed in Table 12.1. In addition to these, a number of others occur more rarely. *Angiostrongylus vasorum* for instance and a filarial parasite, probably a *Dipetalonema* spp., both of which have been found in greyhounds recently imported from Ireland (Jacobs & Prole 1975; Stevenson *et al* 1975). Certainly the latter and possibly both species can be transmitted in Britain. Other parasites are found in imported dogs during or soon after the quarantine period. Among the most common in this category are *Ancylostoma caninum* and *Dirofilaria immitis*, but neither of these have been reported from indigenous dogs and presumably therefore they are incapable of establishing themselves in Britain.

The prevalence and distribution of the helminths varies widely, not only between the species, but also between animals kept under different systems of management.

12.1 Ascarid species

Toxocara canis is at once the most widespread of the nematodes and because of its public health relevance, also the most important. Table 12.2 summarises data on its prevalence in Britain (for a more detailed account see

Table 12.1 The common helminths of cats and dogs in Great Britain.

	Dog	Cat
Toxocara species	+	+
Toxascaris leonina	+	+
Uncinaria stenocephala	+	–
Trichuris vulpis	+	–
Filaroides osleri	+	–
Aelurostrongylus abstrusus	–	+
Dipylidium caninum	+	+
Taenia species	+	+
Echinococcus granulosus	+	–

Table 12.2 Prevalence of *T. canis* and *T. leonina* in dogs.

Reference	Site	Type of dog	*T. canis*	*T. leonina*
Holt (1976)	Oldham	Unwormed puppies	67%	
		Wormed puppies	33%	
Jacobs & Prole (1976)	London	Greyhounds	12%	
Oldham (1965)	London	Street dogs	6%	2%
Read & Thompson (1976)	Leeds	Street dogs	13%	20%
Sloan (1961)	General	Various	18%	12%
Turner & Pegg (1977)	London	Suburban pets	7.2% 44% pups <3 m.o.	2.7%
Weston (1975)	General	Various	26%, 1968 falling to 10%, 1973	
Woodruff (1970)	London	Street dogs	21%, 1963 falling to 2%, 1969	

Jacobs *et al* 1977). In what may be termed street dogs, there are indications that the prevalence may have declined in recent years, perhaps because of the increasing attention focussed upon the public health aspect of the infection. However, the parasite has a marked age prevalence being transmitted prenataly and in colostrum and it continues to be extremely common in puppies.

Second stage larvae may be acquired and remain in the tissues of the adult animal for years and it is from these in particular that the bitch infects her puppies. While in the tissues or while migrating in the body of the puppy however, larvae are insusceptible to the available anthelmintics. There is therefore, as yet, no value in treating the bitch during pregnancy unless she is actually passing *T. canis* eggs. Successful therapy requires the worms to be allowed to re-enter the intestine. This they do from the third day postpartum onward. However, not all of them reach the intestine at once and small numbers may continue to do so for several weeks.

Patent infections in the puppy (i.e. female worms depositing ova) are present from the end of the third week of life. Anthelmintic must therefore be given before this. Since most larvae are in the intestine by the end of the second week the first treatment should be given then, but it must be repeated at least twice at 10–14-day intervals. Since the bitch also has a patent infection as a result of ingesting migrated larvae in the faeces of her pups, she too must be treated at the same time.

For the control of this species an anthelmintic is required which is at once of high efficiency, safe and easy in use. Unfortunately, although a number of excellent products are available, none yet fully satisfy these requirements. The piperazine salts are well known and satisfy the second two criteria, but they are often not fully effective. However, worms surviving the first treatment are usually eliminated following the second.

Two more recent anthelmintics available in Britain are dichlorvos and mebendazole. Both have a high efficacy against *Toxocara* spp. and *Toxascaris leonina*. The latter, however, in common with a number of other recent benzimidazoles, must be given night and morning for 2 days for optimum efficacy in dogs and cats. While this may not tax the memory or present undue problems for the treatment of animals after weaning, it is less convenient when treating suckling puppies. Dichlorvos, having a similar high efficacy, has the advantage that it need be administered only once per treatment. However, as an organophosphorus compound and a potent cholinesterase inhibitor it is relatively toxic and must be treated with respect (see Chapter 13).

All three of the ascarid species are potentially capable of causing visceral larva migrans in man although it is generally agreed that *T. canis* is the most important. It is therefore essential to prevent contamination of the environment and to check the success of therapy by subsequent faecal examination. The survey by Holt (1976), in which he found a continuing patent infection in one in three treated puppies, amply confirms this. The mere observation of expelled worms in the faeces is not enough because expulsion may be incomplete.

Patent infections are often present in mature dogs although usually of smaller magnitude than in puppies. The literature implies that patent infection cannot follow the ingestion of eggs, for in experimental infections of adult dogs, larvae migrate to the tissues. However, Jacobs *et al* (1977) reported finding immature worms in the small intestine of adult greyhounds and it is also the experience of the present author that mature dogs do sometimes acquire patent infections without having access to suitable paratenic hosts (e.g. small rodents), with larvae in their tissues. For this reason, after weaning, dogs should continue to be regularly screened by faecal examination and treated as required until such time as, for the individual animal, it may be considered to be unnecessary.

All three products mentioned are available for use in cats, but the same disadvantages of each are perhaps more pronounced here. Prenatal infection with *Toxocara cati* does not occur and though it can be transmitted through the mammary gland, the age prevalence is less marked, and for this reason, mebendazole, either as a tablet, or given in food or milk, may be the drug of choice in view of its efficacy and safety. Dichlorvos appears to have a relatively high toxicity for cats and may only be used in the tablet form.

12.2 Hookworm

Uncinaria stenocephala is particularly common in kennels where animals share confined exercise areas, especially in grass or earthen paddocks.

Infection is transmitted orally and by penetration of third stage larvae through the skin.

Probably more than 50% of kennelled greyhounds under 2 years of age are infected, but the prevalence declines in older animals (Hovell & Weston 1970; Jacobs & Prole 1976). It is similarly widespread in foxhounds. Although also common in many breeding kennels, the combined effects of anthelmintic treatment, the development of immunity and the absence of reinfection after the sale of puppies, renders it rather rare in companion animals.

In Britain, *Ancylostoma caninum* has only been recorded in dogs after recent importation and treatment is therefore confined to the quarantine period.

The anthelmintics mebendazole and dichlorvos represent great advances in the treatment of these infections. The efficacy of both is almost absolute at recommended rates, but the former must be given for a full 5-day course.

In addition to anthelmintics however, the control of *Uncinaria* requires some attempt to limit reinfection. Jacobs (1976) has shown the kinetics of infective larvae on grass-runs to be comparable to that of many of the strongyloid and trichostrongloid parasites. Peak numbers are reached in late summer and some larvae persist to the following summer. The object therefore, should either be to exercise dogs in clean concrete-runs from which faeces are removed, or to prevent contamination with hookworm ova by the use of anthelmintic administered regularly to all animals, especially in the spring and early summer.

12.3 Trichuris vulpis

Although the need to treat this infection may be infrequent, it has been troublesome in the past because few of the available anthelmintics were effective. Again it is a parasite of kennelled animals, being very infrequent in companion animals.

In the recent past phthalofyne and methyridine have been of value, but these have been superseded by mebendazole and dichlorvos, both with very high efficacy at recommended rates.

12.2 Lungworms

Filaroides osleri is generally an infrequent but widespread parasite of dogs, probably again occurring most commonly in kennelled animals. Hovell and Weston (1970) reported a prevalence of 18% in greyhounds and 6·25% in other dogs, based on faecal examinations of a small sample. Jacobs and Prole (1976) at autopsy found 5 out of 27 greyhounds infected.

A number of treatments have been attempted with varying success, but in a recent report Darke (1976) described good results using oral levamisole at 7·5 mg/kg when continued for 10–30 days.

Infection with another lungworm, *Angiostrongylus vasorum* has also been treated successfully with this drug by a number of authors. Dodd (1973) and Jacobs and Prole (1975) used 10 mg/kg subcutaneously on 3 consecutive days but although their dogs showed no side-effects, it is the general experience that side-effects such as vomiting and diarrhoea are more frequent by this route and the oral route may be preferable.

The lungworm of the cat, *Aelurostrongylus abstrusus* is known to be widespread particularly in country cats where access to rodents and other suitable paratenic hosts is greatest. Its prevalence was reviewed by Hamilton (1963). However, in a subsequent report associating lesions of the pulmonary arteries with this infection, the same author showed that it was even more common than the surveys indicated. Lesions persisted after the spontaneous expulsion of the worms and were present in one in three Glasgow cats (Hamilton 1966). The infection may therefore be a common cause of chronic coughing.

The most successful treatment for this lungworm, as for the canine lungworms, appears to be levamisole. However, the drug is toxic in the cat and it must be used with great care. Whether given orally or parenterally at maximum tolerated doses, repeated daily treatment is required (Hamilton 1968). The drug is unpalatable but apart from the ease of administration, Hamilton found parenteral injection had no other advantages and was much more dangerous. Only at 5 mg/kg was the injection of tetramisole without side-effects and both he and Arundel (1970) recommend the oral route, the latter using 10–15 mg/kg levamisole. Unfortunately, no suitable enteric formulation of the drug is readily available in Britain and because of its unpalatability it may be necessary to have recourse to injection. Probably 4–5 mg/kg levamisole by subcutaneous injection would be safe and equally useful.

It must be added that neither tetramisole nor levamisole are licensed for use in dogs or cats in Britain.

12.5 Cestodes

For the treatment of cestode infections dichlorophen, niclosamide and bunamidine have been available for some years. All three are highly active against *Taenia* species and *Dipylidium caninum* but only the latter has useful activity against *Echinococcus granulosus.* Although against immature worms even the activity of bunamidine is inadequate, it remains the drug of choice for *Echinococcus* species at present. A particular problem with bunamidine is that it appears to sensitise the myocardium to catecholamines

(Alexander 1976), and dangerous interactions with anaesthetic agents may thus arise. However, while in farm dogs, in Wales in particular, *E. granulosus granulosus* is relatively common (Cook & Clarkson 1971; Williams 1976) and in foxhounds the prevalence of *E. granulosus equinus* is high (Thompson & Smyth 1975) the species is otherwise rare in Britain. For this reason efficacy against it, even though it is a serious zoonosis, is less important to most practitioners than that against *Taenia* spp, and the much commoner *D. caninum*.

For the same reason the claim for mebendazole, a broad spectrum anthelmintic having activity against cestodes, must be regarded as inadequate. Against *Taenia* spp. its action is somewhat variable and against *D. caninum* it is generally poor (Hass & Collins 1976). For practical purposes therefore, the cestocidal properties of mebendazole should be regarded as a bonus when the drug is used for nematodes and practitioners will continue for the time being to use the existing compounds for specific action against cestodes.

A number of anthelmintics with very high efficacy against all the important cestode species are at an advanced stage of preparation or are indeed, already available commercially elsewhere. Among these are praziquantel, uredefos (diuredosan), and nitroscanate. At 100 mg/kg *Taenia hydatigena*, *T. ovis* and *D. caninum* are completely elminated by nitroscanate and at 200 mg/kg this is true for *E. granulosus* also (Boray *et al* 1973). The activity of praziquantel is even greater, so that at the recommended rate of 2·5–10 mg/kg, all the common cestodes are eliminated. Even the activity against very young *E. granulosus* is better than 97% (Wikerhauser *et al* 1976). When these drugs become available they will replace the existing cestocidal compounds.

In summary, the situation now, with respect to nematode anthelmintics, is that there are two available with similar spectra and high efficacy against all the common gastrointestinal species of the dog and cat. Dichlorvos is available as resin pellets for use in the dog and as tablets for use in the dog or cat. Pellets can be given in a single dose (27–40 mg/kg) but it is less toxic and more effective if half is given first, followed by the remainder 8–12 hours later. Tablets are given as a single treatment at 10 mg/kg. Puppies or cats of 0·45 kg (1lb) body weight may be treated using a half tablet. Animals should always be weighed for accuracy of dosing. Vomiting may occur but this does not appear to affect the efficacy unless it occurs at once, and animals should never be retreated immediately. Dichlorvos is a potent cholinesterase inhibitor and it must not be used at the same time as insecticides, anaesthetic agents or any other products with similar activity.

Mebendazole is available in tablet form suitable for use in dogs and cats. It is insoluble and poorly absorbed from the gut. Its action is to inhibit the uptake of glucose by the worms but for this reason it has the disadvantage that it must be given night and morning for 2 or 5 days depending on the worm species. The recommended dose rate covers a very wide range from say, 200 mg/kg/day for a small puppy to less than 10 mg/kg/day for a dog between 20 and 30 kg. However, it is still very active at the low rate and it is very safe at the upper limit.

For the future, two other well-known anthelmintics may shortly become available. Haloxon, which has an efficacy similar to dichlorvos against *Toxascaris* and *Toxocara* spp., will be available in tablet form specifically for the treatment of these infections and may be particularly suited for use in puppies. Although like dichlorvos, an organophosphorus compound and a cholinesterase inhibitor, its potency against the mammalian enzyme is much less marked and it is therefore much safer. Its efficacy against *Uncinaria stenocephala* and *Trichuris vulpis* does not compare favourably with the other two drugs.

Pyrantel, better known as an anthelmintic for large animals, may also become available as the pamoate for use in small animal species. Its efficacy against the ascarid species and the hookworms is good but it has little or no activity against *T. vulpis*. The latter is susceptible to oxantel.

For broad-spectrum anthelmintics which have high activity against nematodes and activity against the common cestode species comparable to that of the specific drugs currently available, we must await the arrival of the latest generation of compounds such as nitroscanate. At 50 mg/kg it is highly active against *Taenia* spp. and will also eliminate adult *Toxocara canis* and hookworm.

At 100 mg/kg the activity against *T. canis*, the hookworms, *Taenia* spp., and *D. caninum* is complete. Against *E. granulosus* the activity is also good but not absolute at this dose and against *Trichuris vulpis* it is somewhat variable. Uredefos shows similar promise.

Editors' note

The mode of action of anthelmintics is a complex subject, about which much remains obscure. However, some generalisations can be made. In the case of adult gut-dwelling helminths, at least, the parasite will survive if it can maintain a suitable site for feeding, and use the food which it obtains for the production of metabolic energy. Adult helminths have virtually no other requirements for survival, so anthelmintics must exert their selective toxicity by taking advantage of differences between helminths and their hosts in these two areas. However, it should be said that most of the available anthelmintics have been developed in an empirical fashion rather than by a search for agents with a specific action on vital helminth biochemical functions.

Although fundamental differences exist between some aspects of helminth energy metabolism and that of mammals, there is a wide variety of different metabolic pathways existing in different helminths at different stages of their life cycle: an agent which may be especially powerful in terms of inhibiting a vital stage in one parasite may be relatively ineffective in another, whilst broad-spectrum agents may be correspondingly less powerful in their action on a specific parasite (Rew 1978).

Agents which interfere with helminth neuromuscular co-ordination will compromise the parasite's ability to maintain a suitable feeding site, and the paralysed parasite will be expelled as a result of normal peristalsis, or will die when exposed to an unsuitable intestinal environment. Nematodes appear to have fundamentally different neuromuscular junctions from mammals, although there appear to be some similarities between mammalian smooth muscle and the musculature of the nematode. Sufficient differences exist between neuromuscular co-ordination mechanisms in mammals and helminths (especially nematodes) to allow some agents to exert a selective toxicity for helminths in this respect.

In the case of some anthelmintics the mode of action is unclear. In others, the evidence for the primary mode of action is conflicting. The list below indicates the probable mode of action for several anthelmintics. For further details the reader is referred to reviews by Van den Bossche (1976) and Rew (1978).

Agents which interfere with energy metabolism. Benzimidazole compounds; antimony and arsenic compounds; nitroxynil; niclosamide, rafoxanide and related compounds.

Agents which interfere with neuromuscular transmission. Levamisole; morantel and pyrantel; organophosphorus compounds; piperazine; thenium.

References

Alexander F. (1976) Introduction to Veterinary Pharmacology, p. 321. Churchill Livingstone, Edinburgh.

Arundel J. H. (1970) Control of helminth parasites of dogs and cats. *Aust. Vet. J.* **46**, 164.

Boray J. C., Orelli M. von, & Sarasin G. (1973) *6th Symposium of World Assoc. Adv. Vet. Parasit. Vienna.*

Cook B. R. & Clarkson M. J. (1971) The epidemiology of *Echinococcus* infection in Great Britain. III. *Echinococcus granulosus* and cestodes of the genus Taenia in farm dogs in England in the Lake District, Northern Pennines and East Anglia. *Ann. Trop. Med. Parasitol.* **65**, 71.

Darke P. G. G. (1976) Use of levamisole in the treatment of parasitic tracheobronchitis in the dog. *Vet. Rec.* **99**, 293.

Dodd K. (1973) *Angiostrongylus vasorum* (Baillet, 1866) infestation in a greyhound kennels. *Vet. Rec.* **92**, 195.

Hamilton J. M. (1963) Aelurostrongylus abstrusus infestation of the cat. *Vet. Rec.* **75**, 417.

Hamilton J. M. (1966) Experimental lungworm disease of the cat. Association of the condition with lesions of the pulmonary arteries. *J. Comp. Path.* **76**, 147.

Hamilton J. M. (1968) Treatment of experimentally-induced lungworms of the cat by parenteral administration of tetramisole. *Vet. Rec.* **83**, 665.

Hass D. K. & Collins J. A. (1976) Comparative anthelmintic efficacy in dogs treated with vincofos, ticarbodine or mebendazole. *Proc. Helm. Soc. Wash.* **43**, 135.

Holt P. E. (1976) *Toxocara canis*: an estimation of the incidence of infection in puppies in an industrial town. *Vet. Rec.* **98**, 383.

Hovell G. J. R. & Weston R. (1970) Cramp in greyhounds. Correspondence in Members Inf. Suppl. *Vet. Rec.* **87**, 193.

Jacobs D. E. (1976) Studies on the epidemiology of *Uncinaria stenocephala* infections in British greyhounds: seasonal availability of larvae on grass runs. *Res. Vet. Sci.* **21**, 238.

Jacobs D. E., Pegg E. J. & Stevenson P. (1977) Helminths of British dogs: *Toxocara canis* — a veterinary perspective. *J. Small Anim. Pract.* **18**, 79.

Jacobs D. E. & Prole J. H. B. (1975) *Angiostrongylus vasorum* and other nematodes in British greyhounds. *Vet. Rec.* **96**, 180.

Jacobs D. E. & Prole J. H. B. (1976) Helminth infections of British dogs: prevalence in racing greyhounds. *Vet. Parasit.* **1**, 377.

Oldham J. N. (1965) Observations on the incidence of *Toxocara* and *Toxascaris* in dogs and cats from the London area. *J. Helminth.* **39**, 251.

Read M. A. & Thompson R. C. A. (1976) Research note: prevalence of *Toxocara canis* and *Toxascaris leonina* ova in dog faeces deposited on the streets of Leeds. *J. Helminth.* **50**, 95.

Rew R. S. (1978) Mode of action of common anthelmintics. *J. Vet. Pharmacol. Therap.* **1**, 95.

Sloan J. E. N. (1961) The general incidence of internal parasites affecting the dog. In *Advances in Small Animal Practice 2*, B. V. Jones, Pergamon Press, Oxford.

Stevenson P., Jacobs D. E. & Prole J. H. B. (1975) A filarial parasite of greyhounds. *Vet. Rec.* **97**, 505.

Thompson R. C. A. & Smyth J. D. (1975) Equine hydatidosis: a review of the current status in Great Britain and the results of an epidemiological survey. *Vet. Parasit.* **1**, 107.

Turner T. & Pegg E. J. (1977) A survey of patent nematode infestations in dogs. *Vet. Rec.* **100**, 284.

Van den Bossche H. (1976) In *Biochemistry of Parasites and Host-Parasite Relationships*, p. 553. North-Holland, Amsterdam.

Weston R. (1975) Endoparasites in dogs supplied for laboratory use. 1. The incidence of infestation. *J. Inst. Animal Tech.* **26**, 69.

Wikerhauser T., Brglez J., Kuticic V. & Kozelj B. (1976) [Effects of praziquantel on immature stages of Echinococcus granulosus in dogs] *Acta Parasitologica Iugoslavica* **7**, 33.

Williams B. M. (1976) The epidemiology of adult and larval (tissue) cestodes in Dyfed (UK) I. The cestodes of farm dogs. *Vet. Parasit.* **1**, 271.

Woodruff A. W. (1970) Toxocariasis. *Brit. Med. J.* **3**, 663.

13

Pharmacology and toxicology of organophosphorus pesticides

D. V. ROBERTS

Organophosphorus pesticides are pharmacologically active and so provide valuable therapeutic acids; they have great economic value to world food production but they may also produce serious toxicological effects in man and other animals. Great care is needed in their use, first of all in order to avoid unwanted and possibly toxic effects in animal patients, and secondly in order to avoid bringing these compounds into disrepute, the end result of which may be a restriction in their use, or even a complete withdrawal of organophosphorus compounds from veterinary practice. Such action would not necessarily reduce the toxicological hazards to livestock because new compounds with their own toxic effects would be developed to take the place of the organophosphorus pesticides. This sequence of events has already happened in the case of the organochlorine compounds. As a result of national and international restrictions on the use of organochlorine pesticides, there has been a great increase in the manufacture and use of the anticholinesterase organophosphorus and carbamate pesticides. The long-term toxicological effects of organophosphorus and carbamate compounds have still to be fully evaluated, but it is already clear that the move away from organochlorine pesticides is a change from well-known compounds with relatively little toxicity to mammals, but with long persistence in the environment, to less well known and potentially more toxic compounds, whose main attraction to the ecologists is their shorter persistence. In retrospect, it is reasonable to suppose that with greater care in the use and disposal of organochlorine compounds, the level of environmental contamination might not have been sufficient to provoke such drastic restrictions on their use. More careful use of the very effective organophosphorus compounds in current use as pesticides may do much to extend their useful life.

13.1 Chemical structure

This account of the pharmacology and toxicology of organophosphorus compounds begins with a reference to their basic chemical structure, which is

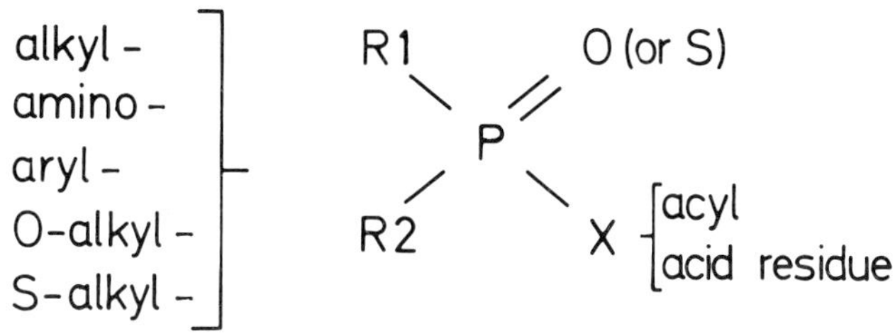

Fig. 13.1 Basic chemical composition of organophosphorus pesticides. Note the functional importance of the alternative O or S groups. Many thiocompounds are relatively inactive against acetylcholinesterase when tested *in vitro*; their anticholinesterase potency is increased *in vivo* after conversion to the oxon-form by liver enzymes (e.g. malathion — inactive, malaoxon — active).

illustrated in Fig. 13.1. The characteristic feature is the centrally placed phosphorus atom, surrounded by four organic chemical groups. The composition of the surrounding groups varies from one pesticide to another, and with it, the biological activity and hence the pesticidal value and also the toxicological effects of a particular compound. Subject to the modifying influences of the various surrounding groups, the mode of action of the organophosphorus pesticides appears to be related, in the main, to their ability to inhibit various enzyme systems of biological importance, not only in the organisms against which the pesticides are directed but also in man and other animals.

13.2 Sites of action

The obvious targets for organophosphorus compounds are the cholinesterase enzyme systems, which are able to hydrolyse acetylcholine and various other esters. These enzyme systems are to be found in many sites in the body, for example in plasma and in erythrocytes. However, a large part of the biological activity of organophosphorus compounds rests on their ability to inhibit acetylcholinesterase, an enzyme which is specific for acetylcholine and which is located at cholinergic synapses in the central, peripheral and autonomic nervous systems. As a result of this inhibition, the duration of action of acetylcholine released from presynaptic nerve terminals is prolonged, its effect on the postsynaptic receptors is enhanced and this in turn leads to the signs and symptoms of acute anticholinesterase poisoning.

The organophosphorus pesticides also react with various liver enzymes in a variety of ways. With some organophosphorus compounds, the liver enzymes act as a detoxification system, removing from the pesticides the particular chemical group which confers on it biological action and toxicity. Liver enzymes react with other compounds in a way which increases their anticholinesterase potential and so makes them more toxic. Both of these effects are subject to modification when liver enzymes are inhibited, for example by other organophosphorus compounds, or when their activity has been increased by previous exposure to a substrate. Under such circumstances it is possible for two organophosphorus compounds administered simultaneously to prove to be more toxic than their individual toxicities would suggest. There is clearly need for more caution when two or more organophosphorus pesticides are given at the same time, or when other drugs with hepatotoxic effects are being administered concurrently.

A third enzyme system, which has recently been recognised as a target for organophosphorus compounds, is contained within the cells of the nervous system, a position which contrasts with that of acetylcholinesterase which is particularly associated with the synaptic connections between cells. The interaction between organophosphorus compounds and this enzyme system is important because, while many organophosphorus compounds inhibit this enzyme to different degrees, in the case of some compounds, inhibition is followed by changes in the structure and function of the affected nerves. These changes result in delayed neurotoxic effects and for this reason, the enzyme has been referred to as neurotoxic esterase (NTE). This effect of inhibition of the neurotoxic esterase by some organophosphorus pesticides is independent of their anticholinesterase properties; in fact, what evidence there is suggests that the ability to inhibit these two enzyme systems is reciprocally related. If a number of organophosphorus pesticides are examined, they may be arranged so that at one extreme they are predominantly anticholinesterase, at the other end they are antineurotoxic esterase, while in the middle there are compounds which exhibit both effects to a significant extent.

13.3 Biochemical mechanisms

(*The reader may care to omit this section at first reading.*)

With these general points in mind, the biochemical basis of anticholinesterase action by organophosphorus compounds may be described. As Fig. 13.2 shows, the starting point of the reaction is the formation of a complex between the inhibitor and the enzyme. If the inhibitor fits suitably at the active site of the enzyme molecule, and if it is sufficiently reactive, a second stage can take place. This consists of phosphorylation of a hydroxy-serine residue on the enzyme by the organophosphorus compound, which loses its X group in the process. The phosphorylated enzyme is unable to accept its normal substrate, acetylcholine, and is said to be inhibited.

From this point, the reaction may go in two different ways, depending on the relative strengths of the bonds between the phosphorus atom and, on the one hand, the groups R_1 and R_2, and on the other, the hydroxy-serine residue

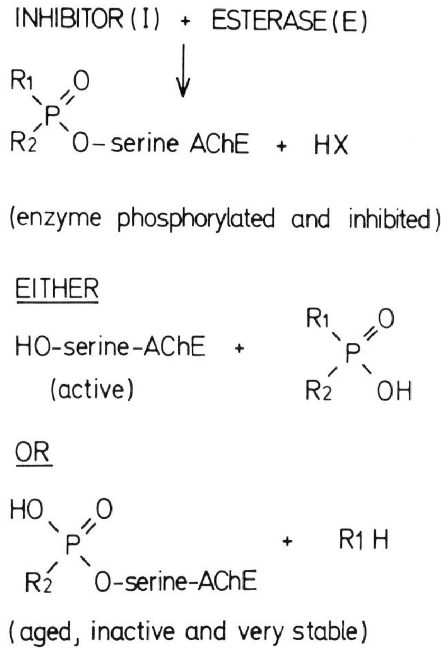

Fig. 13.2 Interactions between acetyicholinesterase and an organophosphorus pesticide which result initially in a phosphorylated inhibited enzyme, followed by either a dephosphorylated and active enzyme, or an 'aged', inactive and stable enzyme-inhibitor complex.

which forms the active site of the esterase. When the phosphorus-R_1, R_2 bonds are relatively stronger, cleavage takes place between the phosphorus and the serine group, the enzyme is said to be dephosphorylated and it regains its former esterase activity. The inactive organophosphorus compound is then free to move away from the site and to undergo metabolism and detoxification. The rate at which this dissociation takes place is relatively fast so that provided no more inhibitor compound is administered, the duration of inhibition of the enzyme is limited.

However, when the phosphorus-R_1, R_2 bonds are relatively weaker, cleavage takes place at the bond between R_1 and the phosphorus. This leaves the hydroxy-serine residue on the enzyme occupied by the rest of the organophosphorus compound and as a result, the enzyme remains inhibited. This combination between enzyme and inhibitor is very stable, and the mechanism of its formation, because it is time-dependent, is known as 'ageing'. Once ageing has occurred, reappearance of cholinesterase activity probably takes place only when new enzyme is synthesised because there seems to be no way of reactivating an 'aged' enzyme. In contrast, dephosphorylation (i.e. cleavage of the phosphorus-serine bond), may be facilitated by the administration of substances, such as pralidoxime, which help to disengage the phosphorus from the hydroxy-serine residue by interaction of the quaternary nitrogen of the oxime molecule with the anionic site of the enzyme. The administration of pralidoxime in cases of organophosphorus poisoning, after the enzyme has been inhibited but before ageing has taken place, is a useful adjunct to atropinisation.

A somewhat similar sequence of events is responsible for the delayed neurotoxic effect of some organophosphorus compounds. Here, the target enzyme is contained within nerve cells and while it has the power to hydrolyse phenyl phenylacetate and phenylvalerate, its physiological function is at present unknown. As with acetylcholinesterase, organophosphorus compounds phosphorylate and so inhibit the esteratic site. With some compounds, the enzyme remains inhibited until dephosphorylation takes place, and in such cases no delayed neurotoxic effects occur. With other organophosphorus compounds, however, fission occurs at the R_1 group leaving the organophosphorus with an additional charge, and attached to the enzyme. By analogy with the organophosphorus-cholinesterase interaction, this process is also termed 'ageing' and it appears to be the trigger for further changes whose nature is at present unknown, which lead ultimately to delayed neurotoxic effects. It should be noted that inhibition of the neurotoxic enzyme does not, by itself, lead to delayed neurotoxicity and in fact, occupation of the esteratic site by a compound which does *not* cause ageing in the enzyme can protect the enzyme against other organophosphorus compounds which have delayed neurotoxic effects.

Thus, in relation to neurotoxic esterase, it is possible to recognise two main groups of organophosphorus compounds. Both groups inhibit the neurotoxic esterase but one results in an 'aged' enzyme and delayed neurotoxicity, while the other only inhibits the enzyme and so may be protective in action (Fig. 13.3). This difference in action is the result of differences in the

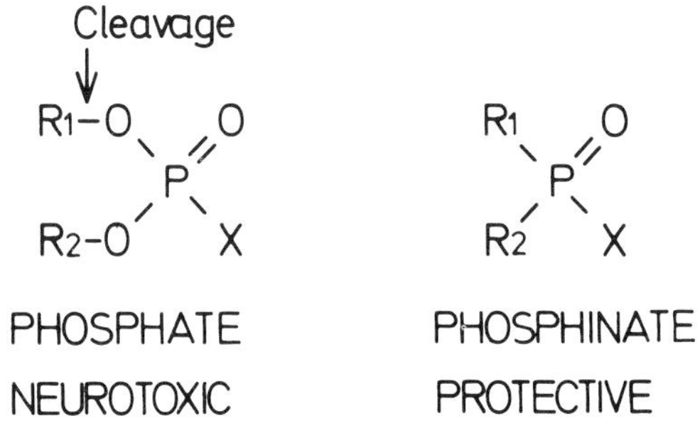

Fig. 13.3 Basic chemical composition of two organophosphorus compounds, both of which inhibit neurotoxic esterase. The phosphate is neurotoxic because of the relative weakness of the R_1-oxygen link, which allows 'ageing' of the inhibited enzyme to take place. In the phosphinate, the more stable R_1-phosphorus link favours dephosphorylation; the inhibited enzyme does not undergo 'ageing' and is protected by the phosphinate from the action of other neurotoxic organophosphorus compounds.

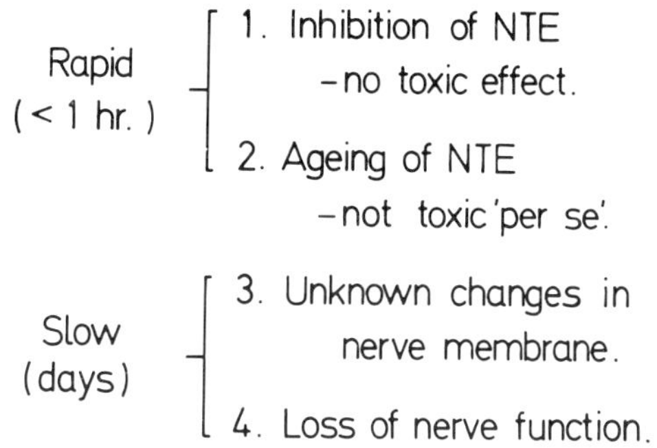

Fig. 13.4 Sequence of changes leading to delayed neurotoxicity. Note the rapid inhibition and 'ageing' of the neurotoxic esterase and the slow development of functional and structural changes in nerve fibres.

strength with which the R_1 and R_2 groups are bound to the phosphorus. For example, a phosphate compound which inhibits neurotoxic esterase and in which the R_1 and R_2 groups are linked to the phosphorus through oxygen atoms is neurotoxic. On the other hand, a phosphinate compound in which R_1 and R_2 groups are linked directly to the phosphorus, while it also inhibits neurotoxic esterase, does not lead to an aged enzyme; delayed neurotoxicity does not occur and the enzyme is protected from attack by 'delayed neurotoxic' organophosphorus compounds.

While the details of the reactions leading to delayed neurotoxicity have still to be worked out, the general sequence of events is depicted in Fig. 13.4.

Of the four stages envisaged in this scheme, the first two are rapid, occurring within 1 hour of the inhibition of neurotoxic esterase, and lead to ageing of the enzyme but not to any signs of delayed neurotoxicity. The third and fourth stages are much slower to take effect, but lead ultimately to some loss of nerve function. This may be observed electroneuromyographically as a reduction in conduction velocity or it may become clinically apparent as ataxia, paresis or paralysis.

It is important to note that once stage 2 has occurred, stages 3 and 4 proceed independently of any further change in enzyme activity, which may indeed be restored to normal before neurotoxic signs and symptoms are observed. It seems as though the ageing process acts as a trigger to subsequent changes which result in the neurotoxic effects but the nature of this trigger mechanism has still to be discovered.

13.4 Clinical effects of exposure

The remainder of this chapter will be concerned with the effects of exposure to anticholinesterase and antineurotoxic esterase compounds, beginning with the acute effects of inhibition of acetylcholinesterase. Predictably, such

Table 13.1 Signs of acute exposure to anticholinesterase compounds.

Muscarinic
Secretion: nasolacrimal glands; bronchial glands; sweat glands; gastrointestinal glands.

Smooth muscle: bronchoconstriction; miosis; impaired visual accommodation; increased intestinal motility.

Cardiovascular: bradycardia; hypotension.

Nicotinic
Skeletal muscle fasciculation; skeletal muscle cramps; skeletal muscle weakness.

Central nervous system
Restlessness; tremor; tonic/clonic convulsions; abnormal reflexes; respiratory and cardiac depression; coma.

effects will occur at cholinergic synapses in the autonomic nervous system, in the peripheral neuromuscular pathways, and in the central nervous system. These effects are many and varied but may be categorised as muscarinic, nicotinic and central signs, as is shown in Table 13.1.

The muscarinic effects have been subdivided in terms of the target tissues, which are principally the exocrine glands, smooth muscle and the cardiovascular system. In certain organs there may be summation of secretory and smooth muscle effects. For example, the increased secretions of the glands of the respiratory tracts and the narrowing of the airway by bronchoconstriction may combine to reduce pulmonary ventilation and gas exchange. Similarly, increased gastrointestinal secretion and motility may together result in a rapid loss of water and salts. In the case of the cardiovascular system, the major effects are the decrease in heart rate brought about by enhanced vagal action on the sinoatrial node and the fall in mean arterial blood pressure which results from cholinergic vasodilatation of the larger precapillary resistance vessels of skeletal muscle. However, both these effects may be modified by the intervention of homeostatic cardiovascular reflexes.

Inhibition of the acetylcholinesterase at skeletal neuromuscular junctions, and the reduced rate of hydrolysis of acetylcholine, are responsible for the nicotinic effects of exposure to organophosphorus compounds. The depolarising action of spontaneously released acetylcholine is increased and may be sufficient to produce asynchronous contractions of skeletal muscle. Alternatively, fasciculation may be produced reflexly by increased muscle spindle activity resulting from inhibition of intrafusal acetylcholinesterase. The larger quantities of acetylcholine released by motor nerve activity, which may be voluntary or induced by electrical stimulation, remain at the endplate for longer than the refractory period of skeletal muscle fibres. As a result, the muscle fibres respond repetitively to each nerve impulse, so that muscle activity is prolonged and increased in amplitude as successive contractions summate. Repetitive activity may also occur in the motor nerve terminals as a result either of the action of the organophosphorus compound or of persistent acetylcholine on presynaptic cholinoreceptors. Eventually, a degree of neuromuscular block may occur, due in part to the desensitisation of postsynaptic cholinoreceptors when exposure to acetylcholine is prolonged.

The variety of central nervous system signs resulting from acute exposure to organophosphorus compounds no doubt reflects changes at many cholinergic synapses. Acetylcholine which persists at these synapses will initially enhance, and later depress transmission from neurone to neurone. The signs are further complicated by the resulting disturbance in the normal balance of excitatory and inhibitory influences operating at different levels of the nervous system.

When exposure is prolonged, a different set of signs may appear. Thus as exposure continues, the initial muscarinic and nicotinic effects may decrease in severity and eventually disappear, and the animal is said to have acquired tolerance to the acute effects of inhibition of cholinesterase. Little is known about the mechanisms which underlie tolerance, but probably desensitisation of acetylcholine receptors plays some part in the process. The development of tolerance is of practical importance for two reasons. Firstly, it makes it possible to give doses in excess of the acute LD_{50} level by a gradual build up from very small initial doses. Secondly, when exposure to an anticholinesterase compound needs to be prolonged for therapeutic reasons, it is important to remember that once tolerance has developed, the muscarinic and nicotinic effects of an acute exposure may no longer serve as effective warning signs of overtreatment.

A second effect of chronic exposure to anticholinesterase compounds, and one which is perhaps related to the development of tolerance, is to be found in the cholinesterase enzyme system itself. There is much experimental and clinical evidence that prolonged inhibition of the enzyme provokes an increase in production of that enzyme. From the point of view of synaptic function, such adaptation has obvious advantages in restoring the hydrolysis of acetylcholine towards the normal level. However, when this adaptation leads to an increase in the total amount of enzyme present in plasma and red cells, the use of these enzyme levels as indicators of exposure may no longer be valid. Any increase in the total amount of enzyme will lead to an underestimation of the degree of inhibition. Indeed, it is possible to obtain normal, and in some cases higher than normal, values for plasma cholinesterase even though an inhibitor substance is present and some of the enzyme is inhibited.

Other effects of chronic exposure to anticholinesterase compounds arise as a result of the increased persistence of acetylcholine at synapses when the rate of enzymatic hydrolysis is reduced by inhibition. Functional and structural changes have been observed in motor nerve endings and in the endplate regions of the skeletal muscle, the ultimate effect of which is to reduce the effectiveness of neuromuscular transmission and so lead to muscular weakness. If similar changes occur in muscle spindles, this could explain the impairment of motor co-ordination which is sometimes a sign of exposure. Evidence of more subtle effects on central nervous system function comes from studies in rats of conditioned reflexes, which are extinguished more rapidly during treatment with organophosphorus compounds.

These effects of chronic exposure to anticholinesterase compounds may be compared with the results of inhibition of the neurotoxic esterase. Here, the end results are functional and structural changes in both peripheral and central nerve fibres, which show first as a reduction in conduction velocity and later as complete failure of transmission. As a consequence of the neuronal lesion, demyelination may also be found and this no doubt contributes to the functional impairment. Recovery from the effects of inhibition of neurotoxic esterase is limited, and when the initial loss of function is extensive, a vicious circle is established in which reduction of food intake leads to loss of muscle mass and eventual death from starvation or respiratory failure. Treatment in these circumstances is symptomatic only, and should be directed towards the maintenance of adequate levels of food and water intake, in order to allow time for recovery or functional compensation to take place.

When the exposure is to an organophosphorus compound which inhibits both acetylcholinesterase and neurotoxic esterase, the pattern of signs may be even more complicated. The initial muscarinic and nicotine anticholinesterase effects may be clear and easily recognisable but may be soon replaced by impairment of neuromuscular transmission. To this is added, after a latent period of up to 14 days, the neuronal conduction defect brought about by the initial inhibition of neurotoxic esterase. The relative severity of these signs and symptoms will depend upon the level of exposure and affinity of the organophosphorus compounds for the two enzymes concerned. Care is particularly required when the exposure is low level but prolonged, because in such circumstances the inhibition of acetylcholinesterase may take place at too slow a rate to give rise to the signs of an acute exposure, although tolerance to these effects as well as the effects of chronic exposure may result; eventually delayed neurotoxicity may become apparent. When the exposure is brief, the animal may exhibit the expected muscarinic and nicotinic signs, whose disappearance after 1 or 2 days may suggest that recovery has taken place. That this is not so will become apparent when the signs of delayed neurotoxicity develop.

13.5 Principles of treatment of organophosphorus poisoning

Prevention is probably the most effective principle to adopt when using organophosphorus compounds; this applies not only to animals under treatment but also to the health and safety of those responsible for administering or applying these toxic compounds. As far as animals are concerned, strict adherence to recommended dose schedules should prevent overtreatment. Nevertheless, the veterinary practitioner should be alert for unexpected reactions, for example in animals rendered more sensitive to the effects of anticholinesterase compounds by disease or concurrent therapy. He should also be aware of the physical and chemical properties of the particular organophosphorus compound he is using and how these properties may modify the amount of drug actually received by the animal or the duration of exposure. For example, dichlorvos flea collars have been found to produce ataxia, CNS depression and death in cats kept in a warm dry environment. No toxic effects were observed when atmospheric conditions of high humidity prevailed, even when two or three collars were used. These differences are attributable to faster release of dichlorvos from collars in warm dry atmospheres, and more rapid hydrolysis and detoxification of free dichlorvos in warm humid conditions. The same compound also has the property of adsorption on the fabric of the room in which it is released; subsequent vaporisation of the compound may prolong exposure of the occupants of the room after the primary source has been removed. No doubt other organophosphorus compounds have their own idiosyncrasies which should be taken into account when they are used.

Hazards to the health of persons applying organophosphorus compounds may be reduced by the use of recommended safety precautions, including the wearing of protective clothing when necessary and the maintenance of a high standard of personal hygiene. The persons concerned should be trained to recognise the early warning of acute intoxication provided by muscarinic signs and symptoms, and appropriate first aid and medical cover should be arranged to deal with severe intoxication. It is worthy of note that in the case of sheep-dipping for example, each animal receives only one dose, whereas the applicator may be potentially or actually exposed for the duration of the dipping operation.

When acute intoxication with an organophosphorus compound with anticholinesterase actions has occurred, treatment should be directed towards restricting further exposure to the compound, reducing the effects of excessive acetylcholine and reactivation of acetylcholinesterase. These objectives may be achieved by the following procedures:

1 If the organophosphorus compound has been administered orally, gastric lavage should be used to prevent further absorption. If exposure has occurred as a result of environmental contamination, the affected animal or person should be decontaminated and removed to a 'clean' situation.

2 Atropine should be given to counter the muscarinic effects of excessive acetylcholine, intramuscularly or for more rapid action, intravenously. Repeated doses may be required, depending on the duration of inhibition of acetylcholinesterase, but the size of each dose and the interval between doses may be reduced as the enzyme recovers its function.

3 While atropine will reduce bronchial constriction and secretion, it may be necessary to ensure that the airways are clear by suction and to maintain adequate levels of gas exchange with assisted ventilation.

4 The effects of inhibition of acetylcholinesterase may be minimised by reducing nervous and muscular activity, if necessary by the careful use of either a barbiturate or diazepam and, to counter excessive neuromuscular activity, a non-depolarising blocking agent together with artificial respiration.

5 In the case of some organophosphorus compounds, it is possible to reactivate the acetylcholinesterase by detaching the phosphoryl group from the enzyme with pralidoxime chloride, TMB-4 dibromide or obidoxime dichloride. These agents have only a short period of action and repeated doses may be necessary as long as an active inhibitor compound is present in the system. However, because an aged enzyme cannot be reactivated in this way, these agents may not be effective if given too long a time after the organophosphorus compound. The degree of reactivation achieved may be assessed, as far as blood enzymes are concerned, if blood samples are taken before and after administration of a reactivator and the levels of enzyme activity measured in erythrocytes and plasma. However, this procedure takes some time, depending on the availability of laboratory facilities, and blood enzyme levels do not accurately reflect changes in tissue enzymes. For these reasons, clinical appraisal is probably the best guide to the need for further reactivation therapy.

6 Measures to maintain normal fluid and electrolyte levels should be used when required, and broad-spectrum antibiotics used to prevent infection, particularly in the lungs.

In the case of chronic organophosphorus (anticholinesterase) intoxication the foregoing measures may be of value, with the exception of reactivation therapy because the enzyme is probably aged as a result of the prolonged inhibition. In general, treatment of chronic intoxication rests on cessation of organophosphorus therapy or exposure, and supportive measures until restoration of normal function, and the same principles will apply to the treatment of delayed neurotoxicity, for which there is as yet no specific therapy.

13.6 Conclusion

From this account of the pharmacology and toxicology of organophosphorus pesticides it will be apparent that the effects of exposure are complex. Each of the many compounds in use may possess several modes of action, and these in varying degrees. Moreover, many of the effects are time-dependent, so that the clinical pattern may change as exposure continues. Perhaps the most appropriate conclusion is to emphasise that these compounds should be used with care and respect and that animals treated with organophosphorus pesticides should be closely monitored for signs of short and long-term ill-effects.

Clinical note (added by editors)

The number of organophosphorus compound products available for the treatment of small ecto-parasite infestations has increased rapidly over the past few years, and certain risks associated with the widespread use of these products are apparent.

The chief risk appears to be that an animal may receive an unduly large cumulative dose by being exposed to several small doses from different sources. Before administering one of these compounds, the veterinary surgeon should ascertain that the animal has not previously been wearing a flea collar, nor been exposed to an atmosphere contaminated with an organophosphorus compound. (The latter circumstance may arise when plastic strips, impregnated with these compounds, are used to control flying insects in the home. Dichlorvos is the compound commonly used, and it is slowly released from the plastic strip, to maintain an atmospheric concentration sufficient to kill flying insects. Such products, are, incidentally, useful for the control of flea populations in buildings, but if the manufacturer's instructions are not carefully adhered to, relatively high atmospheric concentrations may build up.) The veterinary surgeon should also warn the owner of the danger of allowing the animal to come into contact with any organophosphorous source after administration of any of these compounds. These precautions clearly apply most importantly where an organophosphorus compound is given systemically, and especially when relatively high doses are given in the treatment of Demodex infestation. Nonetheless, caution should govern the therapeutic use of any organophosphorus compound. The potential hazard of organophosphorus aerosols should not be forgotten by the veterinary surgeon, and it is probable that such products should be dispensed to clients only after careful consideration, and with written instructions. On the other hand, there is clearly a potential risk to the veterinary surgeon or his staff, if such products are frequently used in the surgery, unless proper precautions are taken. A severe reaction in a person using such an aerosol has been reported to one of the editors (A.Y.) (Smith, pers. comm.).

Anaesthesia

One of the potentially hazardous situations likely to be encountered in small animal practice is the effect of depolarising muscle relaxants in animals which have been receiving organophosphorus compounds. Suxamethonium chloride is the commonest depolarising relaxant in current use, and will provide 15–20 minutes apnoea, when given to dogs at a dose rate of 0:3 mg/kg. Muscle activity returns as a result of the hydrolysis of suxamethonium to an inactive form by cholinesterases.

Conclusion

The use of suxamethonium in animals which have been treated with an organophosphorus compound may therefore result in prolonged, and perhaps irreversible paralysis, because active cholinesterase levels are too low to deactivate the relaxant.

Further reading

Aldridge W. N. & Reiner E. (1975) *Enzyme inhibitors as substrates. Interaction of esterases with esters of organophosphorus and carbamic acids.* North Holland, Amsterdam.

Johnson M. K. (1975) The delayed neuropathy caused by some organophosphorus esters: mechanism and challenge. *Crit. Rev. Toxicol.* **3**, 289.

Karczmar A. G., Usdin E. & Wills J. H. (1970) *International encyclopedia of pharmacology and therapeutics: anti-cholinesterase agents.* Sect. 13, vol. 1. Pergamon, Oxford.

Koelle G. B. (1963) *Handbuch der Experimentellen Pharmacologie.* Vol. 15. Springer-Verlag, Berlin.

Silver A. (1974) The biology of cholinesterases. In *Frontiers of Biology*, vol. 36. North Holland, Amsterdam.

14

Veterinary applications of the pharmacology of neoplasia

A. T. YOXALL

Until comparatively recently surgery has been the only method for attempting to treat malignant disease, and it was not until the end of the nineteenth century that the discovery of X-rays made it possible to offer an alternative form of treatment, which might supplement the straightforward surgical approach and provide some improvement in the prognosis for patients suffering from malignant conditions. In the early part of the present century the foundations were laid for a discipline which has become one of the more sophisticated branches of modern medicine. Cancer chemotherapy has been practised for centuries, and if most of the treatments developed and enshrined in the folklore of centuries were remarkable chiefly for their unpleasantness, the same might be said of the mustard-gas derivatives, developed during World War II and subsequently found to have a potent tumouricidal activity. The compounds of this group were the first agents to have a proven efficacy in the treatment of cancer (Rhoads 1946) and their arrival marked the beginning of an era of investigation and discovery in this field, in which real progress in cancer chemotherapy has gone hand in hand with fundamental discoveries on the structure and biochemistry of normal and malignant cells.

Unfortunately, cancer chemotherapy remains a blunt and rather unpleasant weapon. At the moment, whilst it may be used to produce impressive and sometimes prolonged remissions with a minimum of unwanted effects, there are very few cases in which it can produce a complete cure. There is no effective agent yet discovered which will react only with tumour cells, whilst having no effect at all on any normal cells.

For the veterinarian in practice, radiotherapy is usually impossible unless he can form a working relationship with a local hospital radiotherapy department, or refer cases to a university veterinary school with this facility. Unless the veterinarian is content to remain as helpless in the face of malignant disease as his predecessor in the human field 100 years ago, his only alternative is to turn to chemotherapy, whatever drawbacks may remain in this field. Yet, here again, the general practitioner is faced with tremendous difficulties, for the sum total of veterinary experience in the use of these agents is pitifully small and the range of agents and combinations which have been tried in the treatment of human disease is enormous.

Cancer chemotherapy is a field in which there are few straightforward clinical rules, and the practitioner wishing to embark on this type of treatment would be well advised to begin by approaching some individual with experience in the field, so that a mutually beneficial co-operative approach to the problems involved may be established. For this reason the present chapter contains little in the way of therapeutic instructions, but is intended primarily as a review for those intending to study the subject further.

In spite of the provisos mentioned above, there is no doubt that chemotherapy can be a valuable therapeutic modality in the treatment of some malignant disease in animals, providing useful palliation, with a prolongation of a happy and useful life, in some cases for several years. The most successful approach to the treatment of malignancy undoubtedly is to remove by surgery as much of the tumour as possible, and then plan a concerted programme of treatment, using such resources as may be available, on the basis of a histopathological diagnosis.

14.1 Basic principles of cancer chemotherapy

When one is trying to destroy invading micro-organisms, it is relatively easy to find absolute differences between the organisms which one wishes to destroy and the host cell which one wishes to preserve. For example, bacteria usually have cell walls whilst mammalian cells do not, and we may be able to exploit this difference by using an agent such as penicillin, which has a specific effect on cell wall synthesis in bacteria whilst having little or no deleterious effect on the host.

In cancer chemotherapy this fortunate position does not obtain. One is trying to destroy cells, or at least inhibit the growth of cells, which usually closely resemble the normal tissue cells from which they have arisen. In general, the primary difference between malignant and normal cells is that the former have a propensity to grow in an uncontrolled fashion and to invade and destroy healthy tissues. Attempts at therapy are designed to take advantage of this difference in growth behaviour but in so doing one almost invariably finds that the treatment regime adopted will have some deleterious effect on sensitive normal cells. These sensitive cells will usually be those of the bone marrow, alimentary epithelium and others with a high turnover rate. A knowledge of the nature of cell and tissue growth and the ways in which multiplying normal and malignant cell populations behave is therefore an essential prerequisite for effective chemotherapy.

Whilst the fundamental difference between normal cells and neoplastic cells probably lies in the activity of the genetic mechanism, certain other differences between normal and abnormal cells can be recognised. Since these differences occur as a common feature in different tumour types, there must presumably be a common underlying mechanism. However, it is difficult to isolate any one particular feature of neoplastic cells as being of overwhelming importance, since the nature of intracellular activity is such that a particular biochemical or physical change is likely to set off a chain of secondary changes which will ultimately have a modifying effect on the initiating change, so that cause and effect relationships become difficult to work out.

Definite changes in the cell membrane are present in neoplastic cells and these changes are manifested by loss of contact inhibition of cell multiplication and cell movement, and altered transmembranal transport of various nutrients. These changes are accompanied by changes in the cell membrane structure, in terms of glycolipid and sialic acid content, and/or by changes in the distribution of membrane components over the surface of the membrane (Berlin *et al* 1975). Intracellular control mechanisms are responsible for changes in the behaviour of the cell membrane but changes in membrane permeability and structure may themselves affect the behaviour of important intracellular components. An example is provided by the role of cyclic 3′5′ adenosine monophosphate (cyclic AMP). Fig. 14.1 shows how synthesis of this mediator from ATP is governed by the activity of the membrane bound enzyme adenyl cyclase, the activity of this enzyme is in turn governed by various extracellular factors. It appears that cyclic AMP is able to exert a moderating effect on several aspects of cellular metabolic activity and the administration of cyclic AMP, or agents causing an increased intracellular concentration of cyclic AMP, to neoplastic cells *in vitro* will, in many cases, cause the cells to revert to the behaviour of normal cells (Ryan & Heidrick 1974) whilst many malignant cells in culture are found to have low intracellular cyclic AMP levels. However, this does not appear to be always

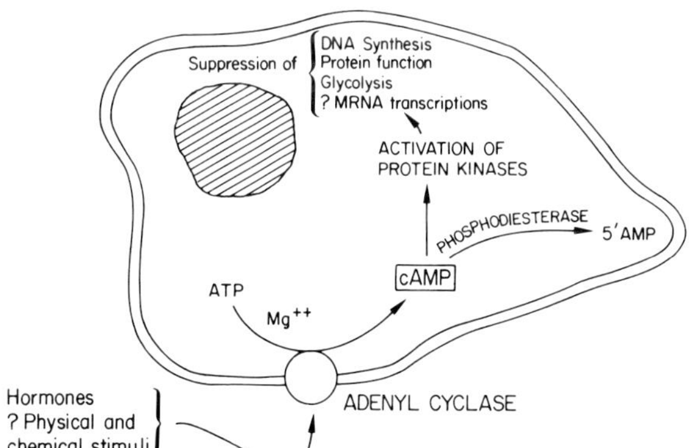

Fig. 14.1 Simplified diagrammatic representation of the possible role of cyclic AMP (cAMP) as a means of controlling some aspects of cellular metabolism.

true of tumour cells *in vivo*. Intracellular cyclic AMP levels amongst many other effects may have an effect on the nature of the cell surface (Roberts *et al* 1973) whilst changes in the nature of the cell surface and thus of the membrane bound enzyme adenyl cyclase which may be associated with neoplastic transformation (Anderson *et al* 1973) may in turn affect cyclic AMP levels. It is likely that future trends in cancer chemotherapy will be directed to some degree towards influencing intracellular control systems, such as that described. Maintenance of intracellular economy may be directed by mediators, such as cyclic AMP, but these mediators must, in turn, exert their effect via various enzyme systems. Differences, both qualitative and quantitative, exist between neoplastic and normal cells in terms of the pattern of enzyme activity. In certain experimental hepatic and renal tumours, at least, the activities of key enzymes governing nucleic acid synthesis and glucose utilisation are increased, with consequent enhancement of these metabolic pathways. These metabolic changes appear to be an integral part of the mechanism by which tumour cells exert a biological dominance over normal cells, so that if the changes are suppressed, the tumour cells may no longer be capable of behaving in a malignant fashion (Weber 1977).

Several of the chemotherapeutic agents in current use affect these key enzymes (see Fig. 14.8) and with recognition of the enzymes involved new agents are likely to be developed with this specific action. However, most of the key enzymes whose activity is grossly increased in malignant cells have a very low level of activity in normal cells, in spite of their key roles in cell metabolism. Therefore, inhibition of their activity may have profound deleterious effects on normal cells.

Other differences between normal and neoplastic cells certainly exist, but their importance at present remains uncertain.

The differences between tumours and normal tissues at a cellular level such as those indicated above, give rise to changes in the behaviour of populations of normal and malignant cells. Normal tissues consist of three cell 'compartments' (Fig. 14.2). The functional cells are normally well differentiated and carry out certain functions specific to that cell type but are not generally capable of further multiplication. These cells gradually die, due to factors such as inherent ageing of the cells, cell removal and other factors related to tissue architecture. Some form of feedback appears to exist whereby the mature cells in this compartment can stimulate cells in the 'stem cell compartment' to divide, to maintain the number of cells in the 'functional cell compartment'. Chemical growth factors, 'chalones', have been implicated as having a role in this feedback system in several tissues (Bullough 1971). In addition to the stem cell and functional cell compartments a third 'maturing cell compartment' must exist, containing cells passing from the stem cell to functional cell compartments. There is some evidence (Metcalf 1973) that failure of normal negative feedback mechanisms, whereby the

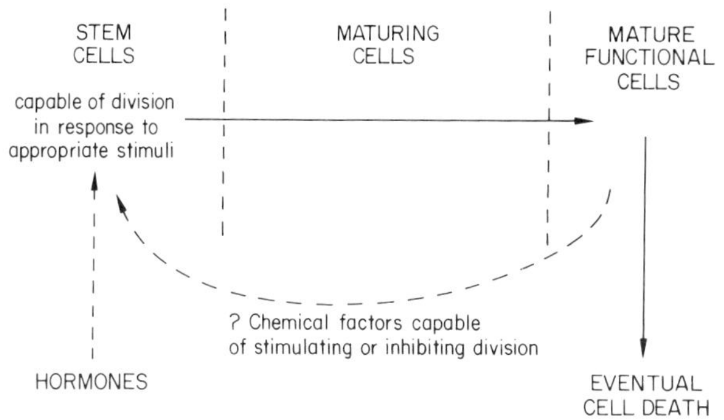

Fig. 14.2 The cell 'compartments' in a population of dividing cells.

functional cells inhibit division of stem cells, may be involved in the genesis of some tumours. The net effect is that tumour cells do not have a faster rate of division than the normal tissues from which they arise, but that tumours contain an increased number of dividing cells.

In order for cells to divide, they have to pass through a series of metabolic steps in specific order between each mitotic division, and this procession of events is known as the cell cycle. Synthesis of DNA is confined to a limited period, the S-phase, of the intermitotic interval, and this phase is separated from the preceding mitosis by a 'gap' period, known as G_1. A second 'gap' phase, G_2, follows DNA synthesis, prior to the onset of mitosis (M) (Fig. 14.3). Hill (1976) reviews the cell cycle, but it is sufficient for the present account to note that replication of chromatin (the chromosomal complex of DNA, RNA, and protein) during the S-phase requires, in addition to the presence of the preformed DNA template and the appropriate precursor nucleotides, the presence of particular RNA species and various proteins and enzymes. Specific RNA synthesis is also required during G_1, if the cell is to progress into S, and in G_2 for progression into mitosis. During G_2 special division-related proteins must also be synthesised.

From the foregoing account it will be apparent that preparation for mitosis is an elaborate process, which occupies the whole of the intermitiotic interval, so that interference with DNA, RNA, or protein synthesis may be sufficient to disrupt the whole process of cell multiplication; Fig. 14.4 indicates the sites of actions of various chemotherapeutic agents in relation to the cell cycle.

In normal tissues a large proportion, and in most malignant tumours usually a small proportion, of the cells leave the reproductive pool to become differentiated, and hence no longer capable of division. Other cells retain the capacity to continue replication, but do not remain actively involved in the cell cycle. Such cells may simply undergo prolongation of the G_2 or G_2 phase, or may enter a 'resting' phase designated G_0. These resting cells form the majority of the stem cell compartment in normal tissues, and whilst the size of

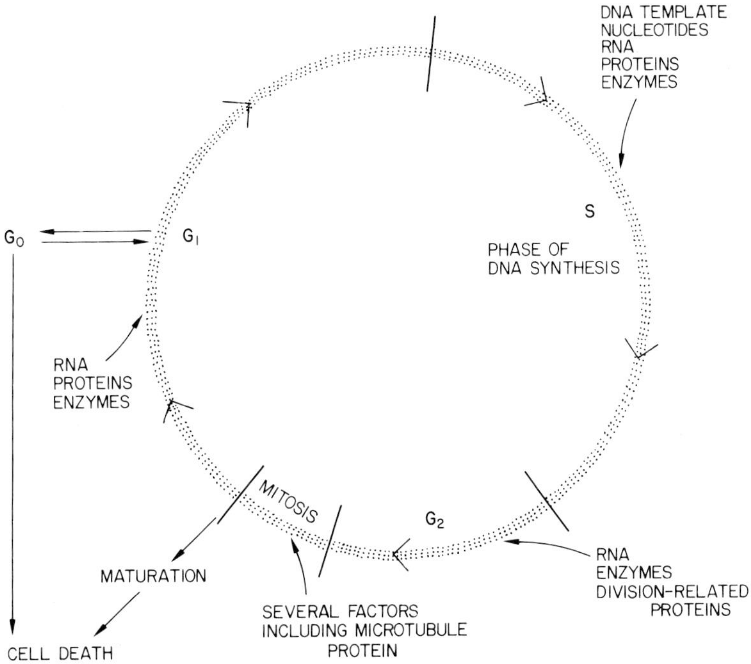

Fig. 14.3 The cell cycle and some of the factors essential for its maintenance.

the G_0 compartment in tumours is probably very variable, it is likely to be large, since tumour cells, which are less inclined to become differentiated, must either remain in the cell cycle or enter G_0 (Fig. 14.3). The importance of this concept lies in the fact that cells in G_0 tend to be resistant to the effects of many cytotoxic drugs. Consideration of the cell kinetic differences between tumours and normal tissue had led to the development of chemotherapeutic techniques designed to take advantage of these differences (Price 1972; Mauer 1975). The principle behind such a kinetically based technique is that tumours contain a high proportion of cells at various stages of the cell cycle which are actively replicating, whilst normal tissues contain a much smaller proportion of dividing cells. If a combination of drugs, all acting on cycling cells, at different phases of the cycle but with *little or no effect on non-cycling cells* are administered as a 'single-shot', the tumour cell population will be reduced to a much greater extent than the normal stem cell populations, since the latter have relatively few susceptible cycling cells. In consequence, many cells will be drawn from the tumour G_0 pool to repopulate the tumour, whilst relatively few cells will be drawn from the stem cell G_0 pool, since a smaller degree of repopulation will be required (Fig. 14.5). Repeated doses of the drugs involved will therefore tend to destroy the whole tumour cell population,

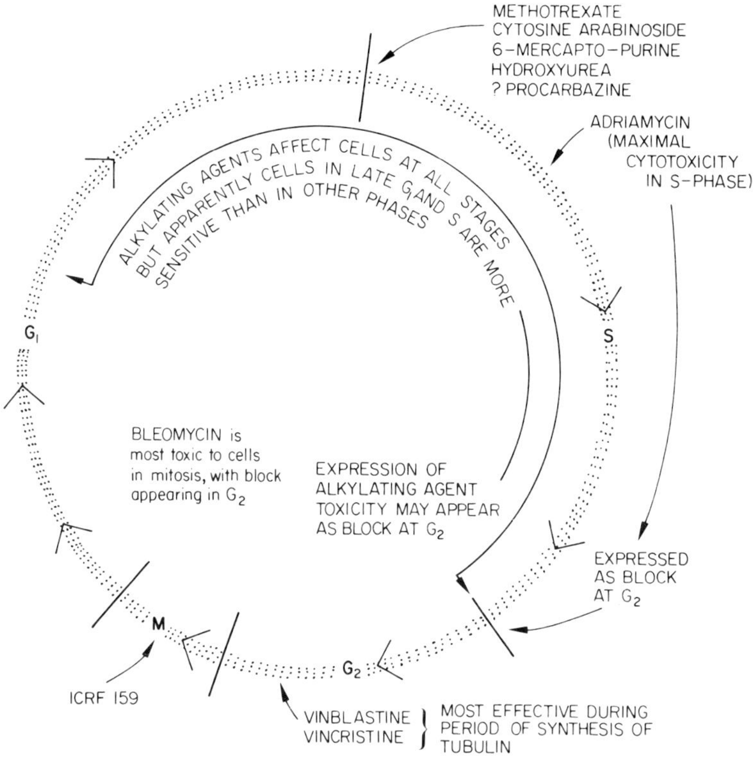

Fig. 14.4 Sites of action of some antitumour agents in relation to the cell cycle; 5-fluorouracil, actinomycin D, DTIC and nitrosoureas affect cells at all stages of the cycle. In devising combination schedules it is logical to avoid using two drugs (e.g. methotrexate and cytosine-arabinoside) which would tend to hold cells in a single stage of the cycle (e.g. G_2 in this case). Conversely, it is logical, but in practice difficult, to give an agent which will block cells at a specific stage of the cycle (e.g. vincristine→block in mitosis; bleomycin→block in G_2) and then to discontinue this agent so that the cells released from the block pass through the cycle in synchrony. A second agent can then be given at the time when the synchronised cells are expected to be passing through a sensitive phase.

whilst leaving a residual normal stem cell G_0 population, which will be available to restore the cycling stem cell pool, thus allowing recovery of normal tissue. The effectiveness of such regimes is not yet proven, but early trials (e.g. Price *et al* 1975) appear promising.

Another significant aspect of the study of cell kinetics is the finding that only tumours with a relatively short cell cycle time and high growth fraction are sensitive to chemotherapy. Most mesenchymal sarcomas, and many adenocarcinomas tend to have long cell cycle times and low growth fractions, and tend to be insensitive (Tubiana & Malaise 1976). However, this is not the whole story, because well-differentiated tumours tend to show similar

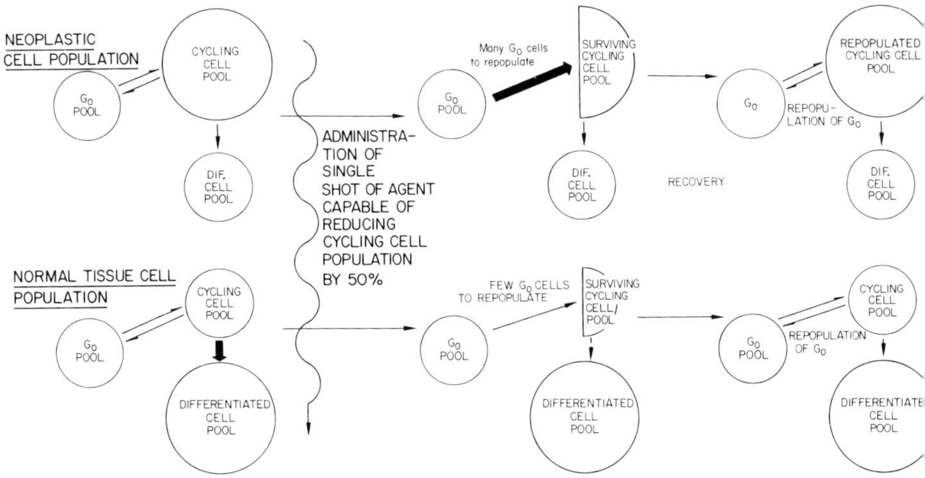

Fig. 14.5 Effect of a single dose of a 'phase-specific' antitumour agent on neoplastic and normal cell populations.

characteristics, but may be chemosensitive, and, once such tumours are caused to go into regression, prolonged freedom from clinical signs of disease may be expected, due to the slow growth rate associated with such kinetic parameters. Unfortunately, it does not follow that poorly differentiated, fast-growing tumours will respond well to treatment. Indeed, it has been shown that tumours with a rapid rate of growth tend to carry a poor prognosis (Steele & Buell 1973).

Tumour growth rate can be expressed in terms of the time taken for the tumour to double in volume, and this doubling time can be very variable. Owen and Steel (1969) found that doubling times for a series of pulmonary metastases of different canine tumours varied from 7 to 150 days. Study of the cell kinetic characteristics described above suggested that the tumours were capable of doubling in periods of 2–16 days, (i.e. the metastatic modules were growing very much more slowly than expected). This is an illustration of the general phenomenon of cell loss, whereby cells are lost from the proliferating tumour mass, thus reducing the rate at which it increases in size. This cell loss factor can account for as much as 90% of the tumour cell production, and several mechanisms contribute to this effect as outlined below.

1 Loss of surface cells to the environment.

2 Loss of cells to body cavities.

3 Migration of cells away from tumour mass in vascular or lymphatic channels, or by amoeboid movement.

4 Death of cells due to:

- **a** Deprivation of oxygen or nutrients, as tumour growth almost invariably outstrips vascular development.

b Secondary infection.
c Host defence mechanisms.
d Failure of cells to complete mitotic division, due to spontaneous derangement of biochemistry or genetic structure.

The cell loss factor clearly militates in favour of the therapist, except insofar as metastasis formation may follow if cells shed from the tumour become implanted in suitable sites. It would seem that one would need only to destroy or incapacitate sufficient tumour cells to increase the cell loss factor beyond the rate of cell proliferation in order to produce tumour regression.

14.2 Resistance to chemotherapy

Tumours are distinguished from normal tissue in terms of having a *relatively* greater sensitivity to most cytostatic agents, and equally resistance must be regarded as a relative term. For example, if a tumour exhibits sensitivity to a particular agent because of a rapid rate of cell proliferation relative to normal tissues, then if the growth rate of that tumour is reduced, the difference in sensitivity to the agent between the normal cells and the tumour will decrease, and the tumour will appear to be relatively more resistant. An example of such resistance is seen in the effects of the drug razoxone. This agent is only effective against rapidly proliferating cells, in which it inhibits cell division, whilst in high doses it also inhibits DNA synthesis. If rapidly proliferating cells are exposed to a high dose of this agent they therefore proliferate more slowly due to inhibition of DNA synthesis, and thereby become less sensitive to the primary cytostatic effect of the drug, which depends upon rapid cell proliferation. Relatively low doses of the drug may therefore be more effective than higher doses (Taylor & Bleehen 1977). This is an example of acquired resistance, in which cells become less sensitive as a result of exposure to the drug in question. Many other mechanisms of acquired resistance are exhibited by tumour cells (see Harrap 1976, for a review). For example, many biochemical processes may follow several alternative routes, so that if one particular route is inhibited, the end result of the inhibited reaction will be achieved by another route if this is possible, and resistance to a particular agent may arise in this way. Many metabolic enzymes are relatively non-specific, and their activity may be induced by presence of substrate, so that increased deactivation of drug may arise due to exposure to that drug. Other changes, such as increased production of target molecules or changes in enzyme specificity may also give rise to acquired resistance (Ball 1969).

Inherent, as opposed to acquired, resistance occurs when tumour cells are insensitive to an agent when first exposed to that agent. For example, 5-fluorouracil is converted to 5-fluorodeoxyuridylate in cells, and this product appears to be the active cytotoxic agent. Because metabolic pathways concerned with DNA synthesis are usually more active in tumour cells, this conversion proceeds more rapidly in tumours than in normal tissues. Some tumours, however, appear to be poor at this conversion, and will therefore be relatively insensitive (Mukherjee *et al* 1963). Many other examples of this type of insensitivity exist (Harrap 1976). Another way in which tumour cells may appear to be insensitive occurs with phase-specific agents. A single dose of such an agent will affect only those cells which pass through the particular sensitive phase of the cell cycle during the period of exposure, whilst a continuous low dose of the drug, or frequent administration, will affect a much higher proportion of the cells, as previously unaffected cells pass into the sensitive phase of the cycle. Table 14.1 illustrates this phenomenon by reference to the work of Skipper *et al* (1967), using a mouse leukaemia model.

Not uncommonly, resistance to chemotherapeutic agents occurs because the agent is not transported across the cell membrane. Membrane transport mechanisms in neoplastic cells have already been mentioned, and cells may acquire resistance to agents such as methotrexate, adriamycin, and the vinca alkaloids, by ceasing to transport these agents across the cell membrane. Daunomycin, adriamycin, vincristine, and vinblastine appear to be able to induce resistance to each other in this way (Danø 1972).

Extracellular factors which may reduce the concentration of active drug reaching the tumour cells include induction of hepatic enzymes and failure of absorption when the drug is administered by an inappropriate route. Another factor is that the structure of solid tumours may limit penetration of the drug to sensitive cells. When Evans Blue Dye is injected intravenously into a tumour-bearing animal, all the tissues will eventually appear grossly blue, as the dye is carried into the small capillaries, and thence to the tissues. If the tumour is then removed surgically, it is often possible to see clearly demarkated zones of staining within the tumour, which are associated with blood vessels, whilst the remainder of the tumour contains no dye. The distribution of those chemotherapeutic agents which have been tested has been

Table 14.1 Effect of dose fractionation with cytosine arabinoside to take advantage of S-phase specificity in L1210 mouse leukaemia cells. From Skipper *et al.* 1967.

Dose (mg/kg)	Times of dosing	Total dose (mg)	No. of animals cured	Leukaemic cells present in animals at end of treatment
240	2, 6, 10 & 14 days	960	0/10	10^9
15	2, 6, 10 & 14 days (8 times daily on these days)	480	10/10	0

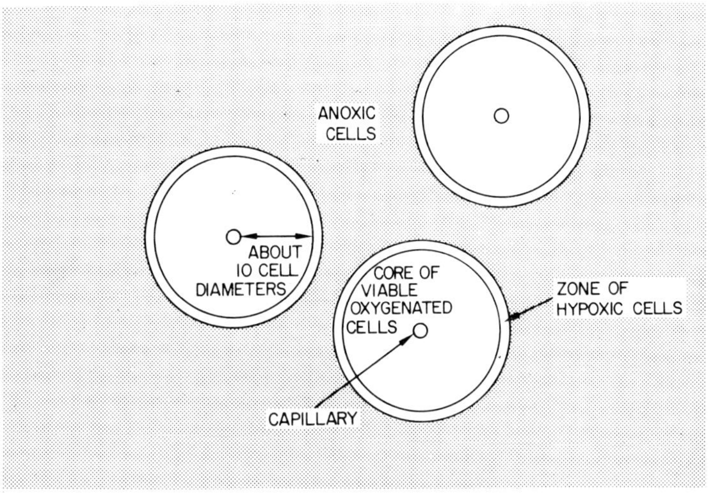

Fig. 14.6 Diagrammatic representation of zones of oxygenation within a tumour (after Thomlinson & Gray 1955).

found to correlate with the distribution of the dye, indicating, even at this gross level, how agents may fail to penetrate into the centre of a tumour mass (A. H. T. Paterson & A. T. Yoxall, unpubl. obs.). At a much finer level, Thomlinson and Gray (1955) were the first investigators to demonstrate the presence of cords of viable tumour cells surrounding small blood vessels, where there is sufficient diffusion of oxygen to maintain metabolic and reproductive activity, whilst cells at some distance from the nearest capillary die due to anoxia (Fig. 14.6). The problem is that some cells will be situated in an hypoxic zone, such that they are neither reproductively active, and are thus resistant to most chemotherapeutic agents, but nor are they dead. If the well-oxygenated cells are destroyed by some therapeutic technique, then the hypoxic cells will come to lie closer to the vessels, and repopulate the tumour. These hypoxic cells may account for 1–10% of the total tumour population. Good perfusion of the tumour is further reduced by a tendency for microthrombi to form within the poorly developed tumour vessels (reviewed by Hilgard *et al* 1977).

14.3 Principles for clinical application of chemotherapeutic agents

As indicated above, most chemotherapeutic agents used in the treatment of malignant disease have a significant degree of toxicity to the patient, and the general principle of treatment is to administer the maximum tolerated dose, which may be given in a particular manner such as to enhance tumour cell damage, whilst minimising damage to normal tissues as far as possible. Drugs are very often given in combination, using agents which have different toxic effects, so that the tumouricidal effect of the combination may be additive, without toxic side-effects of any of the agents in the combination reaching significant levels.

In devising drug combinations consideration also has to be given to interactions which may enhance or diminish tumour cell killing (see Fig. 14.4). If a tumour contains 10^{12} cells initially, four separate agents, each capable of killing 10^3 cells might prove the most effective combination for treatment, but if the tumour should be resistant to one of the drugs in the combination, the patient will be subjected to some degree of toxicity from the agent, without control of the tumour being obtained. Since there is no way of predicting tumour sensitivity, the selection of suitable agents for the combination must be based on an intimate knowledge of the experimental situation and clinical experience, knowing which agents may be effective against the particular type of tumour in question when used on their own. The veterinary oncologist is faced with a dilemma, for this sort of essential information has been collected over the years for many human tumours, but relatively little for tumours of domestic animals, and there is little evidence that tumour sensitivity in man bears any close relationship to the sensitivity of similar tumours in animals. The therapist therefore has the choice of using a single agent, which may well be ineffective, but which will help to produce data on tumour sensitivity; or he may use a combination which is known to be effective treatment in the human patient.

Moreover, we remain almost totally ignorant of the kinetic parameters of animal tumours, and many of the drug combinations used in human medicine are arranged such that one agent may modify these parameters, so that another agent, given subsequently, will exert its maximal effect. Under these circumstances exact timing of the drug sequence becomes all important, and changes of no more than an hour or two may profoundly affect the effectiveness of the treatment. It seems unlikely that there is any possibility of using such sophisticated schedules in veterinary tumour chemotherapy at present.

There is little evidence that the use of combinations does much to delay the onset of acquired tumour cell resistance, except in certain special cases.

The effect of a single treatment with a single agent is proportional to the doubling time of the tumour, and inversely proportional to the tumour mass present. Reduction of the bulk of the tumour by means of surgery or radiotherapy prior to chemotherapy will remove the majority of cells 'protected' by being relatively underperfused, will give host defence mechanisms a better chance to operate, and will reduce the number of cells to be killed by chemotherapy, with a consequent saving in dose and reduction of toxicity. It would be logical to follow a course of chemotherapy with treatment aimed at enhancing the host's cell-mediated immune response, so that this response might be effective in destroying the small number of tumour cells remaining at the end of chemotherapy, especially since most chemotherapeutic agents depress immunological mechanisms. However, immunotherapy is a treatment technique which is in its infancy, although some reports are beginning to appear in the literature describing the very variable results of treatment with non-specific immune stimulants such as BGC (Lamoureux *et al* 1976; Owen *et al* 1977) *Corynebacterium parvum* (Halbern 1975) and levaminsole (Rojas *et al* 1976) either alone or in addition to chemotherapy. Specific immunotherapy, using chemically altered tumour cell extracts as an adjuvant to chemotherapy in the treatment of canine lymphosarcoma has been described by Theilen *et al* (1977b).

14.4 Agents used in the treatment of malignancies

In 1966, W. R. Bruce and his colleagues defined two categories of cytotoxic agents; those which acted at all stages of the cell cycle, and those which acted only at specific stages of the cycle. This is a useful classification since agents in the first category, the 'cycle-specific' agents, are theoretically capable of destroying all the cells in a tumour if given in sufficient quantity, although producing progressive toxicity to sensitive normal cell populations, such as marrow (Fig. 14.7). The 'phase-specific' agents, however, are not able to eliminate the whole population, but will reduce it to a plateau. In general, this plateau level is much lower for tumour cells than for normal tissue cells, when the tumour cells are maximally sensitive to the agent in question (Fig. 14.8). Kinetically based regimes (see above) depend upon the use of

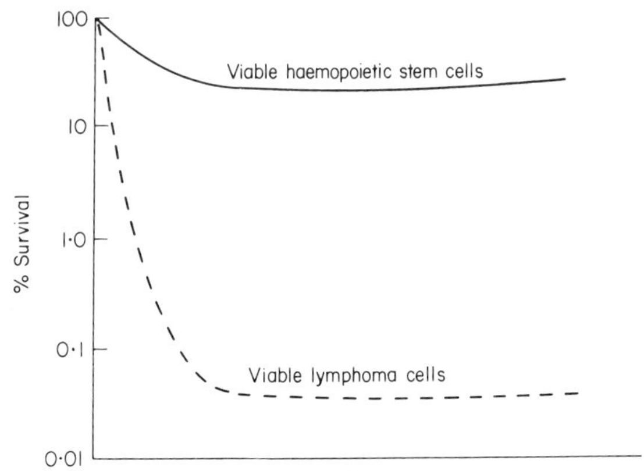

Fig. 14.7 Effect on murine cells of a 24 hour exposure *in vitro* to phase-specific antitumour agents (vinblastine, vincristine, methotrexate, 6-mercaptopurine, cytosine arabinoside). Modified from Bruce *et al* (1966).

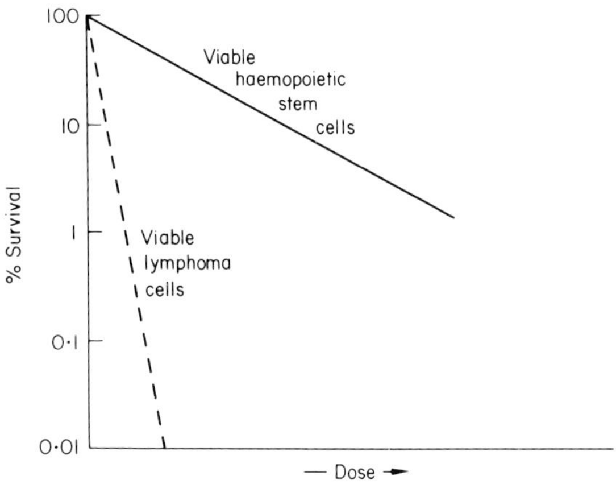

Fig. 14.8 Effect on murine cells of a 24-hour exposure *in vitro* to cycle-specific agents (cyclophosphamide, BCNU, 5FU, actinomycin D). Modified from Bruce *et al* (1966).

phase-specific agents, since these have no effect on cells in G_0, but cycle-specific agents are usually added to enhance the cell-kill, as phase-specific agents will not eliminate all the malignant cells.

14.4.1 Alkylating agents

Alkylating agents are highly chemically reactive compounds, which are capable of binding covalently to cell constituents which are highly negatively charged. They will therefore react readily with many amino acids, enzymes, and nucleic acids, but since they appear to inhibit DNA synthesis rapidly at fairly low dose levels, it is thought that their primary site of action is probably the DNA molecule itself. The most effective alkylating agents have two functional groups, so it is probable that they act by means of forming cross-linkages, possibly between adjacent DNA strands, thus preventing the splitting of these strands for DNA synthesis (Harrap & Gascoigne 1976). Alkylating agents will therefore affect all cells, but in cells which are replicating only slowly, lesions in DNA can be repaired by normal mechanisms before the next cell division, so that the toxic effects of these agents are more apparent in rapidly dividing cells, as in tumours.

Cyclophosphamide is one of the most widely used of the alkylating agents, although the drug is itself inactive, and has to undergo activation in the liver. Tumour cells appear to be less capable of detoxifying the active metabolites of the drug than normal cells, and so some degree of selective killing of tumour cells may be achieved (Connors 1975). However, the pharmacology of cyclophosphamide appears to be different in the dog from that in man, the half-life being much shorter in the dog, with cumulation occurring in the kidneys, liver and spleen (Mellett 1963). In man, cyclophosphamide is usually administered in large doses, given intermittently, but the dog is much less able to tolerate relatively large doses of cyclophosphamide (Hill 1975) and it is usual to give the drug on a continuous low dose basis in this species. Some investigators have used this approach in the treatment of certain human tumours, and have reported a marked reduction in toxicity, with no reduction in efficacy (Mangioni *et al* 1976).

The toxic effects of cyclophosphamide in the dog include myelosuppression, hepatic and renal toxicity, gastrointestinal ulceration, alopecia, and cardiotoxicity at very high dose levels (O'Connell & Berenbaum 1974).

A particular problem with cyclophosphamide is that the unchanged drug and its metabolites are excreted in the urine, and prolonged treatment not infrequently gives rise to a haemorrhagic cystitis, with severe ulceration of the bladder mucosa, these ulcers having proliferating margins, and sometimes progressing to precancerous lesions. *N*-acetylcysteine will prevent development of cyclophosphamide-induced cystitis in experimental animals (Tolley & Castro 1976), and the present author has had limited success in using this agent for the treatment of established cyclophosphamide cystitis in dogs in a small number of cases, 100 mg/kg of the agent being given intravenously, and repeated as required. The most important action however, is to discontinue treatment with cyclophosphamide as soon as there is any evidence of cystitis, and many cases will then subside very slowly spontaneously, although a few may progress to fibrosis and contracture of the bladder.

Chlorambucil is an alkylating agent which has been used in the dog (Bostock & Owen 1972; Theilen *et al* 1977b), and it may be used as an alternative to cyclophosphamide if cystitis occurs during treatment with the latter drug, although in the present author's experience it appears to be rather less effective in maintaining remissions which had previously been well-maintained with cyclophosphamide. Recent experimental work suggests, however, that rather larger doses of this agent may be used, if given in combination with prednisolone (Brandt *et al* 1975).

Both of these alkylating agents have been used with some success in a small number of cases in the treatment of canine squamous cell carcinoma, in combination with methotrexate (A. T. Yoxall, unpubl. obs.), and either alone, or in combination with other agents for the treatment of lymphoreticular tumours (Brick *et al* 1969; Squire & Bush 1973; Cohen *et al* 1975; Theilen 1975; Owen 1976; MacEwan & Hess 1977).

Of the other available alkylating agents, Owen (1964) used ethoglucid for the treatment of osteosarcoma in dogs, by intra-arterial perfusion of the isolated limb, and induced regression in twelve out of fourteen dogs, which was maintained for 2 months or more in five cases. The same author has also used triethylene thiophosphoramide as a 0.3% solution instilled into the bladder for the treatment of transitional cell carcinoma, systemic toxicity being minimised when the drug is given by this route (L. N. Owen, pers. comm.).

14.4.2 Antimetabolites

The antimetabolites bear a structural resemblance to normal metabolites which are essential for cell function, and may act by competing with these metabolites for enzyme binding sites, thus blocking the enzyme in question. Alternatively, they may be incorporated into DNA or RNA, and thus interfere with the genetic code. Fig. 14.9 illustrates the sites of action of some antimetabolites.

One of the most widely used antimetabolites is methotrexate, which exerts its effect by competing with folic acid for the enzyme which converts this precursor to folinic acid. Derivatives of folinic acid are essential constituents in the synthetic pathways of the purines and pyrimidines required for nucleic acid synthesis; therefore interference with folinic acid synthesis will ultimately disrupt nucleic acid synthesis. The primary toxic effect of methotrexate is depression of all bone marrow elements. Gastrointestinal ulceration and hepatic necrosis may also occur in dogs, and vomiting can be a problem. However, most of the effects of methotrexate can be reversed by administration of folinic acid, so that a high dose of the drug may be given to kill tumour cells in the G_1/S phase, and folinic acid may then be given to

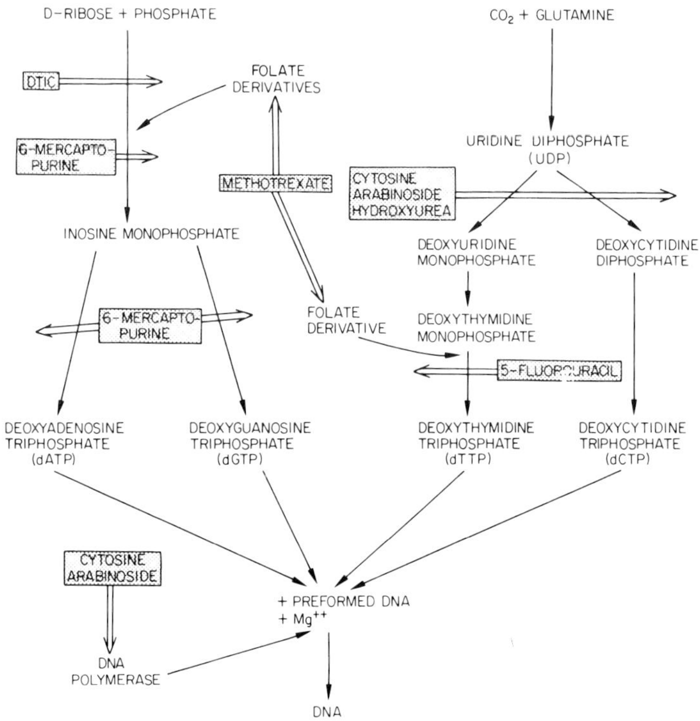

Fig. 14.9 Simplified diagram of pathways of DNA synthesis to illustrate sites of action of some clinically useful antimetabolites.

reduce damage to normal tissues (especially bone marrow), before a large proportion of normal stem cells are drawn from the G_0 pool. This stratagem is necessary because methotrexate has a long plasma half-life. An interesting recent development is the use of purines and pyrimidines to counteract methotrexate toxicity, since it seems that tumour cells may be less effective at taking-up these bases than normal tissue cells, so that some degree of selectivity of action may be achieved (Tew & Taylor 1976).

The high cost of methotrexate and folinic acid limit their use in very high dose schedules in animals, but the present author has used moderately high doses (0·5 g/m^2) with folinic acid rescue in a limited number of cases. The success of this technique in the dog is limited by the toxicity of methotrexate in this species, which is rather greater than in man (Freirich *et al* 1966). Methotrexate can be given rather more successfully on a continuous low dose basis (Theilen *et al* 1977b; Henness *et al* 1977), and the author has used such an approach for the treatment of squamous cell carcinomas, using alternating 1-month courses of cyclophosphamide or methotrexate for 4 months, followed by 2 months' rest, and the whole cycle being repeated continuously. Cyclical therapy of this sort seems to delay the development of resistance, and such a low dose regime can be continued indefinitely, although occasional haematological examinations should be made. It is sometimes possible to prolong the rest periods, but intermittent maintenance therapy is usually required. It is too early to say how long such remissions can be expected to last whilst maintenance is continued, but a few cases have continued for over 2 years on such treatment.

Cytosine arabinoside is an antimetabolite which appears to act by inhibiting the enzyme DNA-polmerase (Fig. 14.9). It has found a place in veterinary chemotherapy in combination with cyclophosphamide, vincristine, and prednisolone in the treatment of canine lymphosarcoma and mast cell tumours (Theilen 1975).

5-fluorouracil (5FU) is an antimetabolite which is widely used in human practice, and which inhibits the synthesis of thymidylic acid. In dogs, however, and more especially in cats, it produces severe CNS side-effects including convulsions, even at low doses. It is available as a cream for topical application, but systemic toxicity can occur by absorption. In the treatment of malignant effusions, 5FU is particularly useful as it persists in high concentrations for prolonged periods (Clarkson *et al* 1975).

Other antimetabolites are available, but clinical experience of their use in animals has not been encouraging (Hess *et al* 1976).

14.4.3 Antitumour antibiotics

ACTINOMYCIN D

This antibiotic is one of a family isolated from various *Streptomyces* species. It has proved to be of particular value in the treatment of Wilm's tumour in children, and in a few other human tumours but it is not known why its spectrum of activity is so limited. However, it has been suggested that many cells are unable to take up the drug. It is mentioned here because it has been the subject of many fundamental studies on modes of antitumour drug action although it has not been used clinically in animals to any great extent, partly, no doubt, due to its significant toxicity. It exerts its action by intercalating into the DNA helix and thereby inhibiting RNA synthesis. *Mithramycin* is similar and although it has been used for the treatment of certain embryonal testicular tumours in man, it is too toxic for use in animals.

ADRIAMYCIN

Adriamycin, also known as doxorubicin, is another antibiotic isolated from a *Streptomyces* and is widely used in the treatment of human malignancies, since it is not only a very effective agent for the treatment of lymphoreticular neoplasia but also has a unique activity against a number of solid tumours, including soft tissue sarcomas and adenocarcinomas, which are otherwise resistant to chemotherapy. Adriamycin appears to exert its effect by intercalating between adjacent bases of a DNA strand, thus disrupting the helical structure of the paired DNA strands and interfering with the DNA template, upon which synthesis of RNA and further DNA depend. The drug appears to be especially tightly bound to myocardial DNA and this may account for the myocardial toxicity which is the feature of adriamycin which limits the dose which may be administered. Moreover, adriamycin bears a structural resemblance to the cardiac glycosides and this may, in part, account for its cardiotoxicity; cardiac glycosides are effective in preventing or reversing adriamycin cardiotoxocity in the dog (Arena *et al* 1972). The antitumour agent ICRF 159 (see below) will protect the heart to some extent from adriamycin toxicity, possibly by chelating cations (Herman *et al* 1974), whilst cyclophosphamide and adriamycin together may be synergistic in terms of production of cardiac toxicity (Denine & Schmidt 1975). Other toxic effects of adriamycin include myelosuppression, lymphosuppression and severe mucositis. In two cases treated by the present author, desquamation of the skin of the entire ventral body surface was sufficiently severe to cause early discontinuation of treatment. Theilen's group in California have found that the most serious toxic effects of adriamycin can be avoided in dogs if the dose is kept below 30 mg/m^2 given one every 3 weeks for a limited period (Theilen *et al* 1977a; Henness *et al* 1977). At this dose, some degree of alopecia occurs, with loss of the undercoat whilst the guard hairs are preserved (A. M. Henness, pers. comm.). This dose is clearly a compromise between efficacy and toxicity and its clinical value remains to be assessed. Adriamycin is claimed to be of value when given intralesionally in isolated tumour nodules in man (Bast *et al* 1976) and this approach may be worth evaluating in animals.

BLEOMYCIN

Certain tissues, such as skin, lung and some malignant tumours are deficient in the ability to synthesise peptidase enzymes, and for this reason the complex of polypeptide antibiotics, known collectively as bleomycin, accumulate in these tissues, and a relatively higher concentration is obtained in such tissues following administration of the drug. Concentration of the drug occurs particularly in squamous cell carcinomas and the chief indication for the use of this drug in man is in the treatment of this particular malignancy, although useful results have also been obtained in the treatment of lymphoreticular malignancies (Shaw 1976).

Bleomycin is particularly noteworthy because it has a minimal suppressive effect on rapidly proliferating normal tissue, such as bone marrow — a feature which is especially important in combination therapy. However, it is not without particular toxicity of its own, and high doses in man will cause cutaneous and pulmonary toxicity, which is presumably related to the high concentration of drug in these tissues. The pulmonary toxicity takes the form of pulmonary fibrosis and is a special problem since it may occur occasionally at very low doses and may be a progressive and lethal complication to the use of this drug in man. Pulmonary fibrosis has been induced in dogs by the administration of large doses of bleomycin, but it has not been reported at more moderate dose rates, such as might be used in the clinical situation (Buhles & Theilen 1973; Ishizuka *et al* 1970).

The same two groups of workers have reported on the clinical use of bleomycin in animals. Buhles and Theilen found that the agent produced rather short-lived and incomplete remissions in three out of four cases of squamous cell carcinoma in the cat and in two out of six such cases in the dog. However, as Chabner and his colleagues (1975) observe, the action of bleomycin appears to be to specifically inhibit the progression of cells through the G_2/M phase of the cell cycle (see Fig. 14.4) and drugs acting specifically at a single stage of the cycle in this way may be most effective if given on a continuous low dose basis, and the author is not aware of any studies in dogs or cats utilising such a schedule.

In spite of its high cost, bleomycin is an agent which should be evaluated further for use in the treatment of small animal malignancies.

MITOGILLIN

Roga *et al* (1971) have reported extremely favourable results in the treatment of several canine tumours with mitogillin, an experimental polypeptide antibiotic produced by *Aspergillus restrictus*. Many of the animals in this series were said to have died due to excessively rapid breakdown of tumour and absorption of toxic products, so rapid was the effect of the drug.

14.4.4 Plant alkaloids and other plant products

VINCA ALKALOIDS

Four active alkaloids can be extracted from the periwinkle plant, but only two of these, *vinblastine* and *vincristine* have been used clinically to any extent. Although these two agents are very similar in structure, their antitumour spectra and toxic effects are quite different in many respects. They act by blocking mitosis in metaphase by binding with the protein *tubulin*, and thereby disrupting its normal structure. This protein is the chief component of the microtubules of the mitotic apparatus and when the microtubules are disrupted in this way the chromosomes are unable to separate and cell death occurs. Other plant products, colchicine and podophyllotoxin (see below), have a similar mechanism of action. Microtubules elsewhere in the cell have several other biological functions in addition to their role in mitosis and most of the toxic effects of the vinca alkaloids can be understood in terms of loss of these various functions. It has been suggested by Berlin and colleagues (1975) that interactions with microtubules may be involved in the cell surface changes characteristic of malignant cells.

The chief toxic effect of vinblastine is bone marrow depression and it is this which limits the dose which may be administered. With vincristine, on the other hand, marrow suppression is less of a problem but peripheral neuropathy may develop, due, apparently, to the role of microtubules in nerve cell function (Creasey 1975). However, at the doses recommended for use in tumour-bearing dogs, the present author has not observed any evidence of toxicity with vincristine. Although the pharmacology of vinblastine in the dog has been investigated (Creasey *et al* 1975), that of vincristine has not; nevertheless vincristine appears to have been more widely used than vinblastine in clinical practice, chiefly because results with vinblastine seem to have been less promising than those with vincristine (Hess *et al* 1976). It is unfortunate that rather little published work has appeared on the use of vincristine as a single agent in the dog and it is more commonly used in combination with cyclophosphamide, prednisone and cytosine arabinoside in the treatment of lymphoreticular tumours and mast cell tumours, a combination which has proved useful in the experience of the present author and other workers (Squire & Bush 1973; Cohen *et al* 1975; Theilen 1975; Owen 1976). The success of combination therapy based on vincristine and prednisolone in the treatment of lymphosarcoma (*op. cit.*) and mastocytoma (Theilen 1975) is one of the few real successes in the use of chemotherapy in animals and such regimes as those suggested by these authors are capable of producing clinical regression in some cases of lymphosarcoma. Although the tumour will recur sooner or later, prolongation of life is usually possible, for long periods in some cases. The median survival of dogs with lymphosarcoma after diagnosis is about 10 weeks if untreated and about 28 weeks on quadruple chemotherapy (D. E. Bostock, unpubl. obs.).

PODOPHYLLOTOXIN

Podophyllum resin B. Vet. C. has been used in an oily base as a topical application for the treatment of warts and may well be worth trying in some cases. The problem is that this preparation is caustic and care must be taken to avoid applying it to unaffected skin and to prevent the animal from licking the treated area.

14.4.5 Enzymes

L-ASPARAGINASE

Some tumour cells are unable to synthesise L-asparagine, an essential cellular nutrient, whilst normal cells are readily able to do so. For this reason L-asparaginase is the only anticancer agent which is specific for neoplastic cells, since it acts by destroying endogenous L-asparagine, without which dependent tumour cells are unable to survive. Unfortunately this drug is not totally without effect on the function of all normal cells and the remissions induced in sensitive tumours appear to be very short-lived. Hardy and Old (1970) have reported on the use of this agent in the dog and Theilen (1975) has used it to maintain remissions induced in cases of lymphosarcoma by means of combination chemotherapy, as described above.

14.4.6 Miscellaneous agents

PROCARBAZINE

Procarbazine is an interesting agent, which has been used in man chiefly in combination regimes, but which has received little veterinary attention. It is less expensive than some other agents and is effective when given orally and has a relatively high therapeutic index, the main toxic effect being bone marrow suppression, although this complication can be minimised by the use of intermittent high doses. Unfortunately, this schedule is difficult to implement, since the drug causes vomiting in dogs rather readily, a problem which may be overcome by starting with a low dose, which is gradually increased. Its mode of action is not well understood, but it appears to cause a prolongation of interphase, with disorganisation of the chromosomes. It has the useful property of being able to cross the blood-brain barrier.

NITROSOUREA-COMPOUNDS

BCNU and CCNU are relatively new agents which have been the subject of extensive study and which have proved effective in the treatment of a wide range of human malignancies, although cost and limited availability have so far precluded their use in veterinary medicine. They appear to act as alkylating agents and produce a wide range of toxic side-effects including bone marrow depression, which may not appear for some weeks after treatment thus making adjustment of the dose difficult.

DACARBAZINE

Dacarbazine (DTIC) is an agent which appears to be especially effective in the treatment of human malignant melanoma. Adequate trials with this agent in the treatment of canine malignant melanoma have not been carried out but it has not been outstandingly successful in the very few cases treated by the author and the death of one dog due to convulsions may have been attributable to the drug. In man, about 20% of cases appear to respond satisfactorily, so a large number of canine cases would need to be treated in order to assess its value in the dog.

HYDROXYUREA

This agent is one of those which inhibits one of the rate-limiting enzymes of DNA synthesis, the activity of which is increased in malignant cells. The enzyme in this case is that which converts ribonucleotides to deoxyribnucleotides (Fig. 14.9). It has produced remission in some human solid tumours, but it is chiefly used in the treatment of chronic granulocytic leukaemia. It has been used in the dog in the successful treatment of a single case of basophilic leukaemia (MacEwan *et al* 1975) and is currently undergoing trial in the treatment of mastocytoma in the USA (Hess *et al* 1976). Its chief toxic effect is bone-marrow suppression but this can be readily reversed by withdrawal of the drug. It is worthy of further trial for veterinary use.

RAZOXANE

Razoxane or ICRF 159 was developed in response to the hypothesis that most drugs which show an antitumour effect are actual or potential chelating agents, although many chelating agents are not tumouricidal — usually because they are unable to pass into cells. It is a phase-specific agent, and cells are most sensitive in G_2/M, although its mode of action has not been fully elucidated. Controversy still exists over the value of this drug in the treatment of human cancer and it does not, at present, appear to have unequivocally fulfilled the promise of initial experimental results in laboratory animals, in which it demonstrated an ability not only to suppress tumour growth, but also to inhibit the development of metastases in some carcinomas at doses which had no effect on the primary tumour. This property has been attributed to an ability on the part of the drug to improve or 'normalise' tumour vasculature (Salusbury *et al* 1974), and this property of the drug may account for its ability to potentiate the tumouricidal effects of irradiation without causing a concomitant increase in side-effects (Ryall *et al* 1974) if it can cause improved oxygenation of tumour cells by improving tumour vascularity, since the presence of hypoxic cells within tumours is probably one of the main causes of failure to obtain local control of tumours by radiotherapy.

14.4.7 Hormones

Steroid hormones have long been used rather empirically in the treatment of malignancies. Pierpaoli *et al* (1977) review the significance of the pre-existing endocrine status of mice in the development of spontaneous or chemically induced lymphoreticular neoplasms and suggest that cells may undergo malignant transformations and remain in a premalignant state for prolonged periods until some alteration in the endocrine environment allows them to proliferate. They further suggest that spontaneous tumours arise more frequently in mice with an hereditary endocrinological imbalance. Steroid hormones appear to exert their effects on cells in general by stimulating production of specific proteins and it has been suggested that adrenocorticosteroids may exert their inhibitory effect on the growth and proliferation of lymphoid cells by stimulating production of an inhibitory or toxic protein (Makman *et al* 1971). Indeed, corticosteroids used alone will produce marked, but short-lived remissions in many cases of canine lymphosarcoma or mastocytoma, but as Owen and Bostock (1972) point out, there is no evidence that such treatment will result in any prolongation of the animal's life.

The treatment of perianal hepatoid tumours (anal adenoma or adenocarcinoma) by means of hormones is based on the concept that these tumours arise in relation to prolonged stimulation of the perianal glands by testosterone, since these glands are a secondary sexual tissue, and neoplasia occurs almost exclusively in the male dog. It is therefore logical and effective to castrate the dog at the same time as the tumour is removed (Nielsen & Aftosmis 1964), or possibly less effectively, to administer oestrogens (Bostock & Owen 1972). Evidence for androgen sensitivity of perianal tumours had been provided by Evans & Pierrepoint (1975a), who demonstrated the presence of receptors for 5α-androstane-3α, 17α-diol, the probable active androgen in the dog (Evans & Pierrepoint 1975b) in tissue from such a tumour. One might expect that less well-differentiated carcinomas arising in these glands would respond less well to hormonal manipulations, since they are less likely to be under hormonal control.

Carcinoma of the thyroid is another special case. Well-differentiated thyroid tumours may well be stimulated to some extent by thyroid stimulating hormone (TSH) and so it is reasonable to administer thyroxine to reduce TSH secretion by a negative feedback effect on the pituitary. Less well-differentiated tumours will clearly respond less well, and such tumours are probably best treated by a combination of radiotherapy and thyroxine. Since iodine is selectively taken-up by the thyroid, radioactive iodine has been used in the treatment of thyroid neoplasia in man. The rationale in this procedure is that the thyroid will concentrate the radioactive iodine, and thereby receive a high dose of radiation relative to the other tissues.

Canine mammary tumours are important not only because of the frequency with which they occur, but also because they are of considerable interest from a comparative point of view, in spite of the differences in reproductive endocrinology between bitches and women. Mammary tumours probably account for around 15–25% of tumours in bitches according to the most reliable estimates (reviewed by Hamilton 1973), and malignant mammary tumours for about 50% of malignant neoplasms (Schneider *et al* 1969). In the cat, about 90% of mammary tumours are adenocarcinomas (Hayden & Nielsen 1971), which metastasise early and widely as in women, but there is some difficulty in ascertaining what proportion of mammary tumours in the dog are malignant, due to the diversity of histological classifications which have been used. Probably about half can be described as malignant, although a much smaller proportion prove themselves to be malignant by metastasing (Cotchin 1958; and see review by Hamilton 1973). About half the canine cases with histologically malignant tumours die as a result of their tumours (Fidler *et al* 1967; Schneider *et al* 1969; Else 1974). However, Bostock (1975) has shown that a fairly accurate prognosis can be given for such cases on the basis of the histological classification of the tumour, whilst Misdorp and Hart (1976) have elucidated other prognostic factors in this disease and have compared these with the prognostic factors in human breast cancer. The high incidence of malignant mammary neoplasia in the bitch and the poor prognosis following surgical excision has stimulated several workers to attempt hormonal therapy in this condition, since hormonal manipulations have proved to be of considerable value in the management of human breast cancer. Beckman (1945) observed complete remission in 37 out of 50 dogs with mammary tumours following administration of orchitic substance, whilst Beard (1961) obtained regressions in four out of six cases by means of treatment with hydroxyprogesterone and St. John (1970) recommended the use of androgens. Although androgens are of proven value in the treatment of human breast cancer (Nicol 1972), adequate evidence to justify the widespread use of testosterone in the treatment of canine mammary tumours in practice (Wilkinson 1971) appears to be lacking, and the only available evidence is the anecdotal evidence summarised above. Controlled trials with adequate histological diagnosis have not been reported and the evidence currently available must be viewed with some reservations, since as Bostock and Owen (1972) point out, mammary tumours may cease to grow for some months, with the animal eventually dying from lung metastases.

There is, however, strong evidence that canine mammary tumours remain under some degree of hormonal control in some instances and that hormonal factors may have a bearing on the development of these tumours. There are two ways in which sex hormones may be of value in the treatment of malignant conditions arising in the secondary sexual organs. In the first place, it may be, as with anal adenomas, that the target tissue has been stimulated to proliferate by continued stimulation from the gonads, or pituitary, mediated by means of the normal physiological trophic hormones. The alternative approach is that the neoplastic development represents a loss of differentiation in the cells of the secondary organs, so that administration of the appropriate hormone should encourage differentiation of such cells, in the same way that ordered growth and development of the tissues occurs during the sexual development of the normal animal. Such simple views are probably naive, and the combined effects of several or all aspects of endocrine function may play a part in a particular case. The two conflicting approaches are illustrated by the use of stiboestrol in the treatment of canine mammary tumours, for whilst Ojemann (1943) claimed regression of such tumours in response to stilboestrol, Owen (1966) warned that oestrogens might cause an acceleration in growth. This apparent contradiction may be related to findings in experimental animals, in which the stimulatory or inhibitory effects of oestrogens are related to the dose administered and the pre-existing hormonal status of the animal.

At a cellular level, information on the hormone-responsiveness of tumours may be obtained by the detection of cytoplasmic protein receptors in tumour cells for the hormone in question. Most steroid hormones exert their effects on cells by binding with a specific cytoplasmic protein, the hormone-receptor complex then migrating to the nucleus, where the mechanisms giving rise to the characteristic effects of the hormone are activated. Peptide hormones, on the other hand, exert their effects via membrane bound receptors on the cell surface. In human carcinoma of the breast, about 50% of cases have significant levels of cytoplasmic oestrogen-binding protein. 70% of cases with demonstrable levels of oestrogen receptor respond to endocrine ablation, but only 5% of cases with no demonstrable oestrogen receptor respond favourably to such treatment (Brennan 1975). Sensitivity to androgens (see above) is restricted to those cases in which oestrogen receptor is present. Evans and Pierrepoint (1975a) have reported the finding of a receptor for oestradiol-17 in tissue from canine mammary tumours of unspecified histological type, whilst Hamilton (1977) has demonstrated the presence of oestrogen receptors in 52% of canine malignant mammary tumours, but only in 25% of benign mammary tumours, whilst in the cat 10% of mammary carcinomas were found to have demonstrable receptors. The rapidly-growing feline mammary carcinomas might be expected to be less under hormonal control, as discussed previously by the same author (Hamilton 1973). Since normal breast tissue and most benign lesions do not have oestrogen receptors, it is postulated that those malignant tumour cells which do contain receptors are to some extent dependent upon the presence of a particular hormonal environment, and if this environment is changed the cells will die (Huggins 1967), although tumours containing such cells eventually become autonomous (i.e. hormone-independent) and this stage may be morphologically apparent by the undifferentiated histological appearance of the tumour. If a number of tumour cells are killed by the removal of the hormone upon which they are dependent, those which remain will tend to become quiescent, or to continue to grow only very slowly. However, if the endocrine environment is restored, they will again grow at the original faster rate. It is therefore imperative that any hormonal treatment which appears to be beneficial is continued for the life of the animal.

There is also epidemiological evidence for an hormonal role in the development of canine and feline mammary tumours, which has been critically evaluated by Hamilton (1973), and he concludes that:

1 Ovariectomy performed before 2 years of age provides considerable protection against the development of mammary neoplasia in bitches. In cats the majority of mammary tumours occur in intact females, or those neutered late in life (Weijer *et al* 1972).
2 Ovariectomy at the time of mastectomy has no value, in terms of prolonging survival.
3 Age at first pregnancy is not significant.
4 Pseudopregnancy is not related to tumour induction.
5 There may possibly be a reduced incidence in bitches which have had a large number of litters, although there is no significant difference between the incidence in maiden bitches, and that in bitches with a small number of litters.

To these points should be added the observations that canine mammary tumours occur almost exclusively in the bitch (Jabara 1969); that established tumours may show accelerated growth at the time of oestrus (Meier 1963), although Jabara (1962) did not observe tumour formation following prolonged administration of oestrogens. On the other hand, prolonged progestogen administration may induce benign or preneoplastic mammary changes (Owen & Briggs 1976).

There is some evidence that steroid hormones are synergistic with prolactin and/or growth hormone in their effects on normal and neoplastic mammary tissue. Prolactin may enhance both the stimulatory and inhibitory effects of steroids on mammary tissue (Pasteels *et al* 1976), and appears to have a direct relationship to the induction and growth of some experimental tumours in rodents (Pearson *et al* 1969). Elevated prolactin levels have been found in the pituitaries of dogs (Hamilton 1973) and the serum of some women (Murray *et al* 1972) bearing mammary neoplasms. Moreover, some human breast tumours have been shown to be dependent on the presence of prolactin (Salih *et al* 1972) and growth hormone (de Souza *et al* 1974) for growth *in vitro*. On the other hand, bromocriptine, an inhibitor of prolactin release, does not appear to be effective in producing remissions in patients with advanced breast cancer, whose cancer cells were prolactin-dependent *in vitro* (Barrett *et al* 1976). The uncertain role of pituitary hormones in mammary carcinogenesis in animals and man has been discussed by Hamilton (1977).

Although various endocrine manipulations have long been an established part of the treatment of human breast cancer, the physiological and biochemical bases for these manipulations are only now becoming understood. It should be possible to devise strategies for the treatment of mammary neoplasia in small animals based to some extent upon the results of work on human breast cancer, whilst the study of spontaneous animal disease may equally well contribute to the acquisition of knowledge in this complex field.

References

Anderson W. B., Johnson G. S. & Pastan I. (1973) Transformation of chick embryo fibroblasts by wild-type and temperature-sensitive Rous sarcoma virus alters adenylate cyclase activity. *Proc. Nat. Acad. Sci. (Washl)* **70**, 1055.

Arena E., D'Alessandro N., Dusonchet L., Gebbia N., Gerbasi F., Sanguedolce R. & Rausa L. (1972) In *International Symposium on Adriamycin*, ed. S. K. Carter, p. 960. Springer-Verlag, Berlin.

Bakowski M. T. (1976) ICRF 159; (±)1,2-di(3,5-dioxopiperazin-1-yl)propane; NSC-129,943; Razoxane. *Cancer Treat. Rev.* **3**, 95.

Ball C. R. (1969) Intracellular factors influencing the response of tumours to chemotherapeutic agents. *Rec. Res. Cancer Res.* **21**, 26.

Barrett A., Morgan L., Raggatt P. R., & Hobbs J. R. (1976) Bromocriptine in the treatment of advanced breast cancer. *Clin.Oncol.* **2**, 373.

Bast R. C., Segerling M., Ohanian S. H., Greene S. L., Zbar B., Rapp H. J. & Borsas T. (1976) Regression of established tumours and induction of tumour immunity by intratumour chemotherapy. *J. Nat. Cancer Inst.* **56**, 829.

Beard D. C. (1961) Hydroxyprogesterone acetate: use in estrogenic and progesterogenic states in the bitch. *Small Anim. Clin.* **1**, 215.

Beckman C. H. (1945) Sexual hormones in the treatment of mammary tumours of aged bitches. *Vet. Med.* **40**, 20.

Berlin R. D., Oliver J. M., Ukena T. E. & Yin H. H. (1975) The cell surface. *New Eng. J. Med.* **292**, 515.

Bloom F. (1952) Effect of cortisone on mast cell tumours of the dog. *Proc. Soc. Exp. Biol. Med.* **79**, 651.

Bostock D. E. (1975) The prognosis following the surgical excision of canine mammary neoplasms. *Europ. J. Cancer* **11**, 389.

Bostock D. E. & Owen L. N. (1972) Chemotherapy of canine and feline neoplasia. *J. Small Anim. Pract.* **13**, 359.

Brandt L., Konyves I. & Moller T. R. (1975) Therapeutic effect of Leo 1031, an alkylating corticosteroid ester in lymphoproliferative disorders. *Acta Med. Scand.* **197**, 317.

Brennan M. J. (1975) Endocrinology in cancer of the breast. *Amer. J. Clin. Path.* **64**, 797.

Brick J. O., Roenigk W. J. & Wilson C. P. (1969) Chemotherapy of malignant lymphoma in dogs and cats. *J. Amer. Vet. Med. Ass.* **153**, 47.

Bruce W. R., Meaker B. E. & Valeriote F. A. (1966) Comparison of the sensitivity of normal haematopoietic and transplanted lymphoma colony-forming cells to chemotherapeutic agents administered *in vivo*. *J. Nat. Cancer Inst.* **37**, 233.

Buhles W. C. & Theilen G. H. (1973) Preliminary evaluation of bleomycin in feline and canine squamous cell carcinoma. *Amer. J. Vet. Res.* **34**, 289.

Bullough W. S. (1971) Ageing of mammals. *Nature* **229**, 608.

Chabner B. A., Myers C. E., Coleman N. & Johns, D. G. (1975) The clinical pharmacology of antineoplastic agents (11) *New Eng. J. Med.* **292**, 1159.

Clarkson B., O'Connor A., Winston L. & Hutchison D. (1964) The physiologic disposition of 5-fluorouracil and 5-fluoro-2′-deoxyuridine in man. *Clin. Pharm. Ther.* **5**, 581.

Cohen H., Schmidt C. E., Lucas S. R. & Palmer J. L. (1975) Combination chemotherapy with vincristine, cyclophosphamide and prednisone. *Amer. J. Vet. Res.* **36**, 1483.

Connors T. A. (1975) Mechanism of action of 2-chloroethylamine derivatives, sulfur mustards, epoxides, and aziridines. In *Antineoplastic and Immunosuppressive Agents*, part. II, eds. A. C. Sartorelli & D. G. Johns, p. 18. Springer-Verlag, Berlin.

Cotchin E. (1958) Mammary neoplasms of the bitch. *J. Comp. Path.* **68**, 1.

Creasey W. A. (1975) Vinca alkaloids and colchicine. In *Antineoplastic and Immunosuppressive Agents*, part II, eds. A. C. Sartorelle & D. G. Johns, p. 670. Berlin, Springer-Verlag, Berlin.

Creasey W. A., Scott I. A., Wei C-C, Kutcher J., Schwartz A. & Marsh J. C. (1975) Pharmacological studies with vinblastine in the dog. *Cancer Res.* **35**, 1116.

Danø K. (1972) Cross resistance between vinca alkaloids and anthracyclines in Erlich ascites tumour *in vivo*. *Cancer Chem. Rep.* **56**, 701.

Denine E. P. & Schmidt L. M. (1975) *Proc. Med. Soc. Toxicol.* Abstracts of papers, p. 81. Quoted in Lenas L. & Page J. A. (1976) Cardiotoxicity of adriamycin and related anthracyclines. *Cancer Treat. Rev.* **3**, 111.

de Souza I, Morgan L., Lewis U. J., Raggatt P. R., Salih H. & Hobbs J. R. (1974). Growth hormone dependence among human breast cancers. *Lancet* ii, 182.

Else R. W. (1974) Letter to the editor. *J. Small Anim. Pract.* **15**, 417.

Evans C. R. & Pierrepoint C. G. (1975a) Tissue-steroid interactions in canine hormone-dependent tumours. *Vet. Rec.* **97**, 464.

Evans C. R. & Pierrepoint C. G. (1975b) Demonstration of a specific cytosol receptor in the normal and hyperplastic canine prostate for 5α-androstane-3α, 17α-diol. *J. Endoc.* **64**, 539.

Fidler I. J., Abt D. A. & Brodey R. S. (1967) The biological behaviour of canine mammary neoplasms. *J. Amer. Vet. Med. Ass.* **151**, 1311.

Freirich E. J., Gelan E. A., Rall D. P., Schmidt L. H., & Skipper H. E. (1966) Quantitative comparison of anticancer agents in mouse, rat, hamster, dog, monkey and man. *Cancer Chem. Rep.* **50**, 219.

Halpern B., Fray A. & Crepin Y. (1973) *Corynebacterium parvum*, a potent immunostimulant in experimental infections and in malignancies. In *Immunopotentiation* Ciba Foundation Symposium, **18**, 217.

Hamilton J. M. (1973) Comparative aspects of mammary tumours. *Adv. Cancer Res.* **19**, 1.

Hamilton J. M., Else R. W. & Forshaw P. (1977) Oestrogen receptors in canine mammary tumours. *Vet. Res.* **101**, 258.

Hardy W. D. & Old L. J. (1970) L-asparaginase in the treatment of neoplastic diseases of the dog, cat, and cow. *Rec. Res. Cancer Res.* **33**, 131.

Harrap K. R. (1976) Resistance to antitumour agents. In *Scientific Foundations of Oncology*, eds. T. Symington & R. L. Carter. Heinemann, London.

Harrap K. R. & Gascoigne E. W. (1976) The interaction of bifunctional alkylating agents with the DNA of tumour cells. *Europ. J. Cancer* **12**, 53.

Hayden D. W. & Nielson S. W. (1971) Feline mammary tumours. *J. Small Anim. Pract.* **12**, 687.

Henness A. M., Theilen G. H., Park R. D. & Buhles W. C. (1977) Combination therapy for canine osteosarcoma. *J. Amer. Vet. Med. Ass.* **170**, 1076.

Herman E. H., Mhatre R. M. & Chadwick D. P. (1974) Modification of some of the toxic effects of daunomycin by pretreatment with the antineoplastic agent ICRF 159. *Toxicol. Appl. Pharmac.* **27**, 517.

Hess P. W., MacEwan E. G. & McClelland A. J. (1976) Chemotherapy of canine and feline tumours. *J. Amer. Anin. Hosp. Ass.* **12**, 350.

Hilgard P., Schulte H., Wetzig G., Schmitt G. & Schmitt C. G. (1977) Oral anticoagulation in the treatment of a spontaneously metastasising murine tumour. *Brit. J. Cancer* **35**, 78.

Hill B. T. (1976) Biochemistry of the cell cycle. In *Scientific Foundations of Oncology*, eds. T. Symington & R. L. Carter, p. 63. Heinemann, London.

Hill D. L. (1975) *A review of cyclophosphamide.* C. C. Thomas, Springfield, Ill.

Huggins C. (1967) Endocrine-induced regression of cancers. *Science* **156**, 1050.

Ishizuka M., Takayama H., Takeuchi T. & Umezawa H. (1970) Activity and toxicity of bleomycin. *J. Antibiotics.* (series A) **20**, 15.

Lamoureux G., Turcotte R. & Portelance V. (eds.) (1976) *BCG in Cancer Immunotherapy. Proceedings of an international symposium.* Grune & Stratton, New York.

Jabara A. G. (1962) Some tissue changes in the dog following stilboestrol administration. *Aust. J. Exp. Biol. Med. Sci.* **40**, 293.

Jabara A. G. (1969) Two cases of mammary neoplasms arising in male dogs. *Aust. Vet. J.* **45**, 476.

MacEwan E. G., Drazner F., McClelland A. J. & Wilkins R. (1975) Treatment of basophilic leukaemia in a dog. *J. Amer. Vet. Med. Assoc.* **166**.

MacEwan E. G. & Hess P. W. (1977) Canine lymphosarcoma and leukaemia. In *Current Veterinary Therapy VI*, ed. R. W. Kirk, p. 473. W. B. Saunders, Philadelphia.

Makman M. H., Dvorkin B. & White A. (1971) Evidence for induction by cortisol *in vitro* of a protein inhibitor of transport and phosphorylation in rat thymocytes. *Proc. Nat. Acad. Sci. (N.Y.)* **68**, 1269.

Mangioni C., Bolis G., Natale N. & Morasca L. (1976) Continuous low-dose cyclophosphamide therapy in advanced ovarian cancer. *Europ. J. Cancer* **12**, 353.

Mauer A. M. (1975) Cell kinetics and practical consequences for therapy of acute leukaemia. *New Eng. J. Med.* **293**, 389.

Meier H. (1975) Cell kinetics and practical consequences for therapy of acute leukaemia. *New Eng. J. Med.* **293**, 389.

Meier H. (1963) Etiological considerations of spontaneous tumours in animals with special reference to the endocrine system. *Ann. N.Y. Acad. Sci.* **108**, 881.

Mellett L. B. (1963) The absorption and fate of tritium labelled cyclophosphamide in dogs. *Fed. Proc.* **22**, 305.

Metcalf D. (1973) *The Nature of Myeloid Leukaemia.* Leukaemia Research Fund, London.

Misdorp W. & Hart A. A. M. (1976) Prognostic factors in canine mammary cancer. *J. Nat. Cancer Inst.* **56**, 779.

Murray R. M L., Mozaffarian G. & Pearson O. H. (1972) Prolactin levels with L-DOPA treatment in metastatic breast carcinoma. In *Prolactin and Carcinogenesis*, eds. A. R. Boyns & K. Griffiths, 4th Tenovus workshop, p. 154. Alpha Omega, Cardiff.

Mukherjee K. L., Currieri A. R., Javid M. & Heidelberger C. (1963) Studies of fluorinated pyrimidines. XVII Tissue distribution of 5-fluoro-uracil-2-CC^{14} and 5-fluoro-2′-deoxyuridine in cancer patients. *Cancer Res.* **23**, 67.

Nicol N. T. (1972) Clinical experience with drostanolone propionate (Masteril) in breast cancer. In *Steroids in Modern Medicine*, eds. G. A. Christie & M. Moore-Robinson, part 1, p. 23. Excerpta Medica, Amsterdam.

Nielsen S. W. & Aftmosis J. (1964) Canine perianal gland tumours. *J. Amer. Vet. Med. Ass.* **144**, 127.

O'Connell T. X. & Berenbaum M. C. (1974) Cardiac and pulmonary effects of high doses of cyclophosphamide and isophosphamide. *Cancer Res.* **34**, 1586.

Ojemann J. G. (1943) Medicamenteuze behandeling van mammatumoren bij den hond. *Tijdsch. diergeeneskunde* **70**, 161.

Owen L. N. (1966) Prognosis and treatment of mammary tumours in the bitch. *J. Small Anim. Pract.* **7**, 703.

Owen L. N. (1976) Neoplasia in domestic animals. In *Advances in Veterinary Science and Comparative Medicine*, eds. C. A. Brandley, C. E. Cornelius & W. I. B. Beveridge, **20**, 239.

Owen L. N., Bostock D. E. & Lavelle R. B. (1977) Studies on therapy of osteosarcoma in dogs using B.C.G. vaccination. *J. Amer. Vet. Radiol. Soc.* **18**, 27.

Owen L. N. & Briggs M. H. (1976) Contraceptive steroid toxicology in the Beagle bitch and its relevance to human carcinogenicity. *Curr. Med. Res. Opin.* **4**, 309.

Owen L. N. & Steel G. G. (1969) The growth and cell population kinetics of spontaneous tumors in domestic animals. *Brit. J. Cancer* **23**, 493.

Pasteels J. L., Henson J-C., Heuson-Steinnon J. & Legros N. (1976) Effects of insulin, prolactin, progesterone, and estradiol on DNA synthesis in organ culture of 7,12-dimethyl(a)-anthracene-induced rat mammary tumours. *Cancer Res.* **36**, 2162.

Pearson O. H., Llerena O., Llerena L., Molina A. & Butler T. (1969) Prolactin-dependent rat mammary cancer: a model for man. *Trans. Ass. Am. Phys.* **82**, 225.

Pierpaoli W., Haran-Ghera N. & Kopp H. G. (1977) Role of host endocrine status in murine leukaemogenesis. *Brit. J. Cancer* **35**, 621.

Price L. A. (1972) The application of a kinetic model to the clinical use of anti-tumour drugs. In *The Vinca Alkaloids in the Chemotherapy of Malignant Disease*, Proc. 3rd Lilly Symposium, p. 35.

Price L. A., Hill B. T., Calvert A. H., Shaw H. J. & Hughes K. B. (1975) Kinetically-based multiple drug treatment for advanced head and neck cancer. *Brit. Med. J.* **3**, 10.

Rhoads C. P. (1946) Nitrogen mustards in the treatment of neoplastic disease. *J. Amer. Med. Ass.* **131**, 656.

Roberts R. M., Walker A. & Cetorelli J. J. (1973) Fucose-containing glycopeptides from the cell surface of Chinese Hamster ovary cells grown in the presence or absence of cyclic-AMP. *Nature New Biol.* **244**, 86.

Roga V., Hedeman L. P. & Olson B. H. (1971) Evaluation of mitogillin (NSC-69529) in the treatment of naturally occurring canine neoplasm. *Cancer Chem. Rep.* **55**, 101.

Rojas A. F., Mickiewicz E., Feierstein J. N., Glait H. & Olivari A. J. (1976) Levamisole in advanced human breast cancer. *Lancet* i, 211.

Ryall R. D. H., Hanham I. W. F., Newton K. A., Hellman K., Brinkley D. M. & Hjertas D. K. (1974) Combined treatment of soft tissue and osteosarcoma by radiation and ICRF 159. *Cancer N.Y.* **34**, 1040.

Ryan W. L. & Heidrick M. L. (1974) Cyclic nucleotides in cancer. *Adv. Cyclic Nucl. Res.* **4**, 81.

Salih H., Brander W., Flax H. & Hobbs J. R. (1972) Prolactin dependence in human breast cancers. *Lancet* ii, 1103.

Salusbury A. J., Burrage K. & Hellman K. (1974) Histological analysis of the antimetastatic effect of (±)1,2-Bis(3,5-dioxopiperazin-1-yl)propane. *Cancer Res.* **34**, 843.

Schneider R., Dorn C. R. & Taylor D. O. N. (1969) Factors influencing mammary cancer development and postsurgical survival. *J. Nat. Cancer Inst.* **43**, 1249.

Shaw N. (1976) Bleomycin in Hodgkin's disease. *Bleomycin Conspectus* 6. Lundbeck Ltd.

Skipper H. E., Schabel F. M. & Wilcox W. S. (1967) Experimental evaluation of potential anticancer agents. XXI Scheduling of arabinosylcytosine to take advantage of S-phase specificity against leukaemic cells. *Cancer Chem. Rep.* **51**, 125.

Squire R. A. & Bush, M. (1973) The therapy of canine and feline lymphosarcoma. In *Unifying concepts of leukaemia*, eds. R. M. Dutcher & L. Chieco-Bianchi, p. 189. Karger, Basel.

Steele J. D. & Buell P. (1973) Asymptomatic solitary pulmonary nodules. *J. Thorac. Cardiovasc. Surg.* **65**, 140.

St. John S. (1970) Treatment of canine mammary tumours. *Vet. Rec.* **86**, 479.

Straw J. H., Talbot D. C., Taylor G. A. & Harrap K. R. (1977) Some observations on the reversibility of methotrexate toxicity in normal proliferating tissues. *J. Nat. Cancer Inst.* **58**, 91.

Taylor I. W. & Bleehen N. M. (1977) Changes in sensitivity to radiation and ICRF 159 during the life of monolayer cultures of EMT 6 tumour line. *Brit. J. Cancer* **35**, 587.

Tew K. D. & Taylor D. M. (1976) Comparative utilisation of 'Salvage' and 'De Novo' DNA precursors in tumour and normal tissue. (Abstract) *Brit. Assoc. Cancer Res.* Swansea, 1976.

Theilen G. H. (1975) Veterinary medical oncology. In *Textbook of Veterinary Internal Medicine*, ed. S. J. Ettinger, p. 127. W. B. Saunders, Philadelphia.

Theilen G. H., Pool R. & Park R. D. (1977a) Treatment of canine osteosarcoma for limb preservation using osteotomy, adjuvant radiotherapy and chemotherapy. *Vet. Med. Small Anim. Clin.* **72**, 179.

Theilen G. H., Worley M. & Benjami E. (1977b) Chemoimmunotherapy for canine lymphosarcoma. *J. Amer. Vet. Med. Ass.* **170**, 607.

Thomlinson R. H. & Gray L. H. (1955) The histological structure of some human lung cancers and the possible implications for radiotherapy. *Brit. J. Cancer* **9**, 539.

Tolley D. A. & Castro J. E. (1976) Observations on the prevention of cyclophosphamide-induced cystitis. *Brit. J. Cancer* **34**, 323.

Tubiana M. & Malaise E. P. (1976) Growth rate and cell kinetics in human tumours: some prognostic and therapeutic implications. In *Scientific Foundations of Oncology*, eds. T. Symington & R. L. Carter, p. 126. Heinemann, London.

Weber G. (1977) Enzymology of cancer cells. *New Eng. J. Med.* **296**, 486, 541.

Weijer K., Head K. W., Misdorp W. & Hampe J. F. (1972) Feline malignant mammary tumours. I Morphology and biology: some comparisons with human and canine mammary carcinomas. *J. Nat. Cancer Inst.* **49**, 1697.

Wilkinson G. T. (1971) The treatment of mammary tumours in the bitch, and a comparison with the cat. *Vet. Rec.* **89**, 13.

15

Agents acting on the central nervous system I. Fundamental pharmacology of CNS

C. A. WILSON

This chapter and the following chapter are concerned with the mechanism of action of tranquillisers and anticonvulsants used in veterinary practice. Since it is hypothesised that most drugs acting on the central nervous system (CNS) exert their effect by altering the activity of neuronal transmitters much of this review will be concerned with the activity of the transmitters themselves.

This chapter discusses the proposed roles of various chemicals as CNS transmitters and the possible mechanism of action of CNS drugs, whilst Chapter 16 deals with the use of drugs acting on the CNS. To some extent the two chapers may be read independently.

15.1 Introduction

In peripheral nerves it is well established that a propagated action potential will release a chemical at the nerve terminal which then crosses the synapse to the innervated organ (or to a second neurone) and acts on specific receptor sites on the surface membrane causing depolarisation if it is an excitatory transmitter or hyperpolarisation if it is an inhibitory transmitter. In addition, there are presynaptic receptors and depolarisation of these inhibit the release of transmitter from the presynaptic neurone. For example, within the CNS, the amino acid γ-aminobutyric acid (GABA) is released from either neurones or glial cells to act on presynaptic receptors and inhibit the release of excitatory transmitters and hence is said to cause presynaptic inhibition (see Fig. 15.7).

The neurotransmitters in the peripheral nervous system are noradrenaline (NA) and acetylcholine (Bowman *et al* 1968). Within the CNS there are many more substances that may act as transmitters although proof of their role is not complete for any of them. The following criteria are used to establish a particular chemical as a transmitter:

1 It should be present in brain tissue, accompanied by metabolising enzymes.
2 It should be located inside neurones of specific nerve tracts.

3 Administration of the chemical should produce the same effect as electrical stimulation of the nerve tract within which it is located.
4 Release of the substance by stimulation or activation of specific nerve tracts should be demonstrable.
5 Compounds known to interact with the substance in the periphery should interact similarly with the substance in the brain (Barchas *et al* 1972).

Evidence of a central transmitter function is almost complete for the catecholamines, adrenaline (AD), noradrenaline (NA), dopamine (DA), 5-hydroxytryptamine (5HT) and acetylcholine (AcC). Other substances are called putative transmitters. Table 15.1 lists some of the substances thought to be involved in neuronal activity within the CNS.

Table 15.1 Putative transmitters in the CNS.

Amines
Catecholamines: dopamine (DA); noradrenaline (NA); adrenaline (AD)
5-hydroxytryptamine (5HT)
Acetylcholine (AcC)
Histamine
Amino acids
Glycine
γ-aminobutyric acid (GABA)
Glutamate
Aspartate
Taurine
β-alanine
Lipids
Prostaglandins
Peptides
Substance P
Enkephalins and endorphins
Angiotensin
Bradykinin-like peptides
Neurotensin
Vasopressin, vasotocin
Adrenocorticotrophin (ACTH)
Melanocyte stimulating hormone (αMSH)
Releasing hormones: thyroid-releasing hormone; LH-releasing hormone; GH-inhibitory releasing hormone
Scotophobin
Ameletin
Delta sleep-inducing peptide
Fc peptides

15.2 Distribution of the transmitters in the CNS

Most of the work on distribution has been carried out on the amines in spite of the fact that they only account for a small proportion of transmission in the CNS. For example, NA accounts for 5% transmission in the hypothalamus and 1% elsewhere; DA, 15% in the corpus striatum and 1% elsewhere (Hokfelt *et al* 1970); acetylcholine, 10% throughout the brain (McLennon 1970); 5HT 5% or less in the hypothalamus and 1% or less elsewhere (Kuhar & Aghajanian 1973). Glycine and GABA are more ubiquitous and each accounts for 25% of the transmission in the spinal cord (Iversen & Bloom 1972), while GABA is also important in the cortex (27%) and hippocampus (45%) (Iversen & Schon 1973).

A given neurohumoral agent may be a transmitter in more than one tract and therefore may be involved in several physiological functions. It may even be present in two neuronal tracts that functionally oppose each other. Fig. 15.1 show the distribution of noradrenergic tracts in the rat brain (Ungerstedt 1971). The cell bodies are present in the midbrain and their axons. pass forward branching into two tracts, the ventral to the hypothalamus and the upper forward to the cortex. A branch also leads out to the amygdala. It is clear therefore that a drug altering noradrenaline activity will affect many parts of the brain and hence will affect also several different functions. Some of the resulting changes may appear as unwanted side-effects of the drug. In the brain, 5HT has a similar distribution to NA and very often these transmitters alter and oppose the activity of each other so that, for instance, inhibiting NA neuronal activity may enhance 5HT activity since the latter is 'disinhibited' (Brodie & Shore 1957; Dement *et al* 1976). Fig. 15.2 shows the dopamingergic nerves in the brain. There are three main tracts: the nigro-stratial tract from the substantia nigra to the corpus striatum; the tubero-

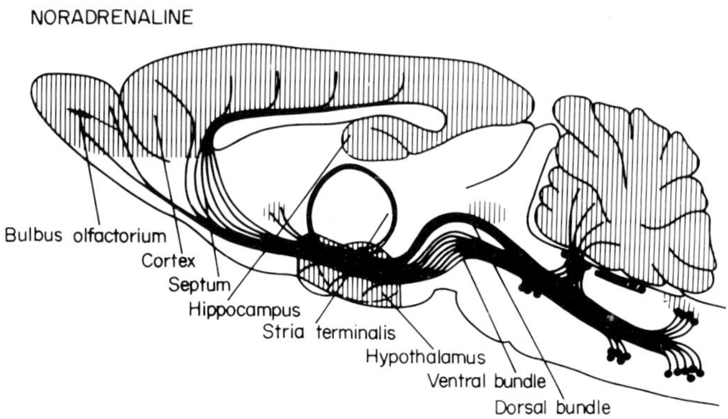

Fig. 15.1 Sagittal projection of the ascending noradrenaline pathways. The descending pathways are not included. The stripes indicate the major terminal areas. The 5HT axons follow closely the noradrenaline pathway. From Ungerstedt (1971) with permission.

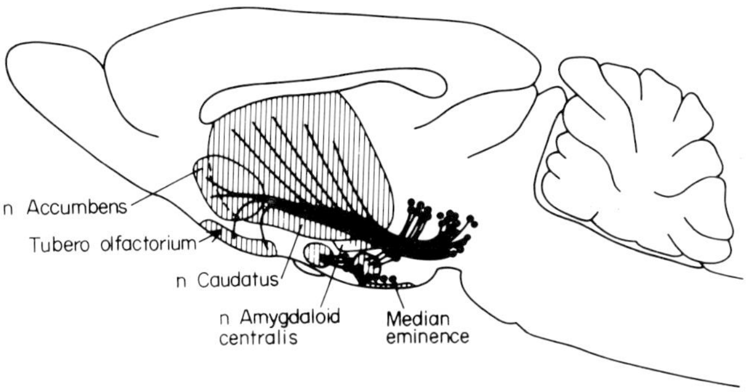

Fig. 15.2 Sagittal projection of the dopaminergic pathways. The stripes indicate nerve terminal areas (Ungerstedt 1971; Bjorkland *et al* 1975).

infundibular tract with cell bodies in the arcuate nucleus and terminals in the median eminence; the incertahypothalamic system which originates in the caudal thalamus and terminates in the preoptic area (Ungerstedt 1971; Bjorkland *et al* 1975).

Specific tracts have not been elucidated for other putative transmitters.

15.3 Neurohumoral control of physiological functions

15.3.1 Mood

Many of the centrally active drugs used in both human and veterinary medicine are given to modify states of hyper or hypoactivity, and it is thought that they act by altering aminergic transmitter activity.

In cases of mental depression in humans, there are low levels of the degradation metabolites of NA, DA and 5HT in either urine or cerebrospinal fluid (McClure 1972; van Praag & Korf 1972; Weissman & Harbert 1972). In manic and aggressive states, on the other hand, high levels of NA and AD are found in the urine (Schildkraut & Kety 1967). Schildkraut and Kety (1967) have hypothesised that the catecholamines are stimulatory transmitters enhancing mood, activity and aggression. 5HT may also be involved in control of mood, producing a feeling of well-being and reducing fear (Coppen 1967; Diaz *et al* 1974). A reduction in the brain level of any one of these transmitters may lead to the production of a depressed state, whilst a manic or hyperexcitable state may ensue if levels rise abnormally high. Acetylcholine may be an inhibitory transmitter since drugs that mimic or enhance its activity tend to cause depression, and it has been suggested that the catecholamine and 5HT systems are suppressed by the cholinergic system, which can antagonise and overcome overactivity of the catecholamine system (Janowsky *et al* 1972).

15.3.2 Arousal and locomotion

Locomotion and alertness are closely allied to mood and may well be controlled by the same neuronal tracts. In general, raising brain NA levels increases arousal, locomotion and exploratory activity in animals. Reducing NA levels, for example, with an inhibitor of NA synthesis, has the opposite effect (Herman 1973a; Dandrya & Potni 1973; Mabry & Campbell 1973; Ahlenius 1974). It is known that the dorsal NA tract (see Fig. 15.1) is concerned with motor activity and this is probably the site at which exogenous NA acts when it is administered intracerebrally.

The nigrostriatal pathway in which DA is the transmitter is also concerned with purposeful locomotion (Papeschi 1972) and is thought, in addition, to control purposeless movement. In humans, lesions of the nigrostriatal tract are associated with low DA levels and manifested as Parkinson's disease, symptoms of which include akinesia, tremors and rigidity. These symptoms also occur in animals after experimental lesions of the nigrostriatal tract (Bolme *et al* 1972). Dihydroxyphenylalanine (DOPA), the precursor of DA, overcomes these symptoms and tranquillisers that block DA receptors (e.g. chlorpromazine, haloperiodol) produce Parkinsonian-like akinesia and rigidity as side-effects when given to animals in high doses (Hornykiewicz 1966).

The role of 5HT in regulating arousal and locomotion is less clear. Intracerebral application of 5HT suppresses arousal behaviour and locomotion, probably by acting on the serotonergic tract in the hippocampus (Mabry & Campbell 1973; Kostowski & Giacolone 1969; Herman 1973b). Lesions in the median raphe nucleus which reduce 5HT levels (particularly in the hippocampus) increase locomotion and active behaviour (Kostowski & Giacalone 1969; Srebo & Lorens 1975). It is suggested that the noradrenergic and serotonergic tracts are in balance and control each other's activity (Costa *et al* 1960; Tanaka *et al* 1972). However, selective depletion of brain 5HT levels by various drugs (5,6-dihydroxytryptamine and 5,7-dihydroxytryptamine) reduces locomotion and exploratory behaviour (Diaz *et al* 1974; Hole *et al* 1976) and rats that have an activity higher than the norm for a given group have a higher brain 5HT turnover (Rosencrans & Schechter 1972) and higher levels of 5HT in the non-telencephalon areas (Kameyama *et al* 1975). It is thus possible that there are several serotonergic tracts which can act in opposite ways.

15.3.3 Sleep

There are two types of sleep, which are controlled by two separate centres. Slow-wave sleep (SWS) is so called because of the pattern of the electroencephalograph (EEG), associated with it, and occupies 75% of sleeping time. Rapid eye movement (REM) or paradoxical sleep (PS) occurs at intervals throughout the sleeping period, and accounts for 20–25% of the total sleeping time. In PS the EEG displays an arousal pattern with small irregular waves and in this period respiration and muscular movement increase while the eyes move rapidly from side to side. It is believed that dreaming takes place during PS periods (Jouvet 1967).

Jouvet has suggested that SWS is controlled from a centre in the midbrain raphe nucleus and that 5HT is the transmitter. Application of 5-hydroxytryptophan (5HTP), a precursor of 5HT, induces either SWS or drowsiness and reduces PS (Jouvet 1969; Ursdin 1976). Reduction of brain 5HT levels with either 5,6-dihydroxytryptamine (56DHT) or p-chlorophenylalanine (PCPA) reduces SWS as do lesions of the midbrain raphe (Kostowski *et al* 1968; Jouvet & Pujol 1974). On the other hand, PS is thought to be controlled by a centre in the pons which is activated by the raphe to induce PS (Jouvet 1972). Jouvet (1972) has suggested that NA controls PS, but there is much evidence against this (Dement *et al* 1976). Another hypothesis proposes that PS occurs when brain levels of the main metabolite of 5HT (5-hydroxyindole acetic acid, 5HIAA) increase above a critical level indicating that 5HT stores need to be replenished (Rechtschaffen *et al* 1973). There are three findings which support this theory: (1) during the PS period 5HT turnover is increased, (2) 5HT precursors reduce PS and this might be because they maintain 5HT levels and (3) MAO inhibitors which prevent the production of 5HIAA are particularly effective in preventing PS (Radulovachi 1974; Jouvet 1969; Ursdin 1976). It is noteworthy that many tryptamine derivatives and drugs acting on 5HT receptors are hallucinogenic (Bowers 1975).

The cholinergic system may also involve the control of PS, since anticholinesterases produce PS immediately while atropine prevents it (Jouvet 1969; Wyatt *et al* 1976).

A completely different line of work has shown that during SWS in rabbits a small peptide is released into the cerebral venous blood which, on intraventricular injection into recipients, induces SWS (Monnier & Schoenenberger 1974). In addition, extracts of the midbrain reticular formation taken from sleeping animals also induce sleep in recipients (Drucker-Colin 1974).

15.3.4 Food intake

The classical theory of control of food intake is that there is a feeding centre in the lateral hypothalamus and if this centre is damaged aphagia occurs, although eventually lower reflexes take over and feeding recommences. In addition, there is a satiety centre in the medial hypothalamus very close to the paraventricular nucleus and if this is lesioned hyperphagia occurs and the animals become obese (Anand 1961).

However, lesions in several areas of the brain can either cause overeating (the mamillary region, frontal and temporal lobes, thalamus, periaquaductal grey of the brainstem and the ventral NA tract in the midbrain), or inhibit eating (globus pallidus, midbrain tegmentum and substantia nigra). Thus Grossman (1975) has suggested that rather than centres, there are two well-defined tracts throughout the brain which can act on and modulate each other's activity. Injection of NA intraventricularly or into the anterior hypothalamus stimulates food intake (Grossman 1962a, 1962b; Booth 1968; Leibowitz 1970; Kruk 1973; Myers 1974). In contrast, NA injection into the lateral hypothalamus inhibits eating, although this occurs only at night (Margules *et al* 1972) and lesions of the ventral NA tract leading to the lateral hypothalamus induce a hyperphagia (Hoebel 1976). It is thus possible that NA is a transmitter in both tracts, inhibiting the action of the 'feeding tract' and also the 'satiety tract'. Amphetamine is an anorexic agent which is known to stimulate both NA and DA receptors directly and enhance endogenous catecholamine release as well. It is inactive after lesioning the noradrenergic ventral tract (Hoebel *et al* 1975), and so it presumably acts by mimicking the inhibitory action of NA in the ventral tract.

Lesions of the substantia nigra also produce aphagia (Oltmans & Harvey 1972; Cooper *et al* 1974) which can be overcome by DA agonist drugs (Ungerstedt 1971). This dopaminergic tract may therefore be involved in stimulating food intake. On the other hand, intraventricular administration of 5HT inhibits food intake (Kruk 1973) as does an inhibitor of 5HT uptake (uptake-inhibitors enhance the action of amine transmitters) (Goudie *et al* 1976). Intraventricular PCPA stimulates eating during the day only (Breisch *et al* 1976) and Hoebel (1976) has suggested that 5HT inhibits food intake at the medial hypothalamus level and acts during the day, while NA inhibits food intake at the midbrain level and is important during the night. It should be noted that this proposal refers to the rat, which is a nocturnal animal. Fenfluramine is an anorexic drug with some central depressant action which is thought to act by releasing endogenous 5HT (Clinesschmidt *et al* 1974; Jespersen & Scheel-Kruger 1973; Kruk 1973).

15.3.5 Water intake

The centre for control of water intake is thought to be the same as or close to the feeding centre (i.e. the lateral hypothalamus), but this may be only part of a whole controlling tract, since lesions in the midbrain near the inter-peduncular nucleus, septal region and zona incerta all inhibit drinking as do lesions in the lateral hypothalamus (Grossman 1975).

The main neurohumoral pathway in this system appears to be cholinergic although adrenergic tracts may also be involved; injection of acetylcholine into the lateral hypothalamus stimulates water intake in rats as does the β agonist isoprenaline (Grossman 1962; Fitzsimmons 1972). On the other hand, the α agonist NA inhibits drinking. Since β agonists and drugs that mimic acetylcholine are both antagonised by β blockers they are probably acting on the same system (Leibowitz 1970, 1971).

15.3.6 Temperature regulation

All the aminergic transmitters listed in Table 15.1 alter body temperature when injected into the brain, particularly the anterior hypothalamus, and there are definite species differences (Table 15.2).

In general, it appears that NA and 5HT act in an opposite manner in a given species and altering ambient temperatures can cause their selective release. For example, when the monkey is placed in the cold, 5HT is released into the cerebrospinal fluid (CSF) at the anterior hypothalamus level, whereas at high ambient temperatures high levels of NA are found in the CSF. CSF from monkeys placed in the cold induces shivering and a rise in body temperature when injected intraventricularly into recipient monkeys kept at normal room temperature (Myers 1974).

Myers has also shown that acetylcholine (AcC) levels alter with ambient temperature, increasing when monkeys are cooled. He has proposed a model for the monkey in which 5HT is released when heat production is required, and this in turn stimulates release of AcC which activates shivering mechanisms. Heat loss may also be controlled by release of NA which acts to

Table 15.2 Effect of amines on body temperature. POA, preoptic area in the brain. (1) Feldberg & Myers 1965; (2) Feldberg 1970; (3) Burks 1972; (4) Rudy & Wolf 1969; (5) Kennedy & Burks 1974; (6) Jacob *et al.* 1972; (7) Quock & Gale 1974; (8) Fitzsimmons 1972; (9) Hellon 1972.

Amine	Route of admin.	Rise	Temperature change fall	No change
NA (Refs 1, 2, 3, 4, 5)	I/ventricular or in POA	Rats, mice in low doses	Cats, dogs, monkeys Rats and mice in high doses	Ox, goats
5HT (Refs 1, 2, 6)	I/ventricular	Cats, dogs, monkeys Rabbits in low doses	Ox, goats, rats, mice, sheep Rabbits in low doses	
DA (Ref. 7)	POA		Cats	
AcC with eserine (Refs 8, 9)	I/ventricular	Sheep, goats, monkeys	Rats, mice	Rabbits

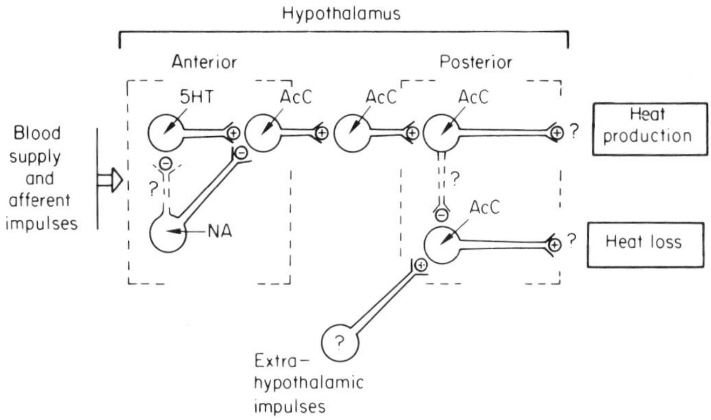

Fig. 15.3 A neuronal model based on the effects on body temperature of microinjections of 5HT, noradrenline or AcC into various hypothalamic regions in monkeys. Cells containing 5HT respond to cooling and activate heat production through a cholinergic pathway to the posterior hypothalamus. Noradrenaline-containing cells respond to warming and this allows the cholinergic heat loss pathway in the posterior hypothalamus to become active, possibly by stimulation from extrahypothalamic sites. From Myers & Yaksh (1969) with permission.

inhibit the heat production pathway (Fig. 15.3) (Myers & Yaksh 1969; Myers & Waller 1975).

In rodents NA and 5HT both seem to have biphasic effects. In low doses NA raises and 5HT lowers temperature (opposite to the monkey) and in high doses or when they are injected into the anterior hypothalamus their affects are reversed (Jacob *et al* 1972; Feldberg 1970).

15.3.7 Anterior pituitary hormone release

The release of anterior pituitary hormones is controlled by releasing hormones in the hypothalamus that pass via the blood vessels of the hypophyseal tract to exert an effect on the pituitary (Harris 1964). The secretion of the releasing hormones is probably controlled by aminergic neurones in the hypothalamus. Table 15.3 summarises the effects of administration of exogenous amines on the release of the pituitary hormones and it is presumed they are simulating the action of the hypothalamic amines.

Drugs altering the activity of hypothalamic transmitters may also alter the secretion of pituitary hormones. Examples include the phenothiazine tranquillisers and reserpine; both reduce DA activity and therefore prevent the inhibitory action of DA on prolactin secretion. This causes the release of prolactin which in humans and rodents leads to psuedopregnancy and possibly galactorrhoea (Clemens *et al* 1974; Barraclough & Sawyer 1969). Recently, a specific DA agonist, bromocriptine, has been used to prevent galactorrhoea in humans since it is known to reduce circulating prolactin levels (Thorner *et al* 1974).

Table 15.3 Effect of amines on the release of anterior pituitary hormones. GT, gonadotrophins.

Amines	GT	ACTH	TSH	Prolactin	GH
NA	↑	↓	↑	↑	↑
DA	*↓↑	↓?		↓	↓?
5HT	↓↑ permissive	↑tonic ↓stress	↓	↑	↑?
AcC	↑	↑		↓?	

*There is a large body of evidence indicating that dopamine inhibits GT release and equally convincing data that it is stimulatory (see also Wilson 1974).

The releasing factors that have been isolated and identified chemically (e.g. LH-releasing hormone, TSH-releasing hormone, GH-inhibitory releasing hormone are small peptides) (Matsuo *et al* 1971; Burgus *et al* 1970; Brazeau *et al* 1973). The exception may be prolactin-inhibitory releasing hormone (PIH) which seems to be DA itself (Shaar & Clemens 1974; Schally *et al* 1976; MacLeod 1976).

15.4 Mechanisms by which drugs alter transmitter activity

15.4.1 Alteration of amine transmission

The synthesis and fate of NA are depicted in Fig. 15.4. The amino acid tyrosine enters the neurone and is converted to DOPA. This is the rate-limiting step in the synthetic pathway. DOPA is then converted to DA, which enters a storage granule or vesicle. Within the granule it is converted by dopamine-β-hydroxylase to NA. It then either remains in a labile, easily releasable form or is stored in a bound form (Blaschko 1957, 1973). When an action potential passes along the nerve, the permeability of the membrane alters, allowing the influx of calcium ions, which attract the granules or vesicles to the membrane wall. The vesicular contents then pass through the membrane wall by exocytosis into the synaptic cleft (Smith 1973). The NA in the synapse can act on the postsynaptic receptors of the innervated organ or, as occurs in the CNS, on a second neurone. Removal of the NA from the synapse occurs rapidly by three mechanisms — approximately 80% returns into the neurone and thence into the storage granule. The reuptake is an active process requiring energy and the presence of certain ions (Iversen 1967, 1973). Of the remaining 20% NA in the synapse, some is degraded to normetanepherine outside the neurone by a membrane bound enzyme called catechol-O-methyl transferase. The rest is degraded within the neurone as it

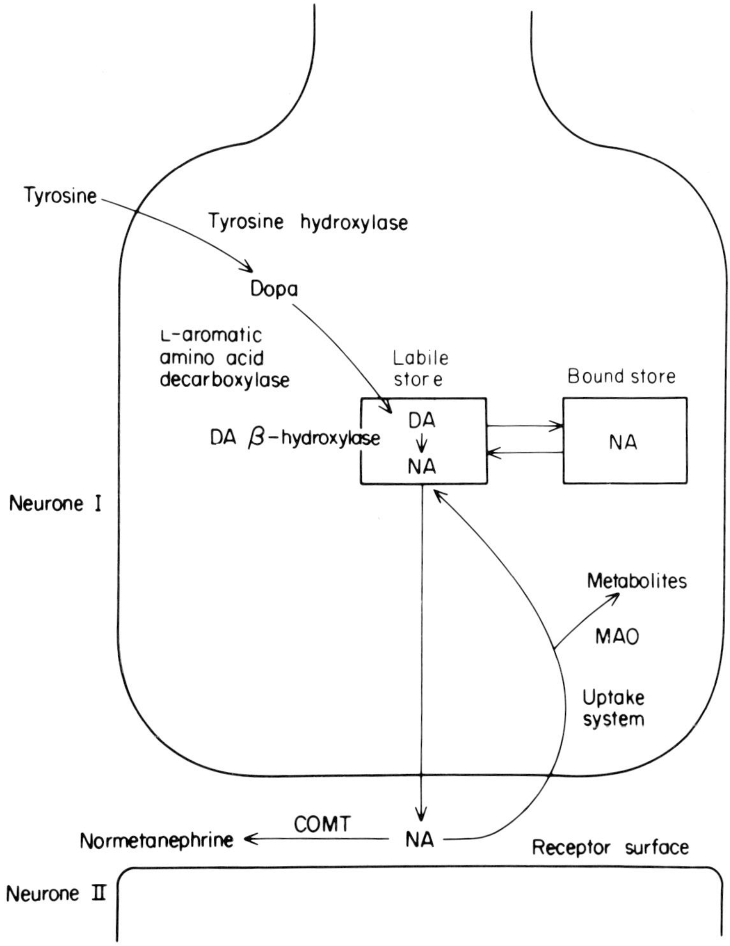

Fig. 15.4 A model of noradrenergic neurone. The presynaptic neurone (neurone I) contains the synthetic enzymes for producing noradrenaline in the storage granule. The labile and strongly bound stores of noradrenaline are in equilibrium. On release, noradrenaline acts on the post-synaptic receptors of neurone II and then approximately 10% is destroyed by membrane bound COMT and 90% is returned to the storage granule by an active uptake mechanism. A small proportion is destroyed by MAO intraneuronally. NA, noradrenaline; DA, dopamine; COMT, catechol-O-methyl transferase; MAO, monoamine oxidase. From Wilson (1974) with permission.

passes through the cytoplasm, by an intraneuronal enzyme monoamine oxidase (von Euler 1958; Sharman 1973). The process is the same in dopaminergic neurones, except the final conversion to NA does not take place.

The synthetic pathway of 5HT from its amino acid precursor tryptophan is shown in Fig. 15.5. Although theoretically the rate-limiting step in this

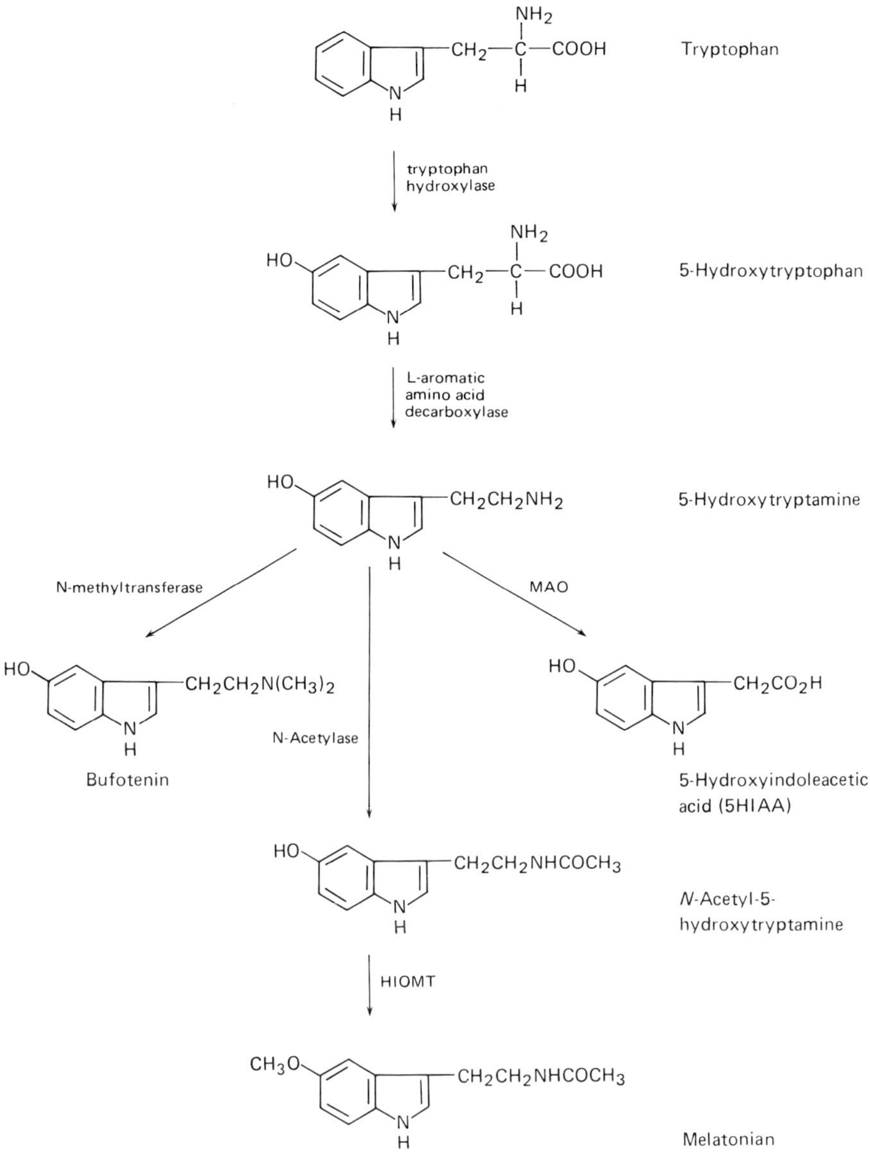

Fig. 15.5 Biosynthesis and metabolism of 5-hydroxytryptamine. From Wilson (1974) with permission.

pathway is the conversion of tryptophan to 5-hydroxytryptophan (5HTP), in practice the rate depends on the availability of dietary tryptophan which is transported from the circulation to the CNS. In normal concentrations tryptophan rarely saturates tryptophan hydroxylase, so that tryptophan concentration is the rate-limiting factor (Grahame-Smith 1971). The 5HT is

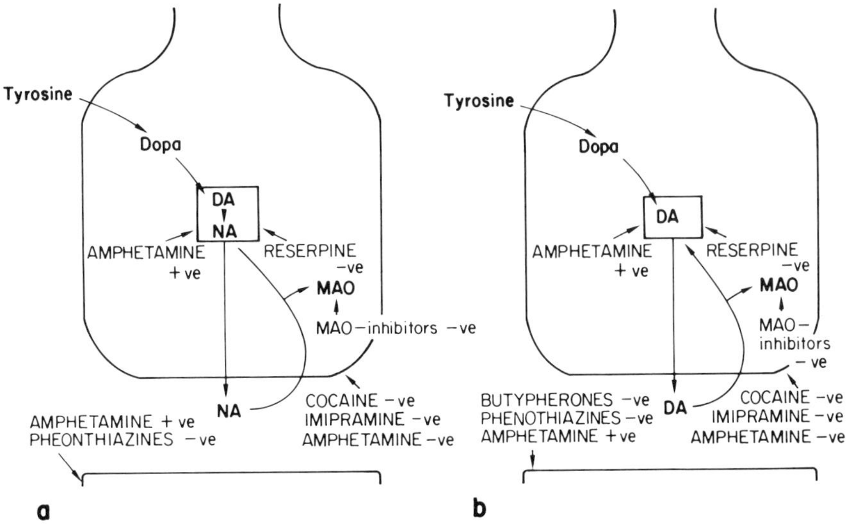

Fig. 15.6 The sites of action of drugs on (a) noradrenergic neurones and (b) dopaminergic neurones.

stored in vesicles which discharge their contents into the synapse by exocytosis after passage of an action potential, and removal from the synaptic cleft is predominantly by reuptake back into the neurone. 5HT is either restored or degraded by monoamine oxidase (Aprison & Hurgtgen 1972).

Figs. 15.6a and 15.6b show the site of action of some centrally active drugs on noradrenergic and dopaminergic neurones within the CNS. It will be seen that the CNS stimulant, cocaine, acts by inhibiting uptake of both NA and DA and therefore enhances their action because they remain in the synapse for a longer period (Hornykiewicz 1966). Amphetamine is another CNS stimulant. It stimulates the release of the catecholamines from the storage granules, inhibits their uptake and also mimics their action on the postsynaptic receptors (Baldessarini 1972).

The tricyclic antidepressants, imipramine and desipramine, inhibit the uptake of catecholamines and also act in a similar way on serotonergic neurones (Carlsson *et al* 1966). Inhibitors of monoamine oxidase (MAOI) prevent the degradation of both the catecholamines and 5HT and they too are used as antidepressants. Certain tranquillisers act on aminergic neurones. For example, the phenothiazines block postsynaptic NA and DA receptors (Anden *et al* 1970) and also increase 5HT synthesis (Bender 1976) and reserpine acts by depleting storage granules in both catecholamine and 5HT neurones (Carlsson *et al* 1957; Shore *et al* 1957). Some CNS stimulants, such as cocaine, have been shown to inhibit 5HT synthesis (Knapp & Mandell 1973, 1976).

15.4.2 Alteration of amino acid transmission

It is believed that the most important amino acid transmitters in the CNS are glycine, which is found mainly in the brainstem and the spinal cord, and GABA which is found in high concentration in most parts of the CNS, (i.e. the cortex, limbic system, cerebellum, midbrain and spinal cord) (Aprison *et al* 1970; de Feudis 1975). Both substances are inhibitory transmitters. Glycine acts only by postsynaptic inhibition causing hyperpolarisation of the postsynaptic receptors, while GABA acts not only postsynaptically in a similar manner, but also presynaptically to produce depolarisation of presynaptic nerve terminals and a consequent inhibition of transmitter release (Fig. 15.7) (Curtis & Johnston 1974; Costa *et al* 1975a).

The metabolic pathway for GABA is as follows:

$$\text{L-glutamic acid} \xrightarrow[\text{glutamic acid decarboxylase}]{} \text{GABA} \xrightarrow[\text{GABA transferase}]{} \text{succinic semi-aldehyde} + \text{glutamic acid}$$

Glycine is involved in transmission in the interneurones of the spinal cord, which are concerned with co-ordination of opposing muscle groups. For example, when extensor muscle neurones are stimulated their collateral nerves will stimulate interneurones to inhibit (via glycine transmission) flexor motor neurones and so suppress flexor muscle movement.

Strychnine is a selective antagonist of glycine. It thus acts by inhibiting inhibition to cause a tetanic convulsion. In strychnine poisoning the extensor and flexor muscles both contract in response to stimulation, and since in most species the extensor muscles are more powerful this results in the typical tonic symmetrical convulsions with extended head and limbs and arched back (Curtis *et al* 1971; Snyder 1975).

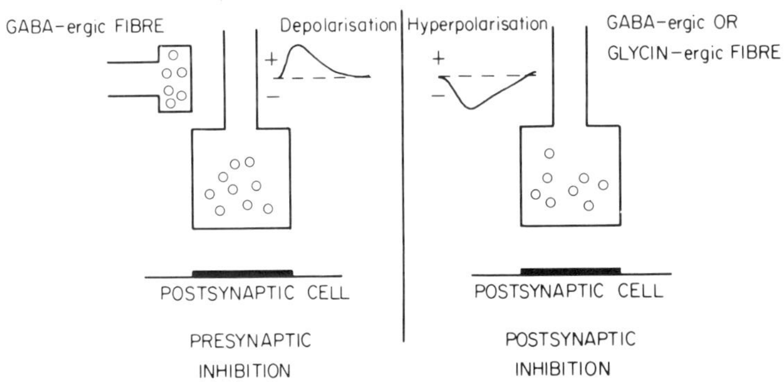

Fig. 15.7 (left) Presynaptic inhibition by a GABA-ergic neurone causing depolarisation of receptors on a stimulatory presynaptic neurone. (right) Postsynaptic inhibition where either glycine or GABA is released from inhibitory neurones and causes hyperpolarisation of the post-synaptic receptors.

One would expect substances which mimic glycine to be muscle relaxants. Mephenesin and guaicol glycerol ether are centrally acting muscle relaxants known to affect transmission in the interneurones of the spinal cord (Bowman *et al* 1968). They may well act to stimulate glycine receptors. They have been used in the treatment of strychnine poisoning and as antitetanus and antiepileptic agents, as well as muscle relaxants in anaesthesia.

GABA is involved in the control of motor activity, particularly by acting on the Purkinje cells in the cerebellum. Substances like isoniazid which inhibit GABA synthesis or which block GABA receptors, such as picrotoxin and bicuculline, cause clonic convulsions. This can be overcome by raising GABA levels with amino-oxyacetic acid (AOAA) which inhibits GABA degradation (Roberts 1974; Costa *et al* 1975b).

The benzodiazapine tranquillisers (e.g. diazepam, chlordiazepoxide and nitrazepam) possess anticonvulsant, muscle relaxant, anxiolytic (in humans) and taming (in animals) properties (Randall & Schalleck 1968; Zbinden & Randall 1967; Wittenborn 1966) and at high dose levels they produce sedative and hypnotic effects (Snyder & Enna 1975). Although there is still some controversy concerning their mechanism of action, there is much evidence to suggest that they act by enhancing both presynaptic and postsynaptic effects of endogenous GABA (Haefely *et al* 1975; Polc & Haefely 1975; Schafener & Haefely 1975). The benzodiazepines selectively antagonise antiGABA convulsant agents and mimic electrophysiological and biochemical effects of GABA in several regions of the CNS (Polc *et al* 1974; Haefely *et al* 1975; Keller *et al* 1976; Costa *et al* 1975a, 1975b). However, they act only if normal levels of GABA and active GABA neurones are present. This indicates that the drugs act by enhancing the action of endogenous GABA and one suggestion put forward is that the drugs stimulate the release of GABA from stores which under normal physiological conditions do not give up their contents (Haefely *et al* 1975; Costa *et al* 1975a).

The benzodiazapines have no affinity for GABA receptors and only bind to glycine receptors in high concentrations well above that required for their therapeutic action (Young *et al* 1974; Snyder & Enna 1975). Recently, however, receptors with a high affinity for benzodiazapines have been demonstrated in the CNS, notably in the frontal and occipital cortex and the limbic system (Squires & Braestrup 1977). The presence of these receptors indicate that the benzodiazapines are mimicking an endogenous substance which enhances GABA activity (Iversen 1977).

The fact that benzodiazepines cause presynaptic inhibition of other neurones means that they will affect the activity of other transmitters in addition to GABA, and indeed, these have been shown to reduce the turnover rates of NA, DA and 5HT as well as inhibiting the release of acetyl choline (Taylor & Laverty 1973; Lidbrink *et al* 1973; Ladinsky *et al* 1973; Fuxe *et al* 1975; Consolo *et al* 1975). It has been suggested that the anxiolytic effect of the benzodiazepines is attributable to a reduction in 5HT activity (Cook & Sepinwall 1975; Stein *et al* 1975) and the sedative action may be due to a decreased NA turnover (Stein *et al* 1975). The muscle relaxation and anticonvulsant effects may be related, in part, to a fall in DA turnover in the limbic system (Fuxe *et al* 1975), and inhibition of acetyl choline release in the striatum has also been associated with muscle relaxation (Consolo *et al* 1975).

15.5 Drugs which alter neuronal membrane permeability within the CNS

The most widely used CNS depressants in veterinary and human medicine are the barbiturates, and members of this chemical group are used as anaesthetics, hypnotics and anticonvulsants. In the latter use, phenobarbitone and primadone (25% of this is metabolised to phenobarbitone *in vivo*) are the primary examples. Another important anticonvulsant is phenytoin. Although the mechanisms of action of these drugs have been studied extensively, they have not been elucidated and so these drugs have been placed in this review under the general category of altering membrane permeability.

The barbiturates are known to act at synapses of both monosynaptic and polysynaptic pathways; the reticular activating system (RAS) is particularly sensitive to their action (Harvey 1975). They do not act directly on any aspect of cerebral metabolism and oxygen consumption etc. is reduced as a secondary functional effect after neuronal depression (Michenfelder 1974).

Both the barbiturates and phenytoin have been shown to act presynaptically inhibiting the release of excitatory transmitters (Weakly 1969; Stratten & Barnes 1971), although it is unlikely that they act by stimulating GABA activity (Costa *et al* 1975a). A possible mechanism of action for these drugs is by altering membrane permeability. Phenytoin reduces neuronal membrane permeability to sodium and calcium ions, thus inhibiting their influx into neurones; it may also stimulate the sodium pump enzyme, ATPase, which would also tend to lower intraneuronal sodium ion concentration (Woodbury & Fingl 1975).

Wakefulness and seizures depend on repetitive activity in multineuronal networks with gradual recruitment of an ever increasing number of neurones until a critical size is attained for regenerative action and self-sustained discharge. In anticonvulsant doses phenobarbitone raises the threshold of electrical activity of neurones in the motor cortex and inhibits the initial discharge. Phenytoin does not alter threshold of activity but appears to depress the subsequent recruited stimuli (Kay & Senner 1977; Harvey 1975).

References

Ahlenius S. (1974) Reversal by L-DOPA of the suppression of locomotor activity induced by inhibition of tyrosine-hydroxylase and DA-beta-hydroxylase in mice. *Brain Res.* **69**, 57.

Anand B. K. (1971) Nervous regulation of food intake. *Physiol. Rev.* **41**, 677

Anden N-E., Butcher S. C., Corrodi H., Fuxe K. & Ungerstedt U. (1970) Receptor activity and turnover of dopamine and noradrenaline after neuroleptics. *Europ. J. Pharmacol.* **11**, 303.

Aprison M. H., Davidoff R. A. & Werman R. (1970) Glycine: its metabolic and possible transmitter roles in nervous tissue. In *Handbook of Neurochemistry* 3rd edn., ed. A. Lajtha, p. 381. Plenum Press, New York.

Aprison M. H. & Hingtgen J. N. (1972) Serotinin and behavior: a brief summary. *Fed. Proc.* **31**, 121.

Baldessarini R. J. (1972) Pharmacology of the amphetamines. *Pediatrics* **49**, 694.

Barchas J. D., Ciaranello R. D., Stolk J. M., Brodie K. H. & Hamberg D. A. (1972) Biogenic amines and behaviour. In *Hormones and Behaviour*, ed. S. Levine, p. 235. Academic Press, New York.

Barraclough C. H. & Sawyer C. H. (1959) Induction of pseudopregnancy in the rat by reserpine and chlorpromazine. *Endocrinology* **65**, 563.

Bender D. A. (1976) The effects of chlorpromazine on serum tryptophan, brain tryptophan uptake and brain serotonin synthesis in the rat. *Biochem. Pharmac.* **25**, 1743.

Bjorkland A., Lindvall O. & Nobin A. (1975) Evidence of an incertahypothalamic dopamine neurone system in the rat. *Brain Res.* **89**, 29.

Blaschko H. (1957) Formation of catecholamines in the animal body. *Brit. Med. Bull.* **13**, 162.

Blaschko H. (1973) Catecholamine biosynthesis. *Brit. Med. Bull.* **29**, 105.

Booth D. A. (1968) Mechanism of action of norepinephrine in eliciting an eating response on injection into the rat hypothalamus. *J. Pharm. Exp. Ther.* **160**, 336.

Bolme P. Fuxe K. & Lidbrink P. (1972) On the function of central catecholamine neurons — their role in cardiovascular and arousal mechanisms. *Res. Comm. Chem. Path. Pharmacol.* **4**, 657.

Bowers M. B. (1975) Serotonin (5HT) systems in psychotic states. *Psychopharm. Comm.* **1**, 655.

Bowman W. C., Rand M. J. & West G. B. (1968) The nervous system. In *Textbook of Pharmacology*, p. 92. Blackwell Scientific Publications, Oxford.

Brazeau P., Vale W., Burgus R., Ling N., Butcher M., Rivier J. & Guillemin R. (1973) Hypothalamic polypeptide that inhibits the secretion of immunoreactive pituitary growth hormone. *Science* **179**, 77.

Breisch S. T., Zemlan F. P. & Hoebel B. G. (1976) Hyperphagia and obesity following serotonin depletion by intraventricular p-chlorophenylalanine. *Science* **192**, 382.

Brodie B. B. & Shore P. A. (1957) A concept for a role of serotonin and norepinephrine as chemical mediators in the brain. *Ann. N.Y. Acad. Sci.* **66**, 631.

Burgus R., Dunn T. F., Desiderio D., Ward D. N., Vale W. & Guillemin R. (1970) Characterization of ovine hypothalamic hypophysiotropic TSH-releasing factor. *Nature* **226** 321.

Burki, H. R., Ruch W. & Asper H. (1975) Effects of clozapine, thioridazine, perlapine and haloperiodol on the metabolism of the biogenic amines in the brain of the rat. *Psychopharmacologia (Berlin)* **41**, 27.

Burks T. F. (1972) Central alpha adrenergic receptors in thermoregulation. *Neuropharmacology* **11**, 615.

Carlsson A., Fuxe K., Hamberger B. & Lindqvist M. (1966). Biochemical and histochemical studies on the effects of imipramine-like drugs and (+)— amphetamine on central and peripheral catecholamine neurones. *Acta Physiol. Scand.* **67**, 481.

Carlsson A., Lindqvist M. & Magnusson T. (1957) 3,4-Dihydroxyphenylalanine and 5-hydroxytryptophan as reserpine antagonists. **Nature 180**, 1200.

Clemens J. A., Smalstig E. B. & Sawyer B. D. (1974) Antipsychotic drugs stimulate prolactin release. *Psychopharmacologia (Berlin)* **40**, 123.

Clinesschmidt B. V., McGuffin J. C. & Werner A. B. (1974) Role of monoamines in the anorexigenic actions of fenfluaramine, amphetamine and p-chloromethamphetamine. *Europ. J. Pharmac.* **27**, 313.

Cook L. & Sepinwall J. (1975) Behavioral analysis of the effects and mechanisms of action of benzodiazepines. In *Advances in Biochemistry and Psychopharmacology* eds. E. Costa & P. Greengard, vol. 14, p. 1. Raven Press, New York.

Cooper B. R., Howard J. L., Grant L. D., Smith R. D. & Breese G. R. (1974) Alteration of avoidance and ingestive behavior after destruction of central catecholamine pathways with 6-hydroxydopamine. *Pharmac. Biochem. Behav.* **2**, 639.

Coppen A. (1967) The biochemistry of affective disorders. *Brit. J. Psychiat.* **113**, 1237.

Consolo S., Garattini S. & Ladinsky H. (1975) Action of the benzodiazepines on the cholinergic system. In *Advances in Biochemistry and Psychopharmacology* eds. E. Costa & P. Greengard, vol. 14, p. 63. Raven Press, New York.

Costa E., Guidotti A., Mao C. C. & Suria A. (1975a) New concepts on the mechanism of action of benzodiazepines. *Life Sciences* **17**, 167.

Costa E., Guidotti A. & Mao C. C. (1975b). Evidence for involvement of GABA in the action of benzodiazepines: studies on rat cerebellum. In *Advances in Biochemistry and Psychopharmacology*, eds. E. Costa & P. Greengard, vol. 14, p. 113. Raven Press, New York.

Costa E., Pscheidt G. R., van Meter W. G. & Himwich H. E. (1960) Brain concentrations of biogenic amines and EEG patterns of rabbits. *J. Pharm. Exp. Ther.* **130**, 81.

Curtis D. R., Duggan A. W. & Johnston G. A. R. (1971) The specificity of strychnine as a glycine antagonist in the mammalian spinal cord. *Exp. Brain Res.* **12**, 547.

Curtis D. R. & Johnston G. A. (1974) Amino acid transmitters in the mammalian central nervous system. In *Reviews of Physiology*, p. 98. Springer-Verlag, Berlin.

Dandrya P. C. & Potni S. K. (1973) Influence of substances acting on the central adrenergic receptor on open field behaviour in rats. *Ind. J. Med. Res.* **61**, 891.

De Feudis F. V. (1975) Amino acids as central neurotransmitters. *Ann. Rev. Pharmac.* **15**, 105.

Dement W., Holman R. B. & Guillemum-Ault C. (1976) The biochemistry of sleep and wakefulness. *Psychopharm. Comm.* **2**, 77.

Diaz J., Ellison G. & Masuoka D. (1974) Opposed behavioral syndromes in rats with partial and more complete central serotoninergic lesions made with 5,6-dihydroxytryptamine. *Psychopharmac.* **37**, 67.

Drucker-Colin R. R. (1974) Possible nature of sleep-inducing brain perfusates: their relationship to seizure-inhibition. In *Neurohumoral Coding of Brain Function*, eds. R. D. Myers and R. R. Drucker-Colin, p. 233 Plenum Press, New York.

Feldberg W. S. (1970) The monoamines of the hypothalamus as mediators of temperature responses. In *Physiological and Behavioural Temperature Regulations*, eds. J. D. Hardy, A. P. Gagge & J. A. J. Stohvijk, p. 493. C. C. Thomas, Springfield, Ill.

Feldberg W. S. & Myers R. D. (1965) Changes in temperature produced by micro-injections of amines into the anterior hypothalamus of cats. *J. Physiol. (London)* **177**, 239.

Fitzsimmons J. T. (1972) Thirst. *Physiol. Rev.* **52**, 468.

Fuxe K., Agnati L. F., Bolme P., Hokfelt T., Lidbrink P., Ljungdahl A., de la Mora M. P. & Ogren S-O. (1975) The possible involvement of GABA mechanisms in the action of benzodiazepines on central catecholamine neurons. In *Advances in Biochemistry and Psychopharmacology*, eds. E. Costa & P. Greengard, vol. 14, p. 45. Raven Press, New York.

Goudie A. J., Thornton E. W. & Wheeler T. J. (1976) Effects of Lilly 10140, a specific inhibitor of 5-hydroxytryptamine uptake, on food intake and on 5-hydroxytryptophan-induced anorexia. Evidence for serotoninergic inhibition of feeding. *J. Pharm. Pharmac.* **28**, 31.

Grahame-Smith D. G. (1971) Studies *in vivo* on the relationship between brain tryptophan, brain 5-HT synthesis and hyperactivity in rats treated with a monoamine oxidase inhibitor and L-tryptophan. *J. Neurochem.* **18**, 1053.

Grossman S. P. (1962a) Direct adrenergic and cholinergic stimulation of hypothalamic mechanisms. *Amer. J. Physiol.* **202**, 872.

Grossman S. P. (1962b) Effects of adrenergic and cholinergic blocking agents on hypothalamic mechanisms. *Amer. J. Physiol.* **202**, 1230.

Grossman S. P. (1975) Role of the hypothalamus in the regulation of food and water intake. *Psychol. Rev.* **82**, 200.

Haefely W., Kulcsár A., Möhler H., Pieri L., Polc P. & Schaffner R. (1975) Possible involvement of GABA in the central actions of benzodiazepines. In *Advances in Biochemistry and Psychopharmacology*, eds. E. Costa & P. Greengard, vol. 14, p. 131. Raven Press, New York.

Harris G. W. (1948) Neural control of the pituitary gland. *Physiol. Rev.* **28**, 139.

Harris G. W. (1964) Sex hormones, brain development and brain function. *Endocrinology* **75**, 627.

Harvey S. G. (1975) Hypnotics and sedatives: the barbiturates. In *The Pharmacological Basis of Therapeutics*, eds. L. S. Goodman & A. Gillman, p. 102. Macmillan, New York.

Hellon R. (1972) Central transmitters and thermoregulation. In *Essays on Temperature Regulation*, eds. J. Bligh & R. E. Moore, p. 71. North-Holland, Amsterdam.

Herman Z. S. (1973a) Influence of noradrenaline, 5-hydroxytryptamine and acetylcholine injected intraventricularly on the rat's behaviour. *Acta Physiol. Pol.* **24**, 87.

Herman Z. S. (1973b) Behavioural effects of dibutyryl cyclic 3′5′ AMP, noradrenaline and cyclic 3′5′ AMP in rats. *Neuropharmacol.* **12**, 705.

Hoebel B. G. (1976) Satiety: Hypothalamic stimulation, anorectic drugs and neurochemical substrates. In *Hunger: Basic Mechanisms and Clinical Implications*, eds. D. Novin, W. Wyrwicka & G. Bray, p. 33. Raven Press, New York.

Hoebel B. G., Hernandez L. & Thompson R. D. (1975) Phenylpropanolamine inhibits feeding but not drinking, induced by hypothalamic stimulation. *J. Comp. Physiol. Psychol.* **89**, 1046.

Hökfelt T., Jonsson G. & Lidbrink P. (1970) Electron microscopic identification of monoamine nerve ending particles in rat brain homogenates. *Brain Res.* **22**, 147.

Hole K., Fuxe K. & Jonsson G. (1976) Behavioral effects of 5,7-dihydroxytryptamine lesions of ascending 5-hydroxytryptamine pathways. *Brain Res.* **107**, 385.

Hornykiewicz O. (1966) Dopamine (3-hydroxytyramine) and brain function. *Pharmacol. Rev.* **18**, 925.

Iversen L. L. (1967) *The Uptake and Storage of Noradrenaline in Sympathetic Nerves*. Cambridge University Press, Cambridge.

Iversen L. L. (1973) Catecholamine uptake processes. *Brit. Med. Bull.* **29**, 130.

Iversen L. L. (1977) Anti-anxiety receptors in the brain? *Nature* **266**, 678.

Iversen L. L. & Bloom F. E. (1972) Studies of the uptake of (3H)-gaba and (3H)-glycine in slices and homogenates of rat brain and spinal cord by electron microscopic autoradiography. *Brain Res.* **41**, 131.

Iversen L. L. & Glowinski J. (1966) Regional studies of catecholamines in the rat brain. II. Rate of turnover of catecholamines in various brain regions. *J. Neurochem.* **13**, 671.

Iversen L. L. & Schon F. E. (1973) The use of autoradiographic techniques for the identification and mapping of transmitter specific neurones in CNS. In *New Concepts in Neurotransmitter Regulation*, ed. A. J. Mandell, p. 153. Plenum Press, New York.

Jacob J., Girault A. & Peindaries R. (1972) Actions of 5-hydroxytryptamine and 5-hydroxytryptophan injected by various routes on the rectal temperature of the rabbit. *Neuropharmacol.* **11**, 1.

Janowsky D. S., El-Yousef M. K., Davis J. M. & Sekerke H. J. (1972) A cholinergic-adrenergic hypothesis of mania and depression. *Lancet* ii, 632.

Jespersen S. & Scheel-Krüger J. (1973) Evidence for a difference in mechanism of action between fenfluramine- and amphetamine-induced anorexia. *J. Pharm. Pharmacol.* **25**, 49.

Jouvet M. (1967) Neurophysiology of the states of sleep. *Physiol. Rev.* **47**, 117.

Jouvet M. (1969) Biogenic amines and the states of sleep. *Science* **163**, 32.

Jouvet M. (1972) The role of monoamines and acetylcholine containing neurons in the regulation of the sleep-waking cycle. *Ergeb. Physiol.* **64**, 166.

Jouvet M. & Pujol J. F. (1974) Effects of central alterations of serotoninergic neurons upon the sleep-waking cycle. *Adv. Biochem. Psychopharmacol* **11**, 199.

Kameyama T., Shigehisa T. & Naheshima T. (1975) Correlation between the 5-hydroxytryptamine contents in the brain and degrees of sensory and locomotor activities in the rat. *Jap. J. Pharmacol.* **25**, 784.

Kay W. J. & Fenner W. R. (1977) Epilepsy. In *Current Veterinary Therapy IV. Small Animal Practice*, ed. R. W. Kirk, p. 853. W. B. Saunders, Philadelphia.

Keller H. H., Schaffner R. & Haefely W. (1976) Interaction of benzodiazepines with neuroleptics at central dopamine neurons. *N.S. Arch. Pharmacol.* **294**, 1.

Kennedy M. S. & Burks T. F. (1974) Dopamine receptors in the central thermoregulatory mechanism of the cat. *Neuropharmacol* **13**, 119.

Knapp S. & Mandell A. J. (1973) Short- and long-term lithium administration: effects on the brain's serotonergic biosynthetic systems. *Science* **180**, 645.

Knapp S. & Mandell A. J. (1976) Cocaine and litium: neurobiological antagonism in the serotin biosynthetic system in rat brain. *Life Sciences* **18**, 679.

Kostowski W., Giacalone E., Garattini S. & Valzelli L. (1968) Studies on behavioural and biochemical changes in rats after lesion of mid-brain raphe. *Europ. J. Pharmacol.* **4**, 371.

Kostowski W. & Giacalone E. (1969) Stimulation of various forebrain structures and brain 5HT, 5HIAA and behaviour in rats. *Europ. J. Pharmacol.* **7**, 176.

Kruk Z. L. (1973) Dopamine and 5-hydroxytryptamine inhibit feeding in rats. *Nature* **246**, 52.

Kuhar M. J. & Aghajanian G. K. (1973) Selective accumulation of (3H)-Serotonin by nerve terminals of raphe neurones: an autoradiographic study. *Nature New Biol.* **241**, 187.

Ladinsky H., Consolo S., Peri G. & Garattini S. (1973) Increase in mouse and rat brain acetyl choline levels by diazepam. In *The Benzodiazepines*, eds. S. Garattini, E. Mussini & L. O. Randall, p. 241. Raven Press, New York.

Leibowitz S. F. (1970) Reciprocal hunger-regulating circuits involving alpha- and beta-adrenergic receptors located, respectively, in the ventromedial and lateral hypothalamus. *Proc. Nat. Acad. Sci.* **67**, 1063.

Leibowitz S. F. (1971) Hypothalamic alpha- and beta-adrenergic systems regulate both thirst and hunger in the rat. *Proc. Nat. Acad. Sci.* **68**, 332.

Lidbrink P., Corrodi H., Fuxe K. & Olson L. (1973) The effects of benzodiazepines, meprobamate and barbiturates on central monoamines neurones. In *The Benzodiazepines*, eds. S. Garattini, E. Mussini & L. O. Randall, p. 203. Raven Press, New York.

Mabry P. D. & Campbell B. A. (1973) Serotonergic inhibition of catecholamine-induced behavioural arousal. *Brain Res.* **49**, 381.

MacLeod R. M. (1976) Regulation of prolactin secretion. In *Frontiers in Neuroendocrinology*, eds. L. Martini & W. F. Gangong, vol. 4, p. 169. Raven Press, New York.

Margules D. L., Lewis M. J., Dragovich J. A. & Margules A. S. (1972) Hypothalamic norepinephrine: Circadian rhythms and the control of feeding behavior. *Science* **178**, 640.

Matsuo H., Baba Y., Nair R. M. G., Arimura A. & Schally A. V. (1971) Structure of the porcine LH- and FSH-releasing hormone. I. The proposed amino acid sequence. *Biochem. Biophys. Res. Comm.* **43**, 1334.

McClure D. J. (1972) Dopamine and depression. *Hormones* **3**, 273.

McLennon H. (1970) *Synaptic Transmission.* 2nd edn., p. 780. W. B. Saunders, Philadelphia.

Michenfelder J. D. (1974) The interdependency of cerebral functional and metabolic effects following massive doses of thiopental in the dog. *Anesthesiol.* **41**, 231.

Monnier M. & Schoenenberger G. A. (1974) Neurohumoral coding of sleep by the physiological factor delta. In *Neurohumoral Coding of Brain Function*, eds. R. D. Myers & R. R. Drucker-Colin, p. 207. Plenum Press, New York.

Myers R. D. (1974) Neurochemical mechanism of temperature regulation and food ingestation. In *Neurohumoral Coding of Brain Function*, eds. R. D. Myers & R. R. Drucker-Colin, p. 99. Plenum Press, New York.

Myers R. D. & Waller M. B. (1975) 5HT and norepinephrine-induced release of ACh from the thalamus and mesencephalon of the monkey during thermoregulation. *Brain Res.* **84**, 47.

Myers R. D. & Yaksh T. L. (1968) Feeding and temperature responses in the unrestrained rat after injections of cholinergic and aminergic substances into the cerebral ventricles. *Physiol. Behav.* **3**, 917.

Myers R. D. & Yaksh T. L. (1969) Control of body temperature in the unanaesthetized monkey by cholinergic and aminergic systems in the hypothalamus. *J. Physiol. (London)* **202**, 483.

Oltmans G. A. & Harvey J. A. (1972) LH syndrome and brain catecholamine levels after lesions of the nigrostriatal bundle. *Physiol. Behav.* **8**, 69.

Papeschi R. (1972) Dopamine, extra pyramidal system and psychomotor function. *Psychiat. Neurol. Neurochir. (Amst.)* **75**, 13.

Polc P., Mohler H. & Haefely W. (1974) The effect of diazepam on spinal cord activities: possible sites and mechanism of action. *N.S. Arch. Pharmacol.* **284**, 319.

Polc P. & Haefely W. (1975) The effect of diazepam on inhibition in the cuneate nucleus of decerebrate cats. *Experientia* **31**, 731.

Quock R. M. & Gale C. C. (1974) Hypothermia-mediating dopamine receptors in the preoptic anterior hypothalamus of the cat. *N.S. Arch. Pharmacol.* **285**, 297.

Radulovachi M. (1974) 5-hydroxyindoleacetic acid in cerebral spinal fluid during wakefulness, sleep and after electrical stimulation of specific brain structures. In *Neurohumoral Coding of Brain Function*, eds. R. D. Myers & R. R. Drucker-Colin, p. 257. Plenum Press, New York.

Randall O. L. L. & Schalleck W. (1968) Pharmacological activity of certain benzodiazepines. In *Psychopharmacology*, ed. D. H. Efron, p. 153. PHSS, London.

Rechtschaffen A., Lovell R. A., Freedman D. X., Whitehead P. K. & Aldrich M. (1973) The effect of parachlorophenylalanine on sleep in the rat: some implications for the serotonin-sleep hypothesis. In *Neurohumoral Coding of Brain Function*, eds. R. D. Myers & R. R. Drucker-Colin, p. 207. Plenum Press, New York.

Roberts E. (1974a) Gamma-aminobutyric acid and nervous system function: a perspective. *Biochem. Pharmac.* **23**, 2637.

Roberts D. (1974b) A model of the vertebrate nervous system based largely on dis-inhibition — a key role of a gaba system. In *Neurohumoral Coding of Brain Function*, eds. R. D. Myers & R. R. Drucker-Colin, p. 419. Plenum Press, New York.

Rosecrans J. A. & Schechter M. D. (1972) Brain 5-hydroxytryptamine correlates of behavior in rats: strain and sex variability. *Physiol. Behav.* **8**, 503.

Rudy T. A. & Wolff H. H. (1969) Receptor selectivity of the hypothermic response to intracerebrally injected catecholamines in cats. *Fed. Proc.* **28**, 443.

Schafener R. & Haefely W. (1975) The effect of diazepam and bicuculline on the stria-nigral evoked potential. *Experientia* **31**, 732.

Schally A. V., Dupont A., Arimura A., Takahara J., Redding T. W., Clemens, J. & Shaar, C. (1976) Purification of a catecholamine-rich fraction with prolactin release-inhibiting factor (PIF) activity from porcine hypothalami. *Acta Endocrinol. (Kbh)* **82**, 1.

Schildkraut J. J. & Kety S. S. (1967) Biogenic amines and emotion. *Science* **156**, 21.

Shaar C. J. & Clemens J. A. (1974) The role of catecholamines in the release of anterior pituitary prolactin *in vitro*. *Endocrinol.* **95**, 1202.

Sharman D. F. (1973) The catabolism of catecholamines: recent studies. *Brit. Med. Bull.* **29**, 110.

Shore P. A., Pletscher A., Tomich D. G., Carlsson A., Kuntzman R. & Brodie B. B. (1957) Role of brain serotonin in reserpine action. *Ann. N.Y. Acad. Sci.* **66**, 609.

Smith A. D. (1973) Mechanisms involved in the release of noradrenaline from sympathetic nerves. *Brit. Med. Bull.* **29**, 123.

Snyder S. H. (1975) The glycine synaptic receptor in the mammalian central nervous system. *Brit. J. Pharmac.* **53**, 473.

Snyder S. H. & Enna S. J. (1975) The role of central glycine receptors in the pharmacologic actions of benzodiazepines. In *Advances in Biochemistry and Psychopharmacology* eds. E. Costa & P. Greengard. vol. 14, p. 81. Raven Press, New York.

Squires R. F. & Braestrup C. (1977) Benzodiazepine receptors in rat brain. *Nature* **266**, 732.

Srebro B. & Lorens, S. A. (1975) Behavioral effects of selective mid-brain raphe lesions in the rat. *Brain Res.* **89**, 303.

Stein L., Wise D. & Belluzzi J. D. (1975) Effects of benzodiazepines on central serotonergic mechanisms. In *Advances in Biochemistry and Psychopharmacology* eds. E. Costa & P. Greengard, vol. 14, p. 29. Raven Press, New York.

Stratten W. P. & Barnes C. D. (1971) Diazepam and presynaptic inhibition. *Neuropharmacol.* **10**, 685.

Tanaka C., Yong-Ja Y. & Takaori S. (1972) Relationship between brain monoamine levels and Sidman avoidance behavior in rats treated with tyrosine and tryptophan hydroxylase inhibitors. *Brain Res.* **45**, 153.

Taylor K. M. & Laverty R. (1973) The interaction of chlordiazepoxide, diazepam and nitrozepam with catecholamines and histamine in regions of the rat brain. In *The Benzodiazepines*, eds. S. Garattini, E. Mussini & L. O. Randall, p. 191. Raven Press, New York.

Thorner M. O., McNeilly A. S., Hagen C. & Besser G. M. (1974) Long-term treatment of galactorrhoea and hypogonadism with bromocriptine. *Brit. Med. J.* **2**, 419.

Ungerstedt U. (1971) Stereotaxic mapping of the monoamine pathways in the rat. *Acta Physiol. Scand.* suppl. 367, 1.

Ursin R. (1976) The effects of 5-hydroxytryptophan and L-tryptophan on wakefulness and sleep patterns in the cat. *Brain Res.* **106**, 105.

Van Praag H. M. & Korf J. (1972) 5-hydroxytryptophan and depression. *Hormones* **3**, 282.

Von Euler U. S. (1958) Distribution and metabolism of catechol hormones in tissues and axones. *Rec. Prog. Horm. Res.* **14**, 483.

Weakly J. N. (1969) Effect of barbiturates on 'quantal' synaptic transmission in spinal motorneurones. *J. Physiol.* **204**, 63.

Weissman A. & Harbert C. A. (1972) Recent developments relating serotonin and behaviour. *Ann. Rep. Med. Chem.* **7**, 47.

Wittenborn J. R. (1966) The clinical psychopharmacology of anxiety. C. C. Thomas, Springfield, Ill.

Wilson C. A. (1974) Hypothalamic amines and the release of gonadotrophins and other anterior pituitary hormones. In *Advances in Drug Research*, eds. A. Simmonds & N. J. Harper, vol. 8, p. 119. Academic Press, New York.

Woodbury D. M. & Fingl E. (1975) Drugs effective in the therapy of the epilepsies. In *The Pharmacological Basis of Therapeutics*, eds. L. S. Goodman & A. Gillman, p. 201. Macmillan, New York.

Wyatt R. J., Dawson S. & Gillin J. C. (1976) REM sleep induction by physostigmine infusion during sleep. *Science* **191**, 1281.

Young A. B., Zukin S. R. & Snyder S. H. (1974) Interaction of benzodiazepines with central nervous glycine receptors: possible mechanism of action. *Proc. Nat. Acad. Sci.* **71**, 2246.

Zbinden G. & Randall L. O. (1967) Pharmacology of benzodiazepines: laboratory and clinical correlations. *Adv. Pharmac. Chemother.* **5**, 213.

16

Agents acting on the central nervous system II. Clinical pharmacology of antiepileptic drugs and tranquillisers

P. LEES

16.1 Antiepileptic drugs

16.1.1 Use of antiepileptic drugs in man

Before considering the animal pharmacology and clinical use of antiepileptic drugs in the dog and cat, a brief description of their clinical pharmacology in man is warranted as a source of background information which remains incomplete in animal studies.

Newer drugs

Several drugs are in common use in man (Table 16.1). Some of these have not yet been used clinically in animals, but they may prove to be of future value. Ethosuximide, carbamazepine, the benzodiazepines and sodium valproate are of particular interest. According to Jeavons (1977) the latter is the drug of first choice for several forms of epilepsy and has proved to be of particular value in petit mal in children. Side-effects are rare. Sedation does not occur with normal dose rates and although thinning or partial loss of hair may occur the effect is temporary. One or two cases of thrombocytopenia have been described. Jeavons (1977) reports that carbamazepine is the drug of choice in psychomotor and sensorimotor (focal) epilepsies and tonic-clonic fits (grand mal). The plasma half-life of 24–46 hours in man following a single oral dose should ensure that once daily therapy is adequate but tolerance develops with chronic usage, and half-life decreases to 8–19 hours. This necessitates the administration of 2–3 doses/day. Side-effects are uncommon and sedation is rare, although skin rashes occur in some 4% of patients. Dizziness has also been reported and toxic doses may produce diplopia or blurred vision. Ethosuximide is the drug of second choice for the treatment of petit mal. It is very effective in this condition but the side-effects of sedation, nausea, vomiting and acute behavioural disturbances make it less suitable than sodium valproate. A number of benzodiazepine derivatives have been used as antiepileptic agents. Diazepam is the drug of choice for patients in *status epilepticus*, while clonazepam and nitrazepam have been used in myoclonic epilepsies (particularly in children) and for infantile spasms. A serious side-effect of all benzodiazepines is their sedative action and this is most pronounced with clonazepam. The carbonic anhydrase inhibitor, acetazolamide, continues to be used as an adjuvant antiepileptic for most forms of epilepsy. Its mode of action is unknown. Its side-effects include metabolic acidosis, hypokalaemia and, on occasions, sedation.

Enzyme induction and dosage requirements

For most of the antiepileptic drugs used in man, the plasma half-life and the optimal range of serum concentrations required for the control of epilepsy have been defined (Table 16.1). Knowledge of these two variables allows prediction of the dose rate and frequency needed to achieve effective control of epilepsy. Whilst it is not possible to transpose this data directly to other species, it does serve to emphasise that the rational use of antiepileptic drugs depends on adjustment of the dose to suit the needs of the individual patient. It should be emphasised that these needs will often change as therapy proceeds. Studies of the clinical pharmacology of antiepileptics in man have revealed that the half-life of drugs is not always constant, even in individual patients. To some extent, this results from the fact that several anticonvulsants including phenobarbitone, primidone, phenytoin and carbamazepine are stimulators of hepatic microsomal enzymes, notably of the mixed function oxidase enzyme system which hydroxylates many drugs (see Chapter 2). This enzyme induction increases the rate of biotransformation, shortens the half-life (note the much shorter half-life of carbamazepine in Table 16.1 associated with its chronic use) and leads to the development of tolerance. The maintenance of plasma concentrations within the optimal range will then require an increase in dose rate and/or frequency. Enzyme induction by one antiepileptic agent may also reduce the half-life of a second drug. For example, in one study the mean half-life of sodium valproate was 9·0 hours in normal subjects and 5·9 hours in epileptics (A. Richens, pers. comm.). This difference was probably caused by enzyme induction in the latter group, who were receiving treatment with other antiepileptic drugs in addition to sodium valproate. By the same mechanism, antiepileptic drugs have been shown to reduce the effects of anticoagulants such as warfarin, the tetracycline derivative doxycycline, and anti-inflammatory agents (Eadi & Tyrer 1974; Laidlow & Richens 1976; Penttila *et al* 1974). Liver enzyme induction by phenytoin, primidone and phenobarbitone has been shown to increase the rate of hepatic biotransformation of vitamin D (Dent *et al* 1970). With low levels of this vitamin serum calcium is reduced, alkaline phosphatase is increased and osteomalacia and/or rickets may result. This

Table 16.1 Clinical pharmacology of antiepileptic drugs in man.

Drug	Half-life (hours)	Optimal serum or plasma concentration (μg/ml)	Dosage**	Principal indications (Jeavons 1977)
Phenobarbitone	36 – 72 (children) 48 – 140 (adults)	15 – 40	Up to 8 mg/kg once daily	Neonatal fits*; grand mal (only in old age)
Phenytoin	9 – 140 (varies with dose)	10 – 20 or 25	Up to 350 mg once daily	Grand mal (males only); psychomotor epilepsy
Primidone	3 – 24	–	Up to 125 mg once daily initially	Grand mal; psychomotor epilepsy
Ethosuximide	24 – 48 (children) 48 – 72 (adults)	40 – 120	500 mg once daily (children)	Petit mal
Sodium valproate	8 – 15	60 – 100	200 mg twice daily initially increase to 400 – 500 mg twice daily	Grand mal*; petit mal*; psychomotor epilepsy; myoclonic epilepsy*; sensorimotor (focal) epilepsy; photosensitive epilepsy*; febrile convulsions*
Carbamazepine	24 – 46 (single dose) 8 – 19 (chronic dose)	4 – 10	20 mg/kg daily in 2 or 3 doses	Grand mal*; psychomotor epilepsy*; sensorimotor (focal) epilepsy*
Diazepam	20 – 42	–	0·15 – 0·25 mg/kg i.v.	*Status epilepticus**; prolonged febrile convulsions*
Nitrazepam	21 – 25	–	0·5 – 1·0 mg/kg once daily (infants and children)	Myoclonic epilepsy (children) infantile spasms
Clonazepam	20 – 40	–	1·0 – 3·0 mg once daily (infants and children)	*Status epilepticus**; prolonged febrile convulsions*; sensorimotor (focal) epilepsy; myoclonic epilepsy
Acetazolamide	4 – 10	–	125 – 250 mg (infants) 250 – 500 mg (children and adults) both once daily	Adjuvant to other agents

has led to the proposal that patient receiving antiepileptic drugs should be given vitamin D supplements prophylactically (Mahn *et al* 1972; Christiansen *et al* 1973). Enhancement of the rate of metabolic conversion of cortisol, androgens and oestrogens to more polar derivatives by phenobarbitone and phenytoin has been described (Kuntzmann 1969).

The opposite of liver enzyme induction (i.e. suppression of activity) has also been demonstrated. The antiepileptic agents sulthiamc and pheneturide, the antituberculous drugs isoniazid and para-aminosalicylic acid, the dicoumarol group of anticoagulants, the oestrogenic component of oral contraceptives, the anti-inflammatory agent phenylbutazone, the ataractics chlorpromazine and chlordiazepoxide, and chloramphenicol have all been shown to suppress phenytoin metabolism and such combinations may potentially lead to the accumulation of toxic levels of phenytoin in the circulation (Hansen 1966; Stockley 1972, 1976). These documented interactions leave one with the impression that they may merely be the tip of the iceberg.

Zero-order and first-order kinetics

Most drugs, including antiepileptic agents, are cleared from the circulation in a biexponential manner. The first phase involves redistribution of the drug and the second excretion and/or metabolism. Excretory and metabolic pathways usually follow first-order kinetics (i.e. the quantity of drug cleared in unit time is proportional to the plasma concentration). At therapeutic dose levels the clearance of phenytoin, in man at least, follows zero-order and not first-order kinetics. This means that a fixed quantity of the drug is cleared in unit time and this has important effects on half-life. For first-order kinetics the half-life remains constant as the dose and plasma concentration change, but with phenytoin half-life increases as the plasma concentration rises. For example, in one human patient, stabilised on low, medium and high doses of phenytoin, the half-lives were 21, 45 and 79 hours respectively (A. Richens, pers. comm.). Because phenytoin is subject to 'saturation kinetics' in man, the plasma concentration rises steeply when the dose is increased by small increments and this makes regulation of plasma levels within the optimal range difficult. The cause of these phenomena is believed to be saturation of the hepatic microsomal enzyme system which hydroxylates the drug by therapeutic dose levels of phenytoin. An alternative proposal is that the p-hydroxyphenyl metabolite feeds back on the enzyme to inhibit further metabolism of phenytoin.

Toxicity

The widespread and long-term use of antiepileptic drugs in man has inevitably led to descriptions of many side-effects, which are sometimes of very low incidence. While similar effects may not have been reported in the veterinary literature, the possibility of their occurrence in animals cannot be discounted. The osteomalacia and rickets which may follow prolonged antiepileptic therapy is a case in point. A coagulation defect, resulting from lack of a vitamin K-dependent coagulation factor, has produced haemorrhage in the first 24 hours of life in babies whose mothers had received phenobarbitone and/or phenytoin during pregnancy (Kohler 1966; Mountain *et al* 1970). The side-effects of hirsutism and coarsening of facial features have been reported with high doses of phenytoin and other antiepileptic agents (Lefebvre *et al* 1972). Peripheral neuropathy, indicated by absent knee, ankle and arm jerks and sometimes associated with impairment of touch and pain sensations, has been described in human (often elderly) subjects receiving high doses of phenytoin over long periods but a definite cause and effect relationship has not been established.

Of special relevance to long-term therapy are potential teratogenic and oncogenic properties. The incidence of congenital malformations, especially cleft palate and hare lip, is probably higher in human mothers who have received phenobarbitone, primidone, trimethadione and phenytoin than in mothers who are not epileptic and have therefore not received such treatment (Pashayan *et al* 1971; South 1972; Speidel & Meadow 1972; Lowe 1973; Monson *et al* 1973; Fredrick 1973; Laughman *et al* 1973). The incidence of malformation is not excessively high; in one study the total malformation rate in 305 children born to epileptic mothers was 10·5%, the figure for non-epileptic mothers being 6·4% (Shapiro *et al* 1976). The corresponding percentage figures for major malformations were 6·6 and 2·7. In another group it was noted that malformation rates were intermediate when fathers of the offspring had epilepsy. These findings indicate that teratogenicity may be linked genetically to the condition of epilepsy itself. However, the antifolic acid properties of anticonvulsant drugs may also be implicated (Reynolds 1973). Whatever the cause of the malformations one authority has claimed that the risk to fetus and mother is greater if drugs are withheld during the first trimester of pregnancy and the teratogenic risk should be ignored (Jeavons 1977). There are fewer reports of oncogenic activity of antiepileptic drugs, although one study found no evidence of such activity in more than 9000 epileptic patients receiving treatment (Clemmensen *et al* 1974).

16.1.2 Treatment of epilepsy in the dog and cat: general considerations

Some general properties and clinical uses of the principal antiepileptic agents used in veterinary medicine are summarised in Table 16.2. The lipid solubility ranges from moderate (phenobarbitone) to high (phenytoin and diazepam). In general, high lipid solubility is associated with rapid and almost complete absorption from the gastrointestinal tract, a high degree of protein binding and low renal excretion of unmetabolised drug.

Table 16.2 Fate in the body and clinical use of antiepileptic drugs.

Drug	Antiepileptic activity of metabolites	Renal excretion of unchanged drug	Degree of binding to plasma protein	Dosage**		Indications
				Dog	Cat	
Phenobarbitone	No	Up to 50%	Low	7·5 – 120 mg per animal 2 – 4 times daily	8 – 32 mg per animal 2 or 3 times daily	Generalised major motor seizures, minor motor seizures, behavioural seizures
				60 – 120 mg per animal i.v. or i.m.	5 – 100 mg per animal i.v. or i.m.	*Status epilepticus* (after diazepam *(if necessary)*)
Primidone	Yes*	Some	Low	8 – 50 mg/kg daily in divided doses	–	Generalised major motor seizures, minor motor seizures
Trimethadione	Yes*	Some	Low	300 – 1000 mg per animal 3 times daily	–	Generalised epilepsies?
Phenytoin	No	Slight	High	Loading dose: 8 – 22 mg/kg Maintenance dose: 6·5 – 11·0 mg/kg 3 times daily	Not recommended	Generalised major motor seizures, minor motor seizures, behavioural seizures
Diazepam	Yes	Slight	High	5 – 35 mg per animal i.v. or i.m.	2 – 10 mg per animal i.v. or i.m.	*Status epilepticus* and acute exacerbation of seizures
				–	2 – 5 mg per animal 2 or 3 times daily	Generalised epilepsies

*Antiepileptic activity attributable mainly or entirely to metabolites;
** Doses for oral administration unless stated.

Whatever agents, alone or in combination, are selected for therapeutic use, there are a number of general considerations which must be outlined before describing the properties of each agent.

Diagnosis of epilepsy

A correct diagnosis of the state of epilepsy and differential diagnosis of the form of epilepsy are important, since many antiepileptic drugs will be of little value in non-epileptic convulsions and the drug of first choice may depend on diagnosis of the type of epilepsy. These matters are outside the scope of this text, but useful accounts have been given by Kay and Fenner (1977), Parker (1973) and Taylor (1958).

Dose levels

Since therapy will commonly be long-term the veterinarian should see the patient at sufficiently regular intervals to ensure that maintenance doses are both effective and non-toxic. The animal to animal variation in dose requirement is usually such that the dose level cannot be fixed on a body weight basis but must be adjusted to the need of the individual patient. Moreover, the quantity of drug required and the frequency of its administration may change in each individual — usually because of the development of tolerance. A useful general approach followed in man is to commence therapy with a small dose of a single drug and increase this at weekly intervals until control is achieved or signs of toxicity appear. A similar approach to animal therapy would seem reasonable, although phenytoin is exceptional (see below); a high loading dose of this agent is given and the level is reduced after a few days. There is a need for experimental and clinical studies in the dog and cat to establish both optimal plasma concentrations of the commonly used anti-epileptic drugs and their half-lives following chronic oral administration. This data will provide a rational basis for dose selection.

Drug combinations

It is common to advise against the use of drug combinations, and it is certainly desirable to commence therapy with a single agent. However, it is not always possible to control seizures with a single drug, and several combinations have been described (Kay & Fenner 1977; Taylor 1958). The former authors use phenobarbitone and phenytoin together routinely in the dog and stress the advantage that the rapid onset of action of phenobarbitone covers the lag period before phenytoin becomes effective. Primidone is used as a third agent when necessary. Pasten (1977) advised against the use of phenobarbitone and phenytoin together on the grounds that the former drug hastens the metabolism of phenytoin, reducing its serum concentration to ineffective levels. This objection could presumably be met, however, by increasing the dose of phenytoin.

If treatment is to be changed from one drug to another, the clinician should allow an overlap of several weeks to ensure that relapse does not occur, the administered dose of the original drug being reduced gradually. This is perhaps particularly important when the new drug is phenytoin or trimethadione.

Route of administration

The requirement for a very rapid onset of action in *status epilepticus* is achieved by intravenous or intramuscular injection of the appropriate agent (diazepam or phenobarbitone). On the other hand, with the need for administration one or more times daily for very long periods in the treatment of less severe epileptic states the oral route is the most suitable.

Failure of therapy

Kay and Fenner (1977) give the principal reasons for partial or complete failure to control epilepsy as non-administration by the owner, prescription of an inadequate dose level, changing drugs with an inadequate period of overlap and the presence of concomitant disease. The control of epilepsy seems to be particularly difficult in certain breeds of dog (German Shepherd, Irish Setter, Great Dane, St. Bernard, Shetland Sheepdog) and Kay and Fenner (1977) often administer high doses of antiepileptics to these breeds.

PHENOBARBITONE (phenobarbital)

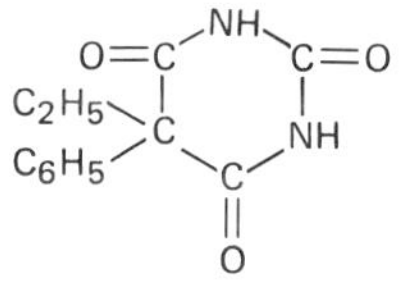

Phenobarbitone

Many barbiturates possess anticonvulsant properties but phenobarbitone is the barbiturate of choice for the treatment of epilepsy since its long duration of action makes administration three or four times daily suitable and its greater specificity relative to other barbiturates as an anticonvulsant ensures that control of epilepsy can be achieved with subhypnotic doses. However, the general depressant action of phenobarbitone on the CNS, as manifested by the sedative action which commonly occurs at therapeutic dose rates, has greatly limited its use in man. Sedation may also occur in the cat and dog, but this is not always a problem. Kay and Fenner (1977) have given doses of up to 450 mg/day to large breeds of dog without causing significant sedation and the drug is still widely used in veterinary medicine (Redding 1969). Kay and Fenner (1977) suggest that it is extremely effective and useful for all forms of epilepsy in the dog. In addition, it is the drug of first choice (a) in the cat for all forms of epilepsy, being given orally two or three times daily (Kay 1975) and (b) in the dog presented during an epileptic attack or in *status epilepticus*. The latter indication emphasises its fairly rapid onset of action. As with other anti-epileptic agents, abrupt withdrawal of phenobarbitone should be avoided to prevent any increase in the frequency of seizures. Animals may become restless and irritable during treatment and polyphagia, polydipsia and polyuria are encountered routinely. Other side-effects, which indicate that the dosage should be reduced, include nystagmus and ataxia. As with phenytoin and primidone, a number of rare toxic reactions have been reported following the use of phenobarbitone in man. These include drug allergies, hypoprothrombinaemia with haemorrhage in newborn infants, megaloblastic anaemia and osteomalacia.

Termination of the action of phenobarbitone is dependent upon both metabolism in the liver and renal excretion of the unchanged drug. Between 10 and 50% may be lost by the latter mechanism. Since phenobarbitone is a weak acid (p*Ka* 7·3) the ratio of ionised to unionised molecules in renal tubular fluid will vary with the pH of the fluid, increasing as the pH rises. Only the unionised molecules can be reabsorbed across the tubular epithelium, so that excretion in the urine rises as pH increases. Theoretically, therefore, alkalinisation of the urine by administering sodium bicarbonate will be of value in the treatment of acute overdosage with phenobarbitone. It is unlikely however that acute overdosage will occur during routine treatment. Some 75% of a given dose is metabolised by hepatic microsomal enzymes to the inactive parahydroxyphenyl derivative (Butler 1956).

The general pharmacology of phenobarbitone is described in standard texts and will not be repeated here. However, the high potency of the drug as an inducer of hepatic microsomal enzymes, involving an increase in enzyme content rather than a change in the properties of the enzymes, must be emphasised (Conney & Burns 1972). This action may lead not only to a need for increasing doses of phenobarbitone itself and other antiepileptic agents used concomitantly, but also to a requirement for more frequent dosing. Since the half-life of phenobarbitone in man ranges from 48 to 140 hours, frequent administration should be unnecessary and dosing once daily is usual. In the dog, however, the normal therapeutic regime involves administration three or four times each day. It would therefore be of some interest to measure the half-life of phenobarbitone in the dog following an initial dose and in the same animals following chronic use of the drug.

Finally, note should be taken of the disinclination of many medical practitioners to prescribe barbiturate drugs at the present time because of the potential for misuse of these drugs. The possibility exists for misuse of phenobarbitone by owners of animal patients.

PRIMIDONE (pyrimidinedione)

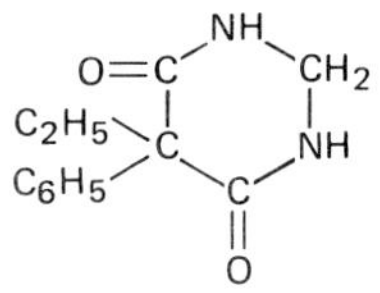

Primidone

This drug is structurally similar to phenobarbitone, a single carbonyl group being replaced by a methylene grouping. It was introduced as an antiepileptic agent in 1952 (Handley & Stewart) and has been used in the dog to treat most forms of epilepsy including generalised major motor, minor motor, sensory and behavioural seizures. In 1965, Oliver and Hoerlein judged primidone to be the most effective agent for the control of epileptic seizures in the dog but it is currently thought to be less useful than phenytoin and phenobarbitone because of the many side-effects produced (Kay & Fenner 1977). Advantages of primidone are said to include a high level of efficacy and a rapid onset of action. It possesses sedative properties, which may become sufficiently severe to incapacitate some animals. However, sedation is often transient, subsiding as therapy continues, and performance may be unimpaired (Higgins 1977). Dosage requirements seem to vary widely (Table 16.2). Polyphagia, polydipsia and polyuria occur in most dogs and irritability, restlessness and personality changes are common. Kay and Fenner (1977) suggest that tests for signs of liver disease should be undertaken periodically if high doses are used.

The effects of primidone are generally similar to those of phenobarbitone. In fact, it has been shown that approximately 25% of the former drug is converted to phenobarbitone in man and the dog. A comparison of the *approximate* daily dose requirements of phenobarbitone (4 mg/kg) and primidone (50 mg/kg) (Kirk 1977) suggests that much of the activity of primidone may be attributable to the barbiturate. This is supported by the findings of Bogan and Smith (1968) in man. These authors calculated that doses of primidone and phenobarbitone in the ratio 5:1 produced similar plasma concentrations of phenobarbitone. In addition, Bogan (pers. comm.) has shown that primidone (60 mg/kg/day for 10 days) produces blood concentrations of phenobarbitone of approximately 15 μg/ml in the dog (Fig. 16.1). If primidone is a pro-drug, its effects being mediated primarily by phenobarbitone, the combined clinical use of the two agents would presumably be of limited value. However, this may be an oversimplification, the picture being further complicated by the fact that primidone is also metabolised to a second biologically active metabolite, PEMA (phenylethylmalonamide) (Woodbury & Fingl 1975). The latter authors suggest that both metabolites and primidone itself contribute to the therapeutic effect. In man, the half-lives of PEMA and phenobarbitone are 24–48 hours and 48–140 hours,

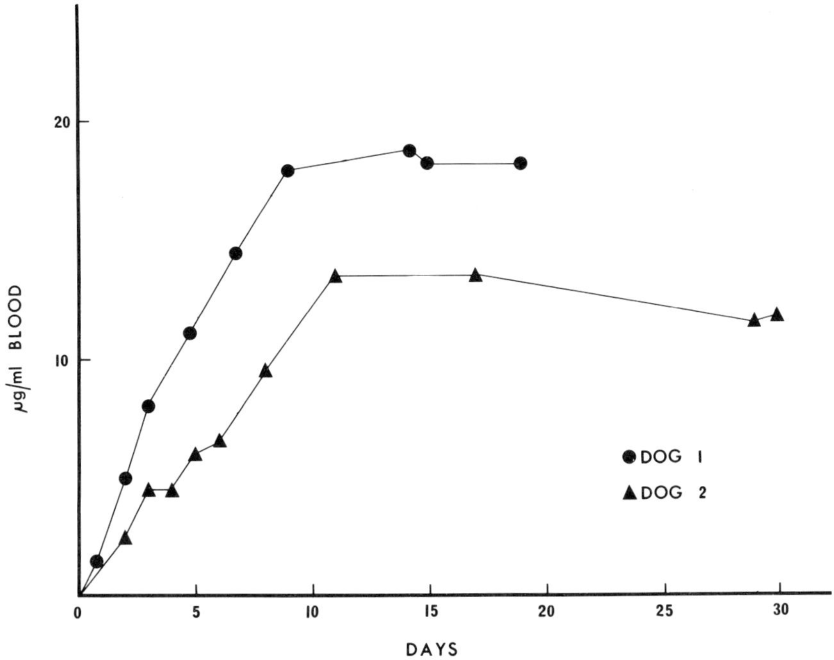

Fig. 16.1 Concentration of phenobarbitone in blood after the administration of primidone (60 mg/kg/day) in two dogs.

respectively, whilst that of primidone is 3–24 hours, so that both metabolites tend to accumulate during chronic medication.

TRIMETHADIONE (troxidone)

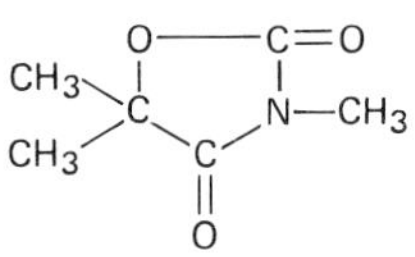

Trimethadione

Trimethadione has been used in man for the treatment of petit mal for more than 30 years. It has also been used in the dog and is presumably best suited to the therapy of absence-like seizures in this species also. It is less potent than phenytoin; in laboratory tests of anticonvulsant activity in mice approximately 100 times the quantity of trimethadione is required to inhibit electroshock and leptazol-induced seizures.

In the liver, significant amounts of the *N*-demethyl derivative of trimethadione, dimethadione, are formed by microsomal enzymes (Butler *et al* 1965). Dimethadione is a more potent anticonvulsant than the parent molecule (Withrow *et al* 1968). Dimethadione is excreted unchanged in the urine, and since its half-life ranges from 6 to 13 days in man, it accumulates during chronic administration to account for much the greater part of the antiepileptic activity. Because of the long half-life, several weeks elapse before plateau levels of the active metabolite in the plasma are reached. This applies both at the start of therapy and when the dosage is altered. Absorption of trimethadione from the gastrointestinal tract is rapid, peak plasma concentrations being attained within 2 hours.

Several side-effects have been reported. Sedation and hemeralopia (blurring of vision in bright light) or photophobia are said to be the commonest (Woodbury & Fingl 1975). The sedative effect generally diminishes with continued medication. A number of blood dyscrasias, allergic responses, and a myasthenic syndrome have also been described, and in some human epileptic patients it has *precipitated* tonic-clonic seizures.

PHENYTOIN SODIUM (diphenylhydantoin sodium)

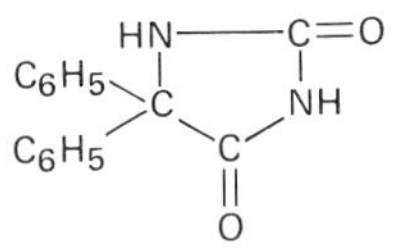

Phenytoin sodium

This agent was introduced by Merritt and Putnam for the treatment of epilepsy in 1938, and is still used extensively in human and veterinary medicine. The property of phenytoin which accounts for most and perhaps all of its biological actions, including its antiarrhythmic effects on the heart, is a membrane stabilising action. The mechanisms whereby it modifies the flux of sodium, potassium and calcium ions across membranes are still undecided (Woodbury & Fingl 1975).

Though structurally similar to phenobarbitone, its mode of action is different (see Chapter 15). Thus, the antiepileptic action of phenytoin is related to its depressant action on the motor cortex, the sensory cortex being little affected. Unlike phenobarbitone, therefore, it is not a general anticonvulsant and is not used to treat poisoning by convulsant drugs or tetanic seizures. (Taylor, 1958, has discussed the differential diagnosis of epileptiform and tetanic convulsions in the dog.) The antiepileptic action of normal therapeutic doses of phenytoin is not accompanied by a sedative effect. Other general advantages are its high degree of efficacy in a large percentage of patients and, although the *range* of side-effects that have been described is high, their incidence and the general toxicity of phenytoin are low.

Chemically, phenytoin is a very weak acid (p*Ka* 8·3) which, like barbiturates, exists as two geometrical isomers (keto and enol) The sodium salt is formed by replacement of the hydroxyl hydrogen of the enolic form. Solutions of the sodium salt are alkaline and irritant to the tissues when injected extravascularly. Thus, in dogs induration, intravascular clotting, adhesions and occlusion have followed intravenous injections, while intramuscular administration produces considerable local damage (Parke Davis, product literature). Moreover, absorption from muscle may be poor, since the drug crystallises out of solution. One study in rabbits demonstrated that half of the administered dose was still present at the injection site after 48 hours. On the other hand, Roye *et al* (1973) obtained similar plasma levels of phenytoin in the dog following oral and intramuscular administration.

In clinical use phenytoin is administered solely by mouth. Absorption from the stomach is very limited because of the poor solubility in acid gastric juice, but intestinal absorption is generally good (Dill *et al* 1956). It is worthy of note, however, that particle size and pharmaceutical formulation can exert profound effects on absorption. In one study the sodium salt of phenytoin was much better absorbed than phenytoin itself, apparently because of the smaller particle size of the former, and in another investigation the replacement of calcium sulphate by lactose as the excipient in oral capsules greatly increased plasma levels of the drug, producing an outbreak of phenytoin toxicity (Tyrer *et al* 1970).

There are several problems relating to the clinical use of phenytoin but it probably remains the drug of choice for the treatment of all types of epilepsy with the exception of *status epilepticus* in the dog (Kay & Fenner 1977). Thus, it is used extensively in the treatment of generalised major motor, minor motor and behavioural seizures. Kay and Fenner (1977) state that it is ineffective in treating *status epilepticus* or an acute exacerbation of seizures. However, phenytoin may be of value in these patients for maintenance therapy once convulsions have been controlled (Oliver & Hoerlein 1965). It has also been recommended for the treatment of nervous excitement in the dog and other nervous conditions manifested by muscular twitching and convulsive seizures. In some cases of early progressive chorea phenytoin has controlled or slowed progression of the condition, while some beneficial effects may be obtained in established cases of chorea with limited muscular involvement.

The recommended dosage schedule has varied. The manufacturers suggest that an initial loading dose of 8·3–16·7 mg/kg be given and this is followed by the same total amount per day in divided doses, the quantity being adjusted on the basis of the patient's response. A similar starting dose (4–8 mg/lb total dose in three or four aliquots) was recommended by Booth (1977). With this schedule several days are normally required to achieve effective levels, so that any preceding therapy should be replaced gradually.

In man, the optimal range of serum concentration of phenytoin is 10–25 μg/ml. Below this range control of epilepsy may be inadequate while signs of toxicity are likely to appear at higher concentrations (Kutt 1971). Only one study of the effective circulating levels of phenytoin in the dog has been reported (Pasten 1977). This author emphasised the necessity of monitoring blood levels rather than 'blindly and intuitively increasing and decreasing the dosage regimen'. The therapeutic range of serum concentration was usually 1·5–3·0 μg/ml (well below the human range) and the dosage schedule most likely to provide these levels was 3–5 mg/lb three times daily. The time required to reach peak levels varied greatly from animal to animal, ranging from 2 to 7 days, although there was no apparent influence of sex, breed or weight, and high levels could be achieved in 12–24 hours by using a loading dose of 10 mg/lb body weight. Serum levels became negligible 1–5 days after terminating therapy. This study demonstrates that the *higher* doses of phenytoin used in the dog than in man produce much *lower* blood levels and this is probably explained by a more rapid rate of biotransformation in the liver of the dog.

The principal metabolite of phenytoin in dogs is 5-(p-hydroxyphenyl)-5-phenylhydantoin (Butler 1957; Toman 1965). This derivative does not possess antiepileptic activity. Its removal from the body is facilitated by conjugation with glucuronic acid (Maynert 1960). The glucuronyl conjugate is polar and thus readily excreted in the urine and the bile. It is well-known that the cat cannot form glucuronides to a significant degree, so that this reaction will not occur in this species. In any event, phenytoin is little used in the cat because it is difficult to achieve a therapeutic effect without producing sedation. The drug also has a longer duration of action in the cat than in the dog and this is reflected in reported values of plasma half-life in the two species. In the kitten intravenous administration yielded a plasma half-life of 41·5 hours (Tobin *et al* 1973), while oral administration of phenytoin (10 mg/kg) to the adult cat gave a half-life of 24–108 hours (Roye *et al* 1973). The long half-life was attributed to an inability to hydroxylate the molecule. In the dog, on the other hand, a relatively high dose rate (50 mg/kg orally) gave a half-life of only 3 hours (Roye *et al* 1973). In an earlier study Dayton *et al* (1967) found the half-life of phenytoin to be 6·0–7·8 hours following a single dose of 50 mg/kg. Pretreatment of the animals with phenobarbitone decreased the half-life to 2·0–2·5 hours. This range is not only much less than the feline half-life but also below the very much wider range of 9–140 hours quoted for man (A. Richens, pers. comm.).

In the rat, hepatic biotransformation of phenytoin was reduced during pregnancy and the time for elimination of the drug was approximately doubled (Buchthal & Lennox-Buchthal 1972). It is not known whether a similar change occurs in the pregnant bitch.

Phenytoin is loosely bound to plasma protein, approximately one-fifth of the total concentration being present as free drug in man, the cat and the dog (Baggot & Davis 1973; Woodbury & Fingl 1975). This high level of binding limits the rate of filtration and hence urinary excretion of the drug. Excretion of the free drug is also limited by good tubular reabsorption, so that clearance by the kidney of the unmetabolised drug is slow. High protein binding also reduces passage of the drug into the CNS. The degree of plasma protein binding is reduced in young animals, in the presence of hypoalbuminaemia and in uraemic patients. In these circumstances the half-life of phenytoin is reduced so that higher doses are required to maintain adequate plasma concentrations.

Signs of acute phenytoin toxicity include ataxia, vertigo, dizziness, nausea, blurred vision, diplopia and nystagmus, but these effects are seen only at high dose rates and indicate that the dose should be reduced. The manufacturers' recommended procedures for treating acute overdosage include emptying of the stomach, provision of airway support, artificial respiration and the administration of oxygen and vasopressor drugs to combat the hypotensive and respiratory depressant effects of excessive doses.

Mild but persistent polyphagia, polydipsia and polyuria are produced by phenytoin (Kay & Fenner 1977). These effects may be related to the hyperglycaemia and glycosuria which have been described and which are probably due to inhibition of insulin secretion (Levin *et al* 1970). A number of additional side-effects, which may occur during initial treatment, include gastric distress, nausea, transient nervousness, weight loss, sleeplessness and unsteadiness. These effects generally diminish with continued use. Several types of allergic reaction have been reported, such as polyarthropathy, fever, hepatitis and skin eruptions. The latter condition usually subsides when therapy ceases. Nash *et al* (1977) described a fatal case of hepatitis in a dog which received phenytoin for 12 days. Death was preceded by refusal to eat, vomiting, loss of weight, dullness, muscular weakness and yellowing of the sclerae. The authors warn against continuing therapy with antiepileptic agents when signs of toxicity are apparent.

Other reported reactions include lupus erythematosus and erythema multiformae. A mild form of gingival hypertrophy is a common side-effect but generally this does not necessitate cessation of phenytoin therapy. High levels of phenytoin occur in saliva and this might be a factor in the genesis of this condition. Excessive motor activity has been encountered on occasions. Reported haematological disturbances include megaloblastic anaemia, leucopenia, agranulocytosis, thrombocytopenia, pancytopenia and aplastic anaemia. Megaloblastic anaemia seems to be caused by folic acid deficiency, which results from the antifolate activity of phenytoin and other antiepileptics (Reynolds 1973; Hawkins & Meynell 1958). Reduced folate absorption and altered folate metabolism may both be involved. Lymphadenopathy is a rare occurrence.

The uncertainties concerning the teratogenic effects of phenytoin in the human female was discussed earlier (see p. 268). It is of interest to note that fetal abnormalities have been produced in mice, but the relevance of this finding is questionable since high doses (150 mg/kg intraperitoneally) were required (Harbison & Becker 1969). It seems that the antivitamin D effect of phenytoin in man may also occur in animals since Villareale *et al* (1974) have reported hypocalcaemia, reduced duodenal transport of calcium and rickets in the chicken.

The wide range of side-effects that have been reported for phenytoin reflect the widespread use of the drug in animals and man for almost 40 years; they are placed in perspective when it is realised that toxicological studies in the dog, involving the administration of daily doses of 22–110 mg/kg body weight for periods of up to 6 months, have not involved weight loss and the animals have produced and nursed young without sign of physical and neurological disturbances (Gruhzit 1939). Cunningham (1971) also reports that the dog tolerates phenytoin well, and even minor side-effects are uncommon.

DIAZEPAM

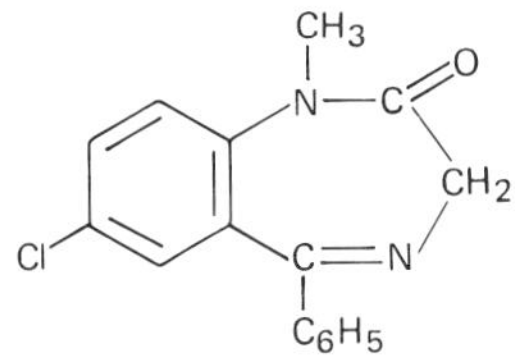

Diazepam

This is both the only benzodiazepine derivative and the only tranquilliser which has been used extensively to treat epilepsy in veterinary medicine. In fact, as Croft (1977) points out, most tranquillisers (e.g. phenothiazines and butyrophenones) are contraindicated in the treatment of primary epilepsy because seizures occur most commonly when animals are relaxed or asleep. Diazepam has been administered orally — very infrequently in the dog and somewhat more commonly in the cat — to control generalised seizure disorders (Kay & Fenner 1977). The main use of diazepam, however, has been in the treatment of *status epilepticus* and exacerbated seizure disorders, when it is given intravenously (Turner 1967; Averill 1970). Averill obtained a satisfactory response in twelve of fourteen dogs in *status epilepticus* with a single dose and in a further animal with three intravenous doses. His procedure is to inject 5·0 mg slowly, repeat this 1–2 minutes later if the *status epilepticus* continues, and administer pentobarbitone (7·5 mg/lb) slowly intravenously if the second dose is also ineffective. Kay and Fenner (1977) recommended the intravenous or intramuscular administration of 10–35 mg diazepam to dogs in *status epilepticus*, to be followed by phenobarbitone (60–120 mg intravenously or intramuscularly) if necessary. If these measures did not suffice, the induction of anaesthesia with minimal doses of a barbiturate or volatile agent was advised. Other agents recommended for intravenous injection were glucose in hypoglycaemic patients and calcium gluconate if hypocalcaemia was present.

The effectiveness of diazepam in *status epilepticus* is related to its rapid onset and short duration of action (explained by the high lipid solubility of diazepam, and hence rapid penetration of the blood-brain barrier), and to its sparing effects on cardiovascular and respiratory functions giving the drug a wide margin of safety. The respiratory and cardiovascular depressant actions of most general anaesthetics (including barbiturates), on the other hand, are likely to be poorly tolerated in patients that may already be unconscious and suffering sufficient hypoxia to cause cyanosis. The efficacy of diazepam may subside after 2–4 hours leading to a recurrence of *status epilepticus*, and the regime may have to be repeated several times. Animals that are unconscious after an attack of *status epilepticus* should receive appropriate intravenous fluid therapy (Kay & Fenner 1977). Finally, oral medication with standard antiepileptic drugs should commence as soon as the animal is able to swallow and the subject monitored for several days to check for the not unlikely possibility of a relapse. For *status epilepticus* in cats, diazepam (2–10 mg intravenously or intramuscularly) and phenobarbitone (5–60 mg intravenously or intramuscularly) have been used (Kay 1975). The recommended procedure is to administer the former drug, wait 10 minutes, and then inject phenobarbitone if necessary. If this also fails, pentobarbitone is administered carefully to induce anaesthesia.

The use of diazepam in cats in other forms of epilepsy may be considered if the animal has reacted unfavourably to phenobarbitone, the oral dose being 2–5 mg per animal two or three times daily (Kay 1975). A. T. Yoxall (pers. comm.) has also used diazepam in the cat. Unconscious animals are sometimes presented in a condition of tetanic opisthotonus of unknown aetiology. The state resembles *status epilepticus* clinically, but it is thought to have a toxic basis. Diazepam, administered intravenously at doses up to 10 mg, produces muscular relaxation and a sleep-like state which lasts for up to 24 hours. On recovering consciousness further treatment is usually unnecessary. The beneficial effects of diazepam were attributed by Yoxall to its sedative effect and to the muscular relaxation produced by action on internuncial neurones in the spinal cord, the latter allowing normal respiratory excursions to occur. Yoxall advises against intramuscular injections since they cause pain at the injection site.

As would be expected from its high lipid solubility, the absorption of diazepam following oral administration is rapid, the degree of binding to plasma protein is high, only small amounts are excreted unchanged in the urine and it is largely metabolised by hepatic microsomal enzymes. Several metabolites have been identified and a number, including the major metabolite in man (the *N*-demethyl derivative), are biologically active. A number of benzodiazepines, including diazepam, have been shown to induce hepatic microsomal enzymes but they are less effective in this regard than barbiturates.

16.2 Tranquillisers

16.2.1 Definitions and drugs

Tranquillisers are normally classified on the basis of their chemical structures into several groups (Table 16.3). There are many similarities but also important differences in the pharmacological properties of these groups (Table 16.4). There may also be significant differences in the actions and side-effects of compounds within a single group. In spite of the availability of so many compounds, the drugs that continue to be used most extensively in small animals are those belonging to the phenothiazine group. Some newer compounds, such as xylazine and the butyrophenone derivative azaperone, are now used extensively in farm animals, the former drug in the cow and the horse and the latter in the pig and the horse. It seems probable that xylazine and the butyrophenones will be used increasingly in small animal medicine. Indeed, there have been several recent reports of the use of xylazine in the dog and cat. The benzodiazepine group of tranquillisers are in widespread use as anxiolytic agents in man. They are used infrequently in veterinary medicine but an increasing number of reports describe indications for the best known member of this group, diazepam. Hence, the properties of this compound will also be reviewed briefly as will those of chloral hydrate. The latter is little used in small animals, but it is perhaps the best known 'classical sedative' in veterinary medicine. Chloral hydrate is a useful drug, therefore, against which newer sedatives and tranquillisers may be compared (Table 16.4). Drugs of minor importance are chlorprothixene, reserpine and meprobamate.

Westhues and Fritsch (1965) refer to tranquillisers (ataractics, neuroplegics) as central nervous system depressants which also depress excitability of the autonomic nervous system, dull consciousness and reduce spontaneous motor activity. Hall (1971) describes tranquillisers as drugs which produce both freedom from disturbance of mind and sedation without at the same time causing drowsiness. Other properties common to most tranquillisers are decreased motor activity, calming and quietening actions and the production of a pronounced taming effect in animals, which by virtue of their individual or species temperament, are naturally vicious.

Some authors have classified tranquillisers into two or three groups according to their potency: minor tranquillisers are said to include the benzodiazepines and some of the least potent phenothiazines; major tranquillisers are the butyrophenones and the more potent phenothiazines; and tranquillosedatives include dithiocarbonate derivatives such as meprobamate. The term neuroleptic is also in common usage, and is usually applied to major tranquillisers of the butyrophenone and phenothiazine groups. For purposes of describing drug actions in animals, these definitions are

Table 16.3 Chemical classification of sedatives and tranquillisers.

Group	Chemical structure	Drugs
Phenothiazines	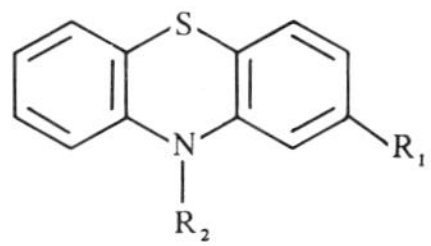	$R_2 = CH_2-CH_2-CH_2-N(CH_3)_2$ and R_1 =H promazine R_1 =Cl chlorpromazine $R_1 = COCH_3$ acepromazine
Thioxanthenes	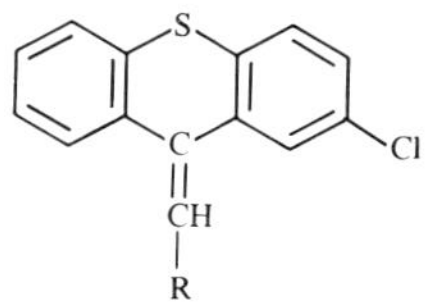	$R = CH_2-CH_2-N(CH_3)_2$ chlorprothixene
Butyrophenones	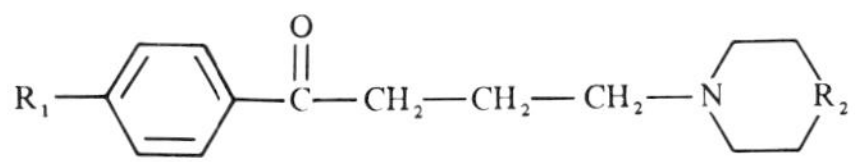	R_1 =F R_2 =N– 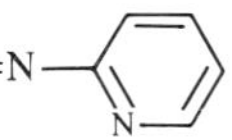 azaperone reserpine

Rauwolfia alkaloids	—	
Benzodiazepines	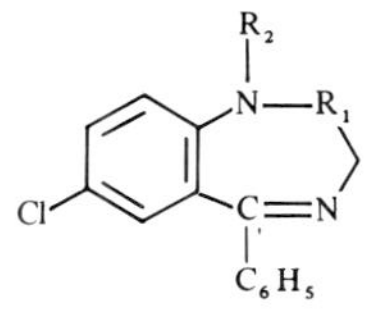	$R_1 = C{=}O$ $R_2 = CH_3$ diazepam
Propanediol carbamates	—	$H_2N{-}\overset{\overset{O}{\parallel}}{C}{-}OCH_2{-}\underset{\underset{CH_3}{\mid}}{\overset{\overset{C_3H_7}{\mid}}{C}}{-}CH_2O{-}\overset{\overset{O}{\parallel}}{C}{-}NH_2$ meprobamate
Xylazine	—	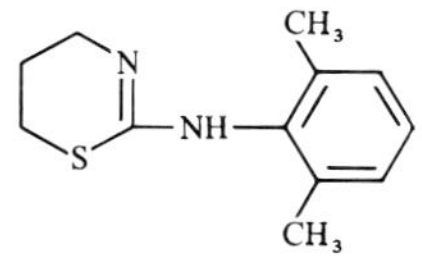

Table 16.4 Comparison of some properties of sedatives and tranquillisers (for comparison of other properties see text)

Property	Chloral hydrate	Diazepam	Xylazine	Acepromazine	Droperidol
Classification	Sedative-anaesthetic	Sedative-anaesthetic	Sedative-anaesthetic	Tranquilliser-sedative	Tranquilliser-sedative
Motor activity	Reduced	Reduced	Reduced	Reduced	Reduced
Body temperature	Reduced	Reduced	Reduced	Reduced	Reduced
Effect of high doses	Anaesthesia	Anaesthesia	Anaesthesia	Catalepsy	Catalepsy
Arousal reaction to sensory stimuli	Sluggish	Sluggish	Sluggish	Possibly normal or enhanced	Possibly normal or enhanced
Leptazol and strychnine-induced convulsions	Suppressed	Suppressed	Suppressed	Not suppressed	Not suppressed
α adrenoceptor blockade	No	No	No	Yes	Yes

unhelpful. Thus, promazine is often described as a minor tranquilliser, while acepromazine is regarded as a major tranquilliser. The latter is certainly more potent but the difference between the drugs does not involve qualitative differences in their actions; a large dose of promazine will exert essentially similar actions and side-effects as a small dose of acepromazine. Furthermore, Soma (1971) has pointed out that tranquilliser definitions which refer solely to states of mental calm and lack of confusion or to the suppression of initiative in humans not only oversimplify the actions of these drugs but are misleading in that they fail to describe the use to which the agents are put in veterinary medicine. This author defines the desired effect in animals as the production of sedation without marked ataxia. The dose levels used in man to achieve antipsychotic effects often produce little sedation, but the choice of drug and dosage employed in veterinary medicine are dictated by the ability of different agents to produce a tractable, sedated animal.

There are many accounts in textbooks of general and veterinary anaesthesia, pharmacology and therapeutics of the actions, fate in the body and uses of sedatives and tranquillisers. Little purpose would be served by repeating information which is already well documented. The present account will therefore be concerned primarily with emphasising both the differences that exist between the various groups of drugs, and those side-effects which are most likely to be deleterious in clinical subjects, as well as with the properties of some of the newer agents.

16.2.2 General properties of tranquillisers and sedatives

Although there are some significant differences in detail, the phenothiazines, butyrophenones, thioxanthenes and rauwolfia alkaloids possess generally similar pharmacological properties. Not only are the tranquillising and sedative actions of the drugs qualitatively alike, other actions often overlap in some degree as well. For example, they are not generally *acutely* toxic in normal animals, and the wide margin of safety as reflected by high therapeutic indices is attributable in all probability to at least two factors. First, high dose levels do not produce anaesthesia or even loss of consciousness but a state of catalepsy — the 'plastic limb' syndrome in which parts of the body may be moulded into unusual positions. Secondly, respiratory function is unchanged or only slightly depressed and there are even reports of respiratory stimulation when the drugs are given either alone or with narcotic-analgesics to produce the state of neuroleptanalgesia (Clarke 1969; Glen 1970). However, a high therapeutic index is not an indication for the indiscriminate use of these agents. The potentially serious cardiovascular side-effects of the phenothiazines and butyrophenones should not be overlooked.

In pharmacological tests phenothiazines, butyrophenones and reserpine depress conditioned reflexes but responses to non-conditioned stimuli are usually unimpaired. Thus, a laboratory rodent trained to recognise an impending punishing shock by the ringing of a bell will, under the influence of subcataleptic doses of a tranquilliser, ignore the warning signal *but* once the shock has been administered the animal may *then* respond. The equivalent situation in clinical practice may be the essentially normal arousal reaction that a sedated animal may show in response to some sensory stimulus. Indeed, the reaction may be exaggerated, so that an excitatory reaction may be seen in response to a mild pain, tactile, visual or noise stimulus.

The distinctive nature of the pharmacological actions of phenothiazine, butyrophenone and rauwolfia derivatives is emphasised when their properties are compared with those of a 'classical sedative' such as chloral hydrate. The latter is a less selective depressant of the CNS. Thus, high dose rates produce not the state of cataleptoid immobility described above but loss of consciousness and general anaesthesia. Respiration is depressed in direct proportion to the dose administered and respiratory failure will ensue with toxic doses. The therapeutic index of chloral hydrate is therefore much lower than that of the tranquillisers. In laboratory animals non-selective sedatives like chloral hydrate are likely to suppress non-conditioned as well as conditioned reflexes and the equivalent of this circumstance in the clinical subject is the more sluggish arousal reaction that is likely under the influence of chloral hydrate. Although non-selective agents like chloral hydrate may also exert effects on peripheral organs and tissues of the body, their action is usually non-specific, in contrast to the specific 'receptor-mediated' actions of phenothiazines and butyrophenones on, for example, the autonomic nervous system (see below). Thus, sedative-anaesthetic agents depress myocardial contractility by reason of their direct negative inotropic actions on the myocardium (see Chapter 10).

Xylazine and diazepam are two agents that have been used in cats and dogs with increasing frequency in recent years. Both have been described as tranquillisers, although xylazine is more commonly referred to as a sedative-analgesic-muscle relaxant drug. Both compounds have more in common with chloral hydrate than the phenothiazines, but their actions are by no means identical with those of the former drug (Table 16.4). Diazepam and xylazine possess centrally mediated muscle relaxant properties, and at high dose levels loss of consciousness and anaesthesia are produced. Indeed, intravenous diazepam is used as an induction agent in man (Baker 1969; Wyant & Studney 1970) and xylazine has been used as a hypnotic in veterinary medicine (see below). In addition, xylazine and diazepam are devoid of the specific effects of butyrophenones, phenothiazines and the rauwolfia alkaloids on the autonomic nervous system. Both drugs may be classified as general anticonvulsants suppressing convulsive seizures regardless of their cause. Phenothiazines, on the other hand, inhibit convulsions induced by certain CNS stimulants, such as nicotine and nikethamide, but not others, including strychnine, leptazol, cocaine and picrotoxin. The antiepileptic action of diazepam also contrasts with the seizure-inducing properties of phenothiazines in epileptic patients.

In view of these differences in the pharmacological actions of the drugs listed in Table 16.1, a classification into two broad groups would seem to be appropriate to their use in veterinary medicine. Chloral hydrate, diazepam, xylazine and meprobamate are grouped as sedative-anaesthetics, while the phenothiazines, thioxanthene, butyrophenones and rauwolfia alkaloids are classed as tranquilliser-sedatives.

Phenothiazines, butyrophenones and to some extent the rauwolfia alkaloids exert a variety of similar actions on peripheral organs and tissues of the body in addition to their selective effects on the CNS. These are exemplified by the multitudinous properties of the most studied phenothiazine tranquilliser, chlorpromazine. It was no mere chance that the trade name Largactil was coined for this drug. Chlorpromazine and, in varying degrees other phenothiazines, possess the following peripheral actions: antihistamine (H_1 receptor antagonist); anti-5-hydroxytryptamine; autonomic ganglion blockade; atropine-like parasympatholytic action; α adrenoceptor antagonism; inhibition of the noradrenaline reuptake process into the noradrenergic neurone (blockade of the $uptake_1$ process); quinidine-like anti-arrhythmic action on the heart (membrane stabilising, local anaesthetic action); spasmolytic action; at high dose levels inhibition of certain enzymes including cytochrome oxidase; antipruritic; anti-inflammatory; and anti-shock.

Some of these peripheral effects are of little clinical consequence, while others may be potentially harmful in either normal or poor risk cases, and yet other actions may be beneficial. These matters will be considered further in relation to the cardiovascular actions of phenothiazines (see below).

There is a good deal of compound to compound variation in the extent to which phenothiazines and butyrophenones possess these peripheral actions. Chlorpromazine is a weak antihistamine and ganglion blocking drug, but moderately potent both in its parasympatholytic action and as a 5HT receptor antagonist. It is also classified as a fairly potent α receptor antagonist. On the other hand, promethazine is a much more potent antihistamine than promazine and its derivatives, and pecazine, in contrast to most phenothiazines which are hypotensive, increases arterial blood pressure (Hall 1971). Moreover, certain phenothiazines possess potent antipsychotic effects but produce little or no sedation. Such drugs are particularly useful for long-term therapy of various psychotic states in man but have little use in veterinary medicine when the sedative action is generally the reason for use of the drug.

In addition to their peripheral effects, the phenothiazines exert other central actions as well as sedation, which may be either harmful or beneficial. For example, depression of the medullary chemoreceptor trigger zone accounts for the potent antiemetic property of phenothiazines when this zone is involved in the production of emesis. Thus, vomiting induced by many drugs, including morphine and ergot alkaloids, is suppressed but that arising from the action of cardiac glycosides and from emetics like copper sulphate which irritate the gastric mucosa is unaffected. There are reports of both depression and stimulation of anterior pituitary hormone secretion by phenothiazines, but such effects are probably of little consequence when the drugs are used on a single occasion. Of greater significance is their hypothermic action, particularly if they are used in cold environments. This is likely to be a greater problem in very small animals because of their high surface area:weight ratio and the consequently greater potential for heat loss from the surface of the body. Hypothermia is probably caused by one or more of the following actions: resetting of temperature regulating mechanisms in the hypothalamus for a lower body temperature; peripheral α adrenoceptor blockade leading to a reduction in vasomotor tone to arteriovenous anastomoses in the skin and hence to an increased blood flow to the surface of the skin; or a reduction in heat production arising from the decline in skeletal muscle activity. The first two factors are probably the more important.

16.2.3 Cardiovascular pharmacology of phenothiazines and butyrophenones

It is probable that antagonism of the action of the postganglionic sympathetic transmitter, noradrenaline, on arteriolar α receptors is the main cause of the hypotensive action of chlorpromazine. However, other actions of the drug may contribute to the fall in arterial blood pressure which usually occurs. The direct spasmolytic effect on vascular smooth muscle may lead to dilatation of arterioles, venules and veins; direct depression of the medullary vasomotor centre may reduce vasomotor outflow from the CNS; peripheral blockade of sympathetic ganglia may provide yet another means of diminishing vasomotor tone. In addition, a direct depressant action on the myocardium, and a dilatation of cutaneous blood vessels, as a result of alteration of thermoregulatory mechanisms in the hypothalamus in the direction of hypothermia, may also explain in part the cardiovascular depressant actions of chlorpromazine.

In general, the peripheral side-effects of promazine and acepromazine are qualitatively similar to those of chlorpromazine. The former drugs are, therefore, also hypotensive agents. In spite of this, the cardiovascular effects of phenothiazines are well tolerated in normovolaemic animals. On the other hand, patients in shock or otherwise hypovolaemic may suffer a precipitous and fatal decrease in arterial blood pressure. In these subjects the compensatory increase in the level of vasomotor tone, which maintains a head of blood pressure sufficient to maintain perfusion of the heart and brain, is reduced possibly to the extent that severe cerebral and myocardial hypoxia arise. In view of these considerations it may seem paradoxical that phenothiazine and butyrophenone tranquillisers and other α adrenoceptor antagonists have been recommended for the *treatment* of shock. The rationale underlying their use involves suppression of the tissue ischaemia and hypoxia resulting from intense peripheral vasoconstriction mediated by the sympathetic nervous system. However desirable this compensatory increase in vasomotor tone may be in tending to restore blood volume and maintain arterial blood pressure in the early stages of shock, as the condition persists the hypoxia of body organs and tissues will lead to cellular damage. Restoration of tissue perfusion with a vasodilator drug is therefore a reasonable therapeutic course of action.

The answer to the paradox lies in restoring circulating blood volume to normal levels or levels slightly above normal. In the absence of appropriate fluid therapy α receptor antagonists are likely to hasten the onset of death, whereas in its presence they will probably delay the onset of acute cardiovascular failure and may increase the chance of survival. The ability of phenothiazines and butyrophenones to provide some degree of protection in shocked patients may be related to their antihistamine, anti-5HT, ganglion blocking and spasmolytic properties but the principal mode of action is probably the prevention of tissue underperfusion by the α blocking effect on arterioles.

A further consequence of the α adrenoceptor blocking actions of phenothiazine and butyrophenone tranquillisers derives from their effect on the venous side of the circulation. Normally, some 40% of the blood volume is contained in the venous capacitance vessels, and the small veins, venules and venous sinuses contain a further 25%. The capacity of the venous reservoir may be reduced by activation of the sympathetic innervation to the vessels; the α receptor mediated constriction of these vessels which results from such activation diminishes the size of the reservoir and increases venous return to the heart. On the other hand, tranquilliser-mediated inhibition of venomotor tone will tend to promote peripheral pooling of blood and therefore lower venous return to the heart. Interference with reflex adjustments to the venous side of the circulation will generally be of little consequence in resting normal subjects. However, the mobilisation of blood in the venous reservoir which may accompany postural changes will be made less readily. (The use in man of α receptor antagonists, adrenergic neurone blocking drugs and ganglion blocking agents, all of which in different ways inhibit the effects of sympathetic nerves on the venous as well as the arterial side of the circulation, is associated with the side-effect of orthostatic hypotension.) This too may be a matter of relatively minor importance in normal animals but in hypovolaemic patients any tendency to promote the peripheral pooling of blood, and hence to reduce venous return, must have potentially serious consequences.

In addition to the direct circulatory effects of phenothiazines and butyrophenones which result from suppression of sympathetic tone to blood vessels, there are indirect reflex responses which also occur. For example, the reduction in arterial blood pressure acts reflexly through carotid and aortic baroreceptor mechanisms to increase heart rate and possibly cardiac output as well. However, hypotension may be long-lasting while the heart rate usually returns to or even falls below control levels within an hour, so that cardiovascular reflexes cannot account entirely for observed changes in cardiac function (Serrano & Lees 1976).

For those derivatives with significant atropine-like actions vagal blockade is a further cause of tachycardia, and the quinidine-like properties of some compounds may explain their known antiarrhythmic actions. On the other hand, the ability of phenothiazines and butyrophenones to prevent or to terminate catecholamine-induced ventricular dysrhythmias, which arise in the presence of 'sensitising' anaesthetic agents such as halothane, chloroform and cyclopropane, is probably attributable to their α adrenoceptor blocking properties. At first sight this may seem paradoxical because it is recognised that all important sympathetic effects on the heart, including the arrhythmogenic actions of catecholamines, are mediated by β adrenoceptors. However, it is also known that certain factors predispose towards catecholamine-anaesthetic arrhythmias. Such factors include the afterload on the heart (i.e. aortic blood pressure) and extracellular potassium concentration. When both of these are high, arrhythmias are more likely to occur. By preventing the rises in blood pressure and plasma potassium concentration which are caused by sympathomimetic amines with α receptor stimulant actions, phenothiazine and butyrophenone tranquillisers can antagonise such arrhythmias as ventricular extrasystoles, bigeminal rhythm and ventricular tachycardia (see also Chapter 10).

A further action of phenothiazine and butyrophenone derivatives that has been well documented is the decrease in packed cell volume and the associated fall in red blood cell count which follows parenteral administration of these agents. This may arise from two actions of the drugs. First, by dilating precapillary vessels (arterioles) relatively less than postcapillary vessels (venules) the capillary hydrostatic pressure will decrease (Fig. 16.2). This will lead to a net transfer of fluid from the interstitial space into the circulation causing haemodilution. In consequence, packed cell volume and plasma protein concentration will decrease. In fact, phenothiazines and butyrophenones do not always reduce plasma protein concentration (Serrano 1974), and the fall in packed cell volume is almost invariably greater than any change in plasma protein levels. From this it seems likely that the second mechanism is a more important cause of the fall in packed cell volume than haemodilution. The second possibility is the uptake of erythrocytes into the splenic reservoir, an action which probably results from inhibition of sympathetic tone to trabecular and capsular muscle of the spleen and a consequent increase in splenic volume (Lees & Serrano 1976). The proposed reduction in sympathetic tone to the spleen could derive from both peripheral and central actions of tranquillisers. However, there is some doubt concerning the validity of the hypothesis since Shepherd (1968) has claimed that there is little or no tonic sympathetic discharge to the capsule of the spleen.

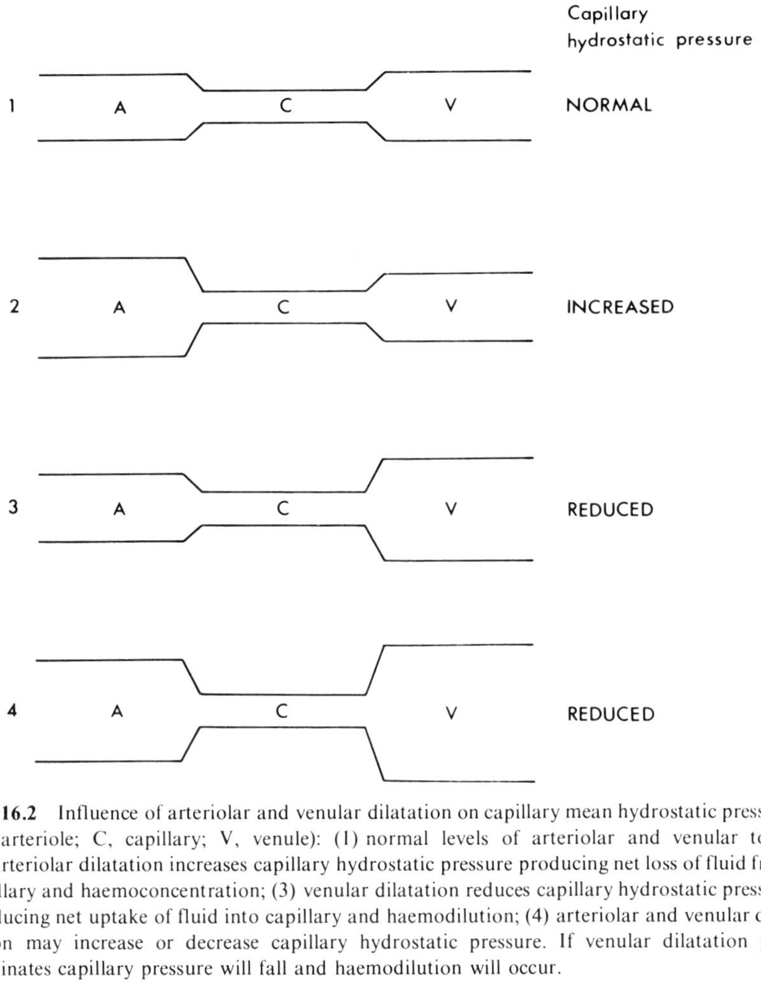

Fig. 16.2 Influence of arteriolar and venular dilatation on capillary mean hydrostatic pressure (A, arteriole; C, capillary; V, venule): (1) normal levels of arteriolar and venular tone; (2) arteriolar dilatation increases capillary hydrostatic pressure producing net loss of fluid from capillary and haemoconcentration; (3) venular dilatation reduces capillary hydrostatic pressure producing net uptake of fluid into capillary and haemodilution; (4) arteriolar and venular dilatation may increase or decrease capillary hydrostatic pressure. If venular dilatation predominates capillary pressure will fall and haemodilution will occur.

There is no reason to believe that the reduced oxygen carrying capacity of blood, which derives from the fall in packed cell volume, presents a serious threat to the healthy subject. However, this may not be so in poor risk patients and, in particular, in animals that are anaemic from any cause. In such cases, special care may be required in using phenothiazines or butyrophenones.

The membrane stabilising and quinidine-like actions of phenothiazine tranquillisers are well documented and may explain in part their anti-arrhythmic actions. However, phenothiazines may also be the *cause* of disturbances of cardiac rhythm if circulating blood levels of the agents are high. This occurs following intravenous administration and most particularly when the injection is given rapidly. Pugh (pers. comm.) has investigated the electrocardiographic changes occurring in dogs following the intravenous administration of clinical dose levels of the phenothiazines, promazine and chlorpromazine, and the thioxanthene derivative, chlorprothixene. With all agents, phases of excitement were a common occurrence. Excitement was associated with tachycardia, T-wave inversion and increased amplitude of the T-wave. The T-wave changes were probably related to the accompanying hyperkalaemia. More seriously, Pugh also recorded a number of rhythm disturbances. Sinus arrhythmia and sinus arrest were sometimes noted and biphasic P-waves, which may have resulted from a wandering pacemaker, occurred. Atrial flutter and premature ventricular beats were observed occasionally, while first and second degree atrioventricular block occurred more frequently. It seems possible that the occasional collapse which follows rapid intravenous injection of phenothiazines could sometimes be due to atrioventricular block and a resultant temporary cessation of left ventricular output (an alternative suggestion is that orthostatic hypotension limits cerebral blood flow). It would seem to be a wise precaution to administer the drugs slowly when the intravenous route is selected, thereby avoiding exposure of the heart to excessive concentrations.

16.2.4 Clinical pharmacology and therapeutic use of tranquillisers

PHENOTHIAZINES

Since their introduction into veterinary medicine in the 1950s, the phenothiazine tranquillisers have held pride of place as the drugs of choice for a variety of purposes, most of which utilise the sedative or 'chemical restraining' properties of the drugs rather than their ataractic effects.

Many compounds are available and although differences in potency and hence therapeutic dosage may be large, equi-effective doses of the commonly employed agents generally produce similar actions. Maximal doses of promazine, chlorpromazine and acepromazine recommended for parenteral administration in the dog are 1·0, 1·0 and 0·2 mg/kg, respectively (Hall 1971). Unfortunately, however, it is not possible to recommend a precise dose rate to suit all animals and circumstances, a significant disadvantage of all phenothiazines being the wide animal to animal variation in the level of sedation achieved with a given dose rate. Moreover, increasing the administered dose does not guarantee that a greater sedative effect will be produced. It would seem rather that an optimal effect is attained at a certain dose rate and that higher doses fail to produce greater sedation, although the onset of action may be more rapid and the duration of effect prolonged. Intravenous and intramuscular routes of admistration are both recommended. The full sedative effects of the drugs are not obtained until 60–90 minutes with the latter route and until 10–15 minutes with the former.

Phenothiazines are used extensively in small animal medicine. They are of particular value when a minimal level of chemical restraint is needed to facilitate handling for diagnostic and other purposes and to minimise the stress of transportation. They are also used with other classes of drug: with analgesics in the technique of neuroleptanalgesia, with local anaesthetics to facilitate minor surgery, particularly in animals regarded as poor risks for general anaesthesia, and as premedicants. It should be noted that potentiation of the actions of induction and general anaesthetic agents by phenothiazines permits reduction in the dose level of the latter drugs. For example, barbiturate dosages are normally reduced by approximately one-third to one-half. The advantages of phenothiazine premedication include the production of a sedated, tractable patient for induction of anaesthesia and minimal excitement and emesis during recovery, although the duration of recovery is usually prolonged. The antiemetic action of phenothiazines is also of value in bitches with pyometra and, more generally, for the prevention of motion sickness. Phenothiazines have been used to alleviate the symptoms of a variety of psychoneurotic conditions in animals; restlessness and noisiness may decrease, while eating, drinking and sleep patterns may be restored to normal (Pugh, pers. comm.). However, as will be discussed later, diazepam may be a more useful agent for these cases. Small animal skin diseases associated with pruritis may benefit from phenothiazine medication. Their action in causing disinclination to interfere with affected sites indirectly assists the healing actions of other primary agents. In addition, the antihistaminic actions of some phenothiazines may contribute to their antipruritic effects.

CHLORPROTHIXENE

This thioxanthene derivative is chemically very similar to chlorpromazine (Table 16.3), and it seems to resemble the latter drug in most of its actions and side-effects. Thus, it has been used as an antipsychotic agent in man, and in addition to its sedative action it is hypotensive and on prolonged administration it produces extrapyramidal effects.

Chlorprothixene has not been used extensively in cats or dogs. Sumner-Smith (1962) advocated the use of doses of 1–2 mg/lb by intravenous or intramuscular injection for the management of intractable dogs and for premedication in this species.

BUTYROPHENONES

In their mode of action, general pharmacological properties and side-effects the butyrophenone tranquillisers are similar to the phenothiazines (Marsboom 1971). Although butyrophenones have not been used extensively in small animals to date, there is no inherent reason why some of them should not prove to be at least as useful as phenothiazines. At this time the three most commonly used drugs in veterinary medicine are azaperone, droperidol and fluanisone, but the former is used only in the pig and the horse (Clarke 1969; Lees & Serrano 1976), while droperidol and fluanisone are used in the dog. They are not usually used alone, however. Both are administered in combination with a potent analgesic agent such as fentanyl to produce the state of neuroleptanalgesia, the droperidol mixture being used in America and the fluanisone combination in Great Britain. (A third combination, comprising the phenothiazine derivative methotrimeprazine and the potent analgesic etorphine, is also available in Great Britain.) Detailed consideration of the state of neuroleptanalgesia is outside the scope of this account but brief comment will be made of the claimed advantages for using analgesics and tranquillisers in combination. These are, summation of the individual depressant actions of each drug on the CNS; enhancement of the analgesic action by the tranquilliser; inhibition by the tranquilliser of the respiratory depressant action of the analgesic; inhibition of the emetic action of the analgesic by the tranquilliser; and, for tranquillisers with significant parasympatholytic actions, suppression of the effects of vagal stimulation which result from the action of the analgesic on the vagal centre in the medulla. It is by no means certain that all of the claimed advantages are justified and there are, moreover, a number of side-effects associated with neuroleptanalgesic drug combinations (Glen 1971; Hall 1971).

The use of droperidol alone in the dog, at tranquillising dose levels, has been associated with bizarre behavioural effects and general depression, which may persist for up to four days (A. T. Yoxall, pers. comm.).

RAUWOLFIA ALKALOIDS

This group of tranquillisers is included solely for the sake of completion, since they are little used in veterinary medicine. Reserpine, which is the principal active substance in extracts of the Indian shrub *Rauwolfia serpentina*, is the best known substance in this group. Although effective as a tranquilliser, its slow onset, long duration of action and toxicity have greatly limited its clinical usefulness. Booth (1977) and Earl (1956) have given detailed descriptions of the many actions of reserpine on several physiological systems, including central and peripheral nervous systems, and circulatory, respiratory, thermoregulatory, ocular, gastrointestinal, endocrinological and reproductive functions.

Reserpine resembles the phenothiazine tranquillisers in its sedative actions. As with phenothiazines a cataleptic response (muscle tremors, rigidity and akinesia) may result, particularly at high dose rates or following chronic administration. It is unsuitable for use as a premedicant because of its slow onset of action (peak effect is attained some two hours after intravenous administration), and subjects receiving long-term reserpine treatment may suffer severe bradycardia and hypotension when general anaesthetics are administered. The limited clinical veterinary uses include chronic sedation of the dog and cat, and as a feed additive to prevent aortic rupture by its antihypertensive action in rapidly growing turkeys (Booth 1977; Earl 1956).

MEPROBAMATE

In human medicine the propanediol derivative, meprobamate, has been classed as a minor tranquilliser. Since it is only sparingly soluble in water, it cannot be given parenterally, administration being confined to the oral route. In addition to its sedative actions, meprobamate possesses central muscle relaxant properties. This mephenesin-like action involves an inhibitory effect at internuncial neurones in the spinal cord to produce relaxation of skeletal muscle without affecting autonomic nervous functions. At high dose levels flaccid muscular paralysis occurs, while heart and respiratory rates are seemingly unchanged (Berger 1954). However, high doses also produce loss of consciousness and anaesthesia, so that meprobamate is not simply equivalent in its actions to the more specific centrally acting muscle relaxants, mephenesin and guaicol glycerol ether. It is somewhat closer in its actions to sedative-anaesthetic agents, such as chloral hydrate. Meprobamate is also distinguished from phenothiazine tranquillisers in possessing general anticonvulsant properties, in failing to produce extrapyramidal effects and in having little or no antipsychotic effects in man.

Booth (1977) recommends oral doses of 100–400 mg, 2–4 times daily as a general sedative in the dog. However, it is not in widespread use.

XYLAZINE

The general pharmacological actions of xylazine are said to include sedation, muscular relaxation and analgesia (Sagner *et al* 1969), although reports of the analgesic potency of the drug are conflicting. Thus, in one study an anaesthetic dose of xylazine (7·7 mg/kg) failed to abolish the response to painful stimuli in 73% of cats (Arbeiter *et al* 1972). Booth (1977) reports that the analgesic effect is pronounced over the head, neck and body but minimal in the extremities.

Xylazine differs from phenothiazine tranquillisers in that it does not seem to cause symptoms of excitement in a small proportion of animals. Moreover, the arousal reaction provoked by sensory stimulation is less likely to be associated with undue excitement with xylazine than with the phenothiazines. However, it has been suggested that animals may be particularly sensitive to noise during recovery from the actions of xylazine. It can be administered intravenously, subcutaneously or intramuscularly in small volumes without apparently producing tissue irritation or other serious adverse effects.

Although the principal use of xylazine to date has been in the chemical restraint of cattle, horses and game animals, there have been several reports of its use in small animals. For example, Amend and Klavano (1973), Haskins *et al* (1975), Moye *et al* (1963) and Müller *et al* (1969) have used xylazine in cats whilst Arbeiter *et al* (1972) have used the drug in both cats and dogs and found it to be a satisfactory sedative and analgesic agent. Müller *et al* (1969) administered xylazine subcutaneously to cats at a dose rate of 2–3 mg/kg. An excellent sedative effect was obtained in more than 200 subjects. Particular advantages were the reliability of the sedative response and its rapid onset of action. The side-effects in dogs and cats are retching, vomiting, defaecation and urination, all of which occur frequently. The time to onset of action in these species is 3–5 minutes after intravenous injection and 10–15 minutes after intramuscular or subcutaneous injection, the sedative state lasting for 1–2 hours and complete recovery occurs within 4 hours (Newkirk & Miles 1974).

Amend *et al* (1972) used xylazine to eliminate the muscular hypertonicity produced by ketamine in cats and several authors have subsequently used these two agents together. For example, Haufman (1976) used xylazine in combination with ketamine at dose rates of 3 and 15 mg/kg, respectively, by either the intravenous or intramuscular route to produce anaesthesia in both dogs and cats. Müller (1976) administered xylazine (1 mg/kg) subcutaneously to dogs 15 minutes before inducing anaesthesia with ketamine. More recently, Cullen and Jones (1977) have described their clinical experiences in the cat with xylazine (1·1 mg/kg intramuscularly) as a premedicant to ketamine (22 mg/kg intramuscularly). In this study xylazine produced a satisfactory sedative effect in all except three animals in a series of 100, and the subsequent period of ketamine anaesthesia lasted for at least 30 minutes. Premedication with atropine was considered to be mandatory for the prevention of ketamine-induced salivation and xylazine-induced bradycardia. The only undesirable effect of this drug combination was considered to be the vomiting which occurred in one-third of the cats. Green (pers. comm.) has noted that full recovery from xylazine/ketamine combinations may take 8–12 hours.

Other reports, for example Müller *et al* (1969), have established that xylazine is compatible with barbiturates and several volatile and gaseous anaesthetics in the cat. However, Haskins *et al* (1975) suggest that extreme caution should be exercised when xylazine is administered before thiamylal because the two drugs act synergistically, and Booth (1977) recommends reduction of the dose rate of barbiturates by one-half for both dog and cat. Xylazine may also be used in combination with narcotic-analgesics in the dog. Green (pers. comm.) has administered pethidine (10 mg/kg) and xylazine (2 mg/kg) intramuscularly to produce a period of neuroleptanalgesia lasting for up to 2 hours. This author has also used a xylazine (1–2 mg/kg) pethidine (2 mg/kg) mixture in the cat for superficial surgery and manipulative procedures.

In cattle, xylazine causes uterine contraction if administered at any time during gestation. This does not appear to be a problem except in the final month of pregnancy when premature birth may occur (Ahlers *et al* 1969). Similar difficulties could presumably also arise in the dog and cat, but they do not seem to have been described to date.

The cardiovascular effects of xylazine have been attributed to 'an initial peripheral sympathomimetic action with a subsequent nicotine-like blockade of transmitter release in both adrenergic and cholinergic autonomic nerve endings' (Haskins *et al* 1975). The latter authors administered xylazine intramuscularly to cats at a dose rate of 4·4 mg/kg and recorded a rise in systolic blood pressure within 1 minute and this persisted for 60 minutes. An immediate bradycardia also occurred and this lasted for at least 100 minutes. The average percentages increase in blood pressure and decrease in heart rate were 31 and 49, respectively. In one cat the heart rate fell to 45 beats/minute. The mean increase in central venous pressure was 9 cmH_2O. Haskins *et al* (1975) suggested that this response might be attributable either to sympathetically mediated constriction of venous capacitance vessels or to decreased myocardial contractility. The latter explanation would seem to be more likely. From these findings it is clear that xylazine is by no means free of side-effects on the feline cardiovascular system. Although Haskins and coworkers used an anaesthetic dose of xylazine, sedative dose levels have produced essentially similar changes (Müller *et al* 1969). Xylazine also modifies cardiac function in the dog; bradycardia, irregular heart rate, A-V dissociation and occasional systolic murmurs have been reported (Green, pers. comm.; Haskins *et al* 1975).

DIAZEPAM

The use of this drug in the treatment of epilepsy was considered earlier. Other veterinary uses include the treatment of anxiety in the dog and cat and for sedation of these species (Booth 1977). Yoxall (pers. comm.) has employed oral diazepam therapy (up to 5 mg per animal per day) over several weeks to combat manifestations of undesirable behaviour, such as fighting and hysterical barking. Howling, compulsive restlessness and other behavioural reactions, which may be precipitated by an emotional event in the life of highly sensitive animals, are also controlled by diazepam and the low dose rates required do not produce gross sedation. The absence of behavioural symptoms often persists when diazepam therapy is terminated. In contrast, phenothiazine tranquillisers are much less useful in these subjects. In spite of their sedative actions they commonly increase the levels of excitement in behavioural disorders.

Martin (1976) has used intravenous doses of 1 or 2 mg diazepam per animal in the dog in combination with the induction agent propanidid, while Müller (1976) injected diazepam intramuscularly in dogs at a dose rate of 0.6 mg/kg 15 minutes before inducing anaesthesia with ketamine. Diazepam has also been administered intravenously at a dose rate of 0·25 mg/lb body weight to abolish ketamine-induced convulsive seizure in the cat (Reid & Frank 1972). In addition, it prevents the excitatory response which sometimes follows the administration of ketamine to miniature swine (Green, pers. comm.). From these reports it would seem that the potential usefulness of benzodiazepine/dissociative anaesthetic combinations, such as diazepam and ketamine, for producing chemical restraint warrants further study. A second combination (tiletamine and zolazepam) has been introduced and assessed in several species with promising results (Green, pers. comm.).

An additional use for diazepam was reported recently by Hall (1976). The occasional need for maintaining sedation in the dog for prolonged periods (2 or more days) was met by the administration of morphine and diazepam. After the appropriate treatment under general anaesthesia, the animal receives 2–10 mg morphine intramuscularly, further doses being given at 6-hourly intervals. Evidence of returning consciousness (indicated by restlessness) is treated by administering diazepam intravenously at a dose rate which restores immobility. The maximal amount given is 5 mg/kg/hour. Hall also stresses the importance of other forms of medication including fluid therapy in these patients.

Yoxall (pers. comm.) has used diazepam postoperatively in dogs. The sedative action of the drug is often useful after major operations. Moreover, it also prevents animals from interfering with their wounds. Similarly, it is a very useful ancillary agent for the treatment of dogs with granulomatous lesions induced by constant licking of an initially small lesion. The primary treatment with corticosteroid and local analgesic creams under an occlusive dressing is facilitated by the action of diazepam which prevents the animal worrying about its condition (Yoxall, pers. comm.).

In contrast to these favourable reports of the actions of diazepam in the dog, are the findings of McKenzie (pers. comm.). She administered diazepam intravenously to four Greyhounds at a dose rate of 2 mg/kg and in three of the animals observed a lack of tranquillisation, marked ataxia and violent struggling which lasted for 2 hours. The dose level used by McKenzie was less than the maximum intravenous dose recommended by Hall (1976) but greater than those used by Martin (1976) and Reid and Frank (1972).

References

Ahlers D., Frerking H. & Treu H. (1969) Trial with the new anaesthetic Rompun in gynaecology and surgery of the udder in cattle. *Vet. Med. Rev.* **2**, 142.

Amend J. F., Klavano P. A. & Stone E. C. (1972) Premedication with xylazine to eliminate muscular hypertonicity in cats during ketamine anesthesia. *Vet. Med. Small Anim. Clin.* **67**, 1305.

Amend J. F. & Klavano P. A. (1973) Xylazine a new sedative-analgesic with predictable emetic properties in the cat. *Vet. Med. Small Anim. Clin.* **68**, 741.

Arbeiter K., Szekely H. & Lovin D. (1972) Results of a 5-year trial of Bay-Va 1470 (Rompun) in the dog and cat. *Vet. Med. Rev.* **3**, 248.

Averill D. R. (1970) Treatment of *Status Epilepticus* in dogs with diazepam sodium. *J. Amer. Vet. Med. Assoc.* **156**, 432.

Baggot J. D. & Davis L. E. (1973) Comparative study of plasma protein binding of diphenylhydantoin. *Comp. Gen. Pharmacol.* **4**, 399.

Baker A. B. (1969) Induction of anaesthesia with diazepam. *Anaesthesia* **24**, 388.

Berger F. M. (1954) The pharmacological properties of 2-methyl-2-n-propyl-1,3-propanediol dicarbamate (Miltown), a new interneuronal blocking agent. *J. Pharmacol. Exp. Ther.*, **112**, 413.

Bogan J. & Smith M. (1968) The relation between primidone and phenobarbitone blood levels. *J. Pharm. Pharmac.* **20**, 64.

Booth, N. H. (1977) Hypnotics, sedatives and anticonvulsants. In *Veterinary Pharmacology and Therapeutics.* 4th edn., eds. L. M. Jones, N. H. Booth & L. E. McDonald, pp. 307–317. Ames, Iowa State University Press.

Buchthal F. & Lennox-Buchthal M. A. (1972) Diphenylhydantoin: relationship of anticonvulsant effect to concentration in serum. In *Anti-epileptic Drugs*, eds. D. Woodbury, K. Penry & R. Schmidt, pp. 169–180, Raven Press, New York.

Butler T. C. (1956) The metabolic hydroxylation of phenobarbital. *J. Pharmac. Exp. Ther.*, **116**, 326.

Butler T. C. (1957) The metabolic conversion of 5:5-diphenylhydantoin to 5-(p-hydroxyphenyl)-5-phenylhydantoin. *J. Pharmacol. Exp. Ther.* **119**, 1.

Butler T. C., Waddell W. J. & Poole D. T. (1965) Demethylation of trimethadione and metharbital by rat liver microsomal enzymes: substrate-concentration-yield relationships and competition between substrates. *Biochem. Pharmac.* **14**, 937.

Christiansen C. Rodbro P. & Kristensen, M. (1973) Effect of Vitamin D on bone mineral mass in normal subjects and in epileptic patients on anticonvulsants: a controlled therapeutic trial. *Brit. Med. J.* **2**, 208.

Clark K. W. (1969) Effect of azaperone on the blood pressure and pulmonary ventilation in pigs. *Vet. Rec.* **85**, 649.

Clemmensen J., Fugkong-Frederikse V. & Plum C. M. (1974) Are anticonvulsants oncogenic? *Lancet* i, 707.

Conney A. H. & Burns J. J. (1972) Metabolic interactions among environmental chemicals and drugs. *Science* **178**, 576.

Croft, P. G. (1977) Treatment of epilepsy in the working dog. *Vet. Rec.* **101**, 394.

Cullen L. K. & Jones R. S. (1977) Clinical observations on xylazine/ketamine anaesthesia in the cat. *Vet. Rec.* **101**, 115.

Cunningham J. G. (1971) Canine seizure disorders. *J. Amer. Vet. Med. Assoc.* **158**, 589.

Dayton P. G., Cucinell S. A., Weiss M. & Perel J. H. (1967) Dose dependence of drug plasma level decline in dogs. *J. Pharmacol. Exp. Ther.* **158**, 305.

Dent C. E., Richens A., Rowe D. J. E. & Stamp T. C. B. (1970) Osteomalacia with long-term anticonvulsant therapy in epilepsy. *Brit. Med. J.* **4**, 69.

Dill W. A., Kazenko A., Wolf L. M. & Glazko A. J. (1956) Studies on 5,5-diphenylhydantoin (Dilantin) in animals and man. *J. Pharmac. Exp. Ther.* **118**, 270.

Eadie M. J. & Tyrer J. H. (1974) *Anticonvulsant Therapy. Pharmacological basis and practice.* Churchill Livingstone, Edinburgh.

Earl A. E. (1956) Reserpine (Serpasil) in veterinary practice. *J. Amer. Vet. Med. Assoc.* **129**, 227.

Fredrick J. (1973) Epilepsy and pregnancy: a report from the Oxford Record Linkage Study. *Brit. Med. J.* **2**, 442.

Glen J. B. (1970) Neuroleptanalgesia with 'Thalamonal Vet' in the dog. *Proc. Ass. Vet. Anaes.* **1** 38.

Gruhzit O. M. (1939) Sodium diphenylhydantoinate. Pharmacologic and histopathological studies. *Arch. Path.* **28**, 761.

Hall L. W. (1971) *Wright's Veterinary Anaesthesia and Analgesia*. 7th edn. Bailliere Tindall, London.

Hall L. W. (1976) Prolonged anaesthesia. *J. Small Anim. Pract.* **17**, 661.

Handley R. & Stewart A. S. R. (1952) Mysoline: a new drug in the treatment of epilepsy. *Lancet* i, 742.

Hansen J. M. (1966) Dicoumarol-induced diphenylhydantoin intoxication. *Lancet* ii, 265.

Harbison R. D. & Becker B. A. (1969) Relation of dosage and time of administration of diphenylhydantoin to its teratogenic effects in mice. *Teratology* **2**, 305.

Haskins S. C., Peiffer R. L. & Stowe C. M. (1975) A clinical comparison of CT 1341, ketamine and xylazine in cats. *Amer. J. Vet. Res.* **36**, 1537.

Haufman P. (1976) Anaesthesia of the dog and cat with a combination of ketamine and xylazine. *Animal de Compagnie* **11**, 361.

Hawkins C. F. & Meynell M. J. (1958) Macrocytosis and macrocytic anaemia caused by anti-convulsant drugs. *Quart. J. Med.* **27**, 45.

Higgins G. (1977) Treatment of epilepsy in the working dog. *Vet. Rec.* **101**, 335.

Jeavons P. M. (1977) Choice of drug therapy in epilepsy. *The Practitioner* **219**, 542.

Kay W. J. (1975) Epilepsy in cats. *J. Amer. Anim. Hosp. Assoc.* **11**, 77.

Kay W. J. & Fenner, W. R. (1977) Epilepsy. In *Current Veterinary Therapy VI. Small Animal Practice*, ed. W. B. Kirk, pp. 853–867. W. B. Saunders, Philadelphia.

Kirk R. W. (1977) *Current Veterinary Therapy VI. Small Animal Practice.* pp. 1380–1381. W. B. Saunders, Philadelphia.

Kohler H. G. (1966) Haemorrhage in the newborn of epileptic mothers. *Lancet* i, 267.

Kuntzmann R. (1969) Drugs and enzyme induction. *Ann. Rev. Pharmacol.* **9**, 21.

Kutt H. (1971) Biochemical and genetic factors regulating Dilantin metabolism in man. *Ann. N.Y. Acad. Sci.* **179**, 704.

Laidlaw J. & Richens A. (1976) *A Textbook of Epilepsy.* Churchill Livingstone, Edinburgh.

Laughman P. M., Gold H. & Vance J. C. (1973) Phenytoin teratogenicity in man. *Lancet* i, 70.

Lees P. & Serrano L. (1976) Effects of azaperone on cardiovascular and respiratory functions in the horse. *Brit. J. Pharmacol.* **56**, 263.

Lefebvre E. B., Haining R. G. & Lanne J. (1972) Coarse faces, calvarial thickening and hyperphosphatasia associated with long-term anticonvulsant therapy. *New Eng. J. Med.* **286**, 1301.

Levin S. R., Booker J. Jr., Smith D. F. & Grodsky G. M. (1970) Inhibition of insulin secretion by diphenylhydantoin in the isolated perfused pancreas. *J. Clin. Endocr. Metab.* **300**, 400.

Lowe C. R. (1963) Congenital malformations among infants born to epileptic women. *Lancet* i, 9.

Mahn T. J., Hendin B. A., Scharp C. R. & Haddad J. G. (1972) Effect of chronic anti-convulsant therapy on serum 25-hydroxy-calciferol levels in adults. *New Engl. J. Med.* **287**, 900.

Marsboom R. (1971) The development and pharmacology of butyrophenones. *Proc. Ass. Vet. Anaes.* **2**, 81.

Martin H. (1976) Anaesthesia in the dog: combined use of diazepam and propanidid for short operations. *Kleinter Praxis* **21**, 219.

Maynert, E. W. (1960) The metabolic fate of diphenylhydantoin in the dog, rat and man. *J. Pharm. Exp. Ther.* **130**, 275.

Merritt H. H. & Putnam T. J. (1938) Sodium diphenylhydantoin in the treatment of convulsive disorders. *J. Amer. Med. Assoc.* **111**, 1038.

Monson R. R., Rosenberg L., Hartz S. C., Shapiro S., Heinonen O. P. & Slone D. (1973) Diphenylhydantoin and selected congenital malformations. *New Eng. J. Med.* **289**, 1049.

Mountain K. R., Hirsch J. & Gallus A. S. (1970) Neonatal coagulation defect due to anti-convulsant drug treatment in pregnancy. *Lancet* i, 265.

Moye R. J., Pailet A. & Smith M. W. (1973) Clinical use of Xylazine in Dogs and Cats. *Vet. Med. Small Anim. Clin.* **68**, 236.

Müller R. (1976) Anaesthesia of dogs with ketamine-xylazine diazepam with special reference to the effect on respiration and blood circulation. *Inaugural Dissertation, Fachbereich Tiermedizin*, München.

Muller A., Weibel K. & Furukawa R. (1969) Rompun as a sedative in cats. *Berliner Muenchener tierarzt. Woch.* **82**, 396.

Nash A. S., Thompson H. & Bogan J. A. (1977) Phenytoin toxicity: A fatal case in a dog with hepatitis and jaundice. *Vet. Rec.* **100**, 280.

Newkirk H. L. & Miles P. G. (1974) Xylazine as a sedative-analgesic for dogs and cats. *Mod. Vet. Pract.* **55**, 677.

Oliver J. E. Jr. & Hoerlein B. F. (1965) Convulsive disorders of dogs. *J. Amer. Vet. Med. Assoc.* **146**, 1126.

Parker A. J. (1973) Epilepsy in the dog. Causes classification and diagnosis. *Illinois Vet.* **16**, 5.

Pashayan N., Pruzansky D. & Pruzansky S. (1971) Are anticonvulsants teratogenic? *Lancet* ii, 702.

Pasten L. J. (1977) Diphenylhydantoin in the canine: clinical aspects and determination of therapeutic blood levels. *J. Amer. Anim. Hosp. Assoc.* **13**, 247.

Penttila O. (1974) Interaction between doxycycline and some antiepileptic drugs. *Brit. Med. J.* **2**, 470.

Redding R. W. (1969) The diagnosis and therapy of seizures. *J. Amer. Anim. Hosp. Assoc.* **5**, 79.

Reid J. S. & Frank R. J. (1972) Prevention of undesirable side reactions of ketamine anaesthesia in cats. *J. Amer. Anim. Hosp. Assoc.* **8**, 115.

Reynolds E. H. (1973) Anticonvulsants, folic acid and epilepsy. *Lancet* i, 1376.

Roye D. B., Serrano E. E., Hammer R. M. & Wilder B. J. (1973) Plasma kinetics of diphenylhydantoin in dogs and cats. *Amer. J. Vet. Res.* **34**, 947.

Sagner G., Hoffmeister F. & Kroneberg G. (1969) Pharmacological principles of a new preparation for analgesia, sedation and relaxation in veterinary medicine (Bay Va 1470). *Vet. Med. Rev.* **3**, 226.

Serrano L. (1974) *Investigations of the actions of some centrally active drugs on cardiovascular, respiratory and metabolic functions in the horse.* PhD Thesis, University of London.

Serrano L. & Lees P. (1976) The applied pharmacology of azaperone in ponies. *Res. Vet. Sci.* **20**, 316.

Shapiro S., Hartz S. C., Siskind V., Mitchell A. A., Slone D., Rosenberg L., Monson R. R., Heinonen O. P., Idenpaan-Heikkila J., Haro S. & Saxen L. (1976) Anticonvulsants and parental epilepsy in the development of birth defects. *Lancet* i, 272.

Shepherd J. T. (1968) Personal communication to Folkow B. & Neil E. (1971) Gastrointestinal and liver circulations. In *Circulation*, p. 483. Oxford University Press, New York.

Soma L. R. (1971) Preanesthetic medication. In *Textbook of Veterinary Anaesthesia*, ed. L. R. Soma, p. 121. Williams & Wilkins, Baltimore.

South J. (1972) Teratogenic effect of anticonvulsants. *Lancet* ii, 1154.

Speidel B. D. & Meadow S. R. (1972) Maternal epilepsy and abnormalities of the foetus and newborn. *Lancet* ii, 839.

Stockley I. (1972). Interactions with phenytoin, phenobarbitone and other antiepileptic agents. *Pharmaceutical J.* **209**, 105.

Stockley, I. (1976) Interactions with oral contraceptives. *Pharmaceutical J.* **216**, 140.

Sumner-Smith G. A. (1962) A preliminary report on the clinical use of chlorprothixene as a sedative, narcotic and premedicant in the dog. *J. Small Anim. Prac.* **3**, 13.

Taylor H. C. (1958) Canine convulsions. Epileptiform vs. Tetanic (Diagnosis and treatment). *North American Veterinarian* **39**, 128.

Tobin T., Dirdjosudjono S. & Baskin S. I. (1973) Pharmacokinetics and distribution of diphenylhydantoin in kittens. *Amer. J. Vet. Res.* **34**, 951.

Toman J. E. P. (1965). Drugs effective in convulsive disorders. In *The Pharmacological Basis of Therapeutics*, 3rd edn., eds. L. S. Goodman & A. Gilman, pp. 215–224. Macmillan, New York.

Turner T. (1967) Treatment of convulsion in dogs. *Vet. Rec.* **81**, 386.

Tyrer J. H., Eadie M. G., Sutherland J. M. & Hooper W. D. (1970) Outbreak of anticonvulsant intoxication in an Australian city. *Brit. Med. J.* **4**, 271.

Villareale M., Gould L. V., Wasseman R. H., Barr A., Chiroff R. T. & Bergstrom W. H. (1974) Diphenylhydantoin: effects on calcium metabolism in the chick. *Science* **183**, 671.

Westhues M. & Fritsch R. (1965) *Animal Anaesthesia, Vol. II, general anaesthesia*, p. 135. Oliver Boyd Ltd, Edinburgh.

Withrow C. D., Stout R. J., Barton L. J., Beacham W. S. & Woodbury D. M. (1968) Anticonvulsant effects of 5,5-dimethyl-2,4-oxazolidinedione (DMO). *J. Pharmac. Exp. Ther.* **161**, 335.

Woodbury D. M. & Fingl E. (1975) Drugs effective in the therapy of the epilepsies. In *The Pharmacological Basis of Therapeutics*, 5th edn. eds. L. S. Goodman & A. Gilman, pp. 201–226. Macmillan, New York.

Wyant G. M. & Studney L. J. (1970) A study of diazepam (Valium) for induction of anaesthesia. *Canad. Anaes. Soc. J.* **17**, 166.

Index